KV-451-355

IMMUNOLOGICAL ASPECTS OF THE LIVER AND GASTROINTESTINAL TRACT

EDITED BY

Anne Ferguson, Ph.D., F.R.C.P., M.R.C.Path.

Gastrointestinal Unit, Western General Hospital Edinburgh and University of Edinburgh

and

Roderick N. M. MacSween, M.D., F.R.C.P., M.R.C.Path.

Department of Pathology, Western Infirmary, Glasgow, and University of Glasgow

WITH A FOREWORD BY

Geoffrey Watkinson, M.D. (London), F.R.C.P.

Consultant Physician and Gastroenterologist, Western Infirmary, Gartnavel General Hospital and Southern General Hospital; Honorary Lecturer in Medicine, University of Glasgow

President of the World Organisation of Gastroenterology (O.M.G.E.)

MTP

Published by
MTP Press Ltd.
St. Leonard's House
Lancaster, England

ISBN 0 852 00 128 2

First published 1976

PRINTED IN GREAT BRITAIN BY
THE GARDEN CITY PRESS LIMITED
LETCHWORTH, HERTFORDSHIRE

Contents

Preface

We have been privileged to start our academic careers at the beginning of the decade in which the immunological roles and hypersensitivity diseases of the gastrointestinal tract and liver have been defined. In the early 1960s IgA was reported to be the main secretory immunoglobulin, immunoblasts were shown to home to the intestinal mucosa and certain serum autoantibodies were described in patients with chronic liver disease. Shortly thereafter IgE and Australia antigen were discovered. Parallel advances in clinical investigation, in particular closed biopsy techniques, facilitated correlation of morphological changes with immunological mechanisms in disease of the gastrointestinal tract and liver. Only 10 years later, the concepts of immunity and hypersensitivity are regularly applied to the pathogenesis, diagnosis, treatment and prognosis of many chronic diseases in these organs.

In designing this book we have attempted to integrate theorectical and clinical immunology as they pertain in 1975; our ultimate aim is aptly described by Brachet as quoted by Professor Paronetto (page 319). We would like to think that this review provides a basis for the next major advances in the fields of gastrointestinal and hepatic immunology. As we see it, the outstanding problem in both sites is how to produce protective immunity without hypersensitivity.

The contributors to this book have most admirably met our requirements and we thank them for producing this series of authoritative reviews. We are grateful to our respective secretaries, Margaret Campbell and Anne Macleod, who have retyped all the edited manuscripts and ungrudgingly undertook this added commitment; and to Mr. Rogers and his staff of the library of the Royal College of Physicians and Surgeons of Glasgow, who checked the many references. Mr. Martin Lister of MTP has been most helpful at all stages of the preparation of the book, and we have drawn freely from his experience. Our spouses, John and Marjory, have not only accepted many hours of solitude during the gestation of this book but also have given considerable help in the final proof reading and indexing.

Little research is now carried out in isolation. We have benefited from free access to many groups of patients; from skilled labotatory assistance and from continued and stimulating discussions, all provided by colleagues and friends. In particular we thank Geoffrey Watkinson who has been a guide and mentor over the years and who has done us the further honour of writing a foreword to this book.

Edinburgh — Anne Ferguson
Glasgow — Roderick N. M. MacSween

List of contributors

MARVIN E. AMENT, M.D.
Associate Professor, University of California Center for Health Sciences, Department of Pediatrics, Division of Gastroenterology, Los Angeles, California, U.S.A.

HERVE BAZIN, D.V.M., D.SC.
Research Scientist, Experimental Immunology Unit, Faculty of Medicine, University of Louvain, Brussels, Belgium.

P. A. BERG, M.D., PH.D.
Privatdozent, Department of Medicine, University of Tübingen, West Germany.

JOHN BIENENSTOCK, M.B., B.S., M.R.C.P.
Professor of Medicine, McMaster University Medical Centre, Hamilton, Ontario, Canada.

M. BJORNEBOE, M.D.
Professor, Physician-in-Chief, Bispebjerg Hospital, Med. Dept. B, Copenhagen, Denmark.

ROBERT L. CLANCY, PH.D., F.R.A.C.P.
Consultant in Clinical Immunology, Department of Clinical Immunology, Royal Prince Alfred Hospital, Camperdown, N.S.W. Australia.

ADRIAN L. F. W. EDDLESTON, D.M., M.R.C.P.
Senior Lecturer in Medicine and Consultant Physician, Liver Unit, King's College Hospital and Medical School, London.

ANNE FERGUSON, PH.D., F.R.C.P., M.R.C.PATH,
Senior Lecturer and Consultant Physician, University of Edinburgh and Gastrointestinal Unit, Western General Hospital, Edinburgh.

H. J. F. HODGSON, M.A., M.R.C.P.
Research Fellow, Academic Department of Medicine, Royal Free Hospital, London.

D. P. JEWELL, M.A., D.PHIL., M.R.C.P.
Senior Lecturer, Academic Department of Medicine, Royal Free Hospital, London.

R. N. M. MACSWEEN, M.D., F.R.C.P., M.R.C.PATH.
Reader in Pathology and Consultant Pathologist, University of Glasgow and Western Infirmary, Glasgow.

HANS D. OCHS, M.D.
Associate Professor, University of Washington School of Medicine, Department of Pediatrics Division of Immunology, Seattle, Washington, U.S.A.

FIORENZO PARONETTO, M.D.
Professor of Pathology; Chief, Laboratory Service, Mt. Sinai School of Medicine and Veterans Administration Hospital, Bronx, New York, U.S.A.

DELPHINE M. V. PARROTT, D.SC.
Professor, University Department of Bacteriology and Immunology, Western Infirmary, Glasgow.

HANNE PRYTZ, M.D.
Research Fellow, Bispebjerg Hospital, Med. Dept. B, Copenhagen, Denmark.

RALPH WRIGHT, M.A., M.D., D.PHIL., F.R.C.P.
Professor of Medicine and Consultant Physician, University of Southampton and Royal South Hants Hospital, Southampton.

CHAPTER 1

The gut-associated lymphoid tissues and gastrointestinal immunity

DELPHINE M. V. PARROTT

Introduction

Lymphoid cells of a variety of types are to be found in the mucosa along the whole length of the gastrointestinal tract, some in the loose connective tissue, the lamina propria, others between the epithelial cells and at various sites there are organized lymphoid tissues, e.g. tonsils, Peyer's patches and appendix.

There is now ample evidence that antigen within the lumen of the gut can stimulate an immune response which is manifest both locally in the lamina propria and systemically throughout the body. Complete coverage of the morphological basis of gastrointestinal immunity should thus, in theory, include not only all lymphoid cells from mouth to anus but also other lymphoid tissues such as the spleen and mesenteric lymph node, which certainly contribute to gastrointestinal immunity, and the liver, which plays an important role in processing antigen from the gut lumen. In this chapter, however, I propose to cover in detail only the lymphoid population of the mucosa of the small intestine and Peyer's patches and appendix, laying particular emphasis on lymphoid cell traffic studies between the gut-associated lymphoid tissues, the rest of the lymphoid system and the lamina propria, in the hope of defining some general principles of gastrointestinal immune mechanisms which will be applicable to the whole length of the gut.

The nature of the cellular infiltrate in the intestinal mucosa

Over recent years, much emphasis has been placed on the importance of localized humoral immunity in the gut and the predominance of IgA producing cells in the gut mucosa[1]. The gastrointestinal tract is, however, subjected to a wide range of complex and often proliferating antigenic stimuli from food (usually protein), microbes, parasites and tumours. All these stimuli can provoke both humoral and cell-mediated immunity and in consequence, a whole range of different effector mechanisms involving many different cell types, all of which would be proceeding at the same time. Thus, one would expect to find not only antibody secreting plasma cells but also effector T-cells either acting on their own or in collaboration with macrophages, monocytes or polymorphs and, in the presence of some parasites, eosinophils or tissue basophils (mast cells). All these cell types have now been demonstrated in the gut mucosa.

Large numbers of macrophages, lymphoctyes, plasma cells and occasionally mast cells and eosinophils are seen in the loose connective tissue of the mucosa, the lamina propria. There are also large numbers of lymphocytes between the columnar epithelial cells (intraepithelial lymphocytes) which on the basis of electronmicroscopy studies can be seen to have crossed the basement membrane[2,3]; just a few mast cells and eosinophils may also cross the basement membrane but not apparently plasma cells. None of these cells are present at birth, plasma cells appearing at about 10 days in the mouse[4] and intraepithelial lymphocytes at 2–3 weeks of age[5], a timing which equates with their being a response to antigenic challenge. Also significant, and for the same reason, is the reduction in numbers of plasma cells[4] and intraepithelial lymphocytes[5] which occur in germfree rats and mice and in 'antigen free' gut grafts.

Until recently most studies in classification of lymphoid cell types were concerned with identifying the type of immunoglobulin produced by the numerous plasma cells in the lamina propria and only very recently has it become evident that there are T- as well as B-lymphocytes in the mucosa.

The predominant immunoglobulin-producing effector cell in the lamina propria of several species including man is IgA secreting (see Bazin[1] for references) although there are also cells containing IgM or IgG, and in ruminants IgG specific plasma cells may be predominant[6]. IgE forming cells have also been found in the gastrointestinal tract[7].

Oral immunization provokes the appearance of large numbers of IgA specific antibody forming cells in the lamina propria although both IgM and IgG producing cells are also formed, and they are not necessarily restricted to the lamina propria. Specific antibody containing cells of all three classes of immunoglobulin are also found in the mesenteric node[8,9] and the spleen[9]. There is controversy as to whether the cells in the mesenteric node and spleen have arisen *in situ* or have migrated from the lamina propria although on present evidence it is equally possible that oral immunization induces formation of specific antibody containing cells in the organized lymphoid tissues and these then migrate to the lamina propria. This topic will be returned to later.

The identification and function of intraepithelial lymphocytes is also a subject of controversy. They are slightly larger than normal lymphocytes, and in electron microscopy studies have been seen crossing the basement membrane; occasionally the processes of these lymphocytes make contact with lamina propria macrophages[2,3]. It has been disputed that these cells are lymphocytes, mainly because small metachromatic granules are present in many of the cells and this has led to the suggestion that they may be degranulated or degenerated mast cells[10]. A very different postulate is that of Fichtelius[11] who suggested that intraepithelial lymphocytes function as a 'bursa-equivalent' or inducer of B-lymphocyte differentiation. This postulate is, however, incompatible with the timing of the first appearance of intraepithelial lymphocytes, i.e. well after birth, with their fluctuation in numbers with respect to intraluminal antigen[5] and with their recent identification as T-lymphocytes (see below). Others have suggested that intraepithelial lymphocytes are discarded or 'dumped' lymphocytes on their way to the grave in the intestinal lumen. Recent attempts[12] to demonstrate this by overloading the lymphoid system with multiple thymus grafts or injections of lymph node lymphocytes so as to push up the number of intraepithelial lymphocyte numbers have not been successful, nor is there any support for this theory from the examination of the debris which accumulates in the lumen of isolated gut grafts[13] since this contains only epithelial cells and not lymphocytes.

Recently evidence has accrued which supports the conclusion that intraepithelial lymphocytes are effector T-cells and a manifestation of ongoing cell-mediated immune responses to intraluminal antigen[14]. The presence of antigen in the lumen of the gut has a considerable influence on the numbers of intraepithelial lymphocytes[5] as it does on

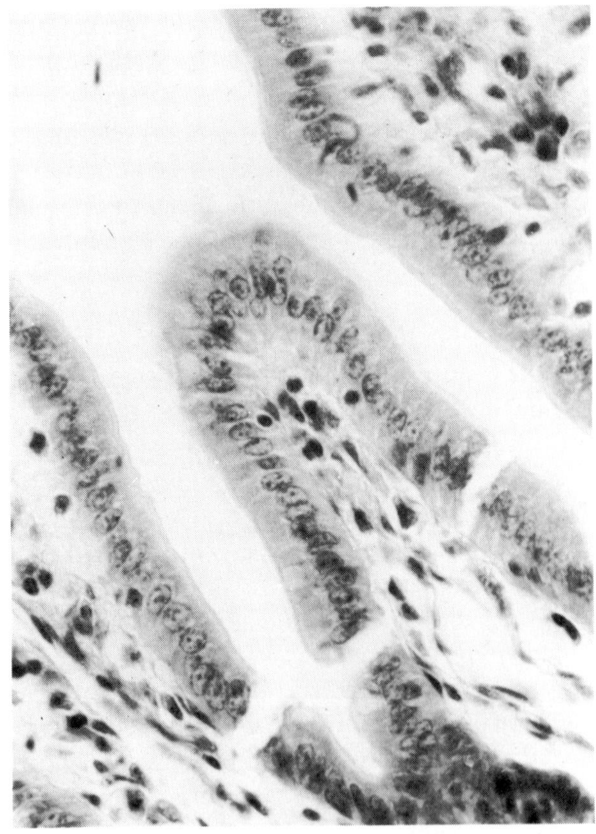

FIGURE 1.1 Section of villi from gut of normal heterozygous (nu/+) mouse. Note normal number of intraepithielial lymphocytes. Stained H & E. × 630

immunoglobulin-containing cells [4]. Both cell types are much reduced in the gut of germ free animals and in grafts of fetal gut implanted under the kidney capsule[5]; such gut grafts develop normally but remain devoid of all antigenic stimulus from the lumen. It was also observed that there were significantly fewer intraepithelial lymphocytes in T-deprived mice, and the reduction in numbers was much greater in gut exposed to antigen than in germ free or antigen free gut.

At first sight this reduction could be interpreted as a straightforward reflection of the reduction in the numbers of circulating T-lymphocytes; from this it could be concluded that in a normal mouse there would be both T and B intraepithelial lymphocytes, and in a T-deprived animal only B intraepithelial lymphocytes. But this conclusion does not take account of the fact that normal circulating T- and B-lymphocytes do not gain access to the mucosal layer of the intestine; only activated immunoblasts enter therein (see below). Moreover, there are virtually no intraepithelial lymphocytes in the epithelium of the congenitally athymic nude mice[15] (Figures 1.1 and

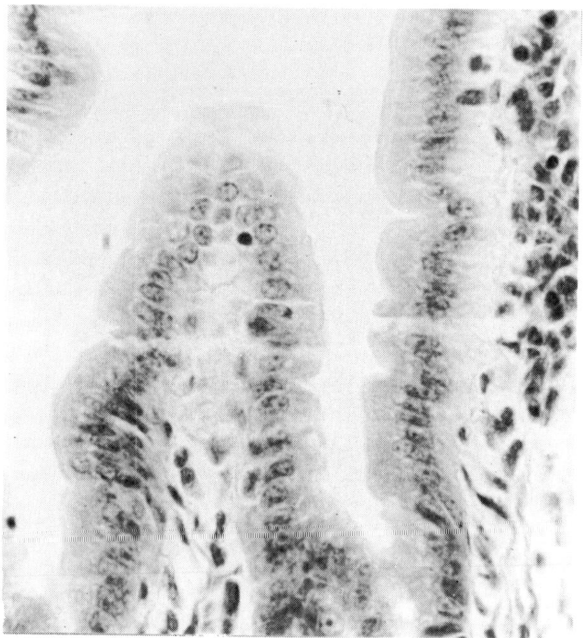

FIGURE 1.2 Section of villi from gut of athymic nude (nu/nu) mouse. Note scarcity of intraepithelial lymphocytes. Stained H and E. × 630

1.2). This weakens the argument that there are B as well as T intraepithelial lymphocytes, for nude mice are not deficient in B-cells, but it substantiates the conclusion that the cellular infiltrate into the intestinal mucosa is a manifestation of a T-dependent immune reaction[14]. Definitive identification of T-cell antigen on the surface of all intraepithelial lymphocytes by immunofluorescence and specific antisera directed against T-cells has been reported recently by Guy-Grand, Griscelli and Vassalli[16] (Figure 1.3). The presence of some intraepithelial lymphocytes in neonatally thymectomized mice is, however, not surprising, for many authors have reported the presence of residual T-cells in these animals, and the presence of higher numbers of intraepithelial lymphocytes in adult, irradiated, thymus deprived mice is still less surprising for it is known that activated T-lymphocytes are very resistant to the effects of X-irradiation[17] and could easily survive the T-cell deprivation process.

Where does sensitization occur?

If it is conceded that both the major lymphoid cell types within the intestinal mucosa, the intraepithelial lymphocytes and plasmablasts

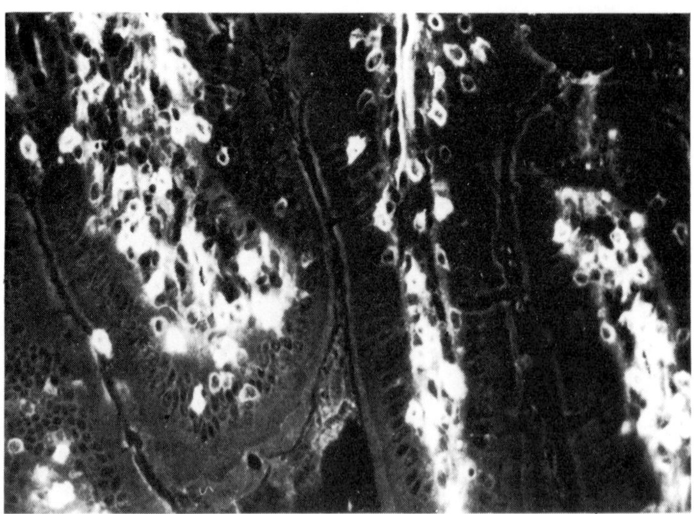

FIGURE 1.3 Fluorescence demonstration of T-cell surface antigens on lymphocytes in lamina propria and between epithelial cells. Section stained with fluorochrome labelled rabbit anti-MSLA (mouse specific lymphocyte antigen–a T-lymphocyte antigen). × 540. (Picture by permission of Dr Delphine Guy-Grand)

and plasma cells, are effector cells carrying out immune responses the next problem is, where does primary sensitization occur? Many authors have considered it likely that sensitization takes place in the lamina propria and that effector cells arise *in situ* not only because of the very high accumulation of IgA forming cells but also because an antigen trapping mechanism[18] has been demonstrated in the lamina propria and there is adequate evidence that orally administered antigen does cross the mucosa. Cornell, Walker and Isselbacher[19] have shown that horse-radish peroxidase passes between epithelial cells into the lamina propria and Bienenstock and Dolezel[20] have identified BSA within

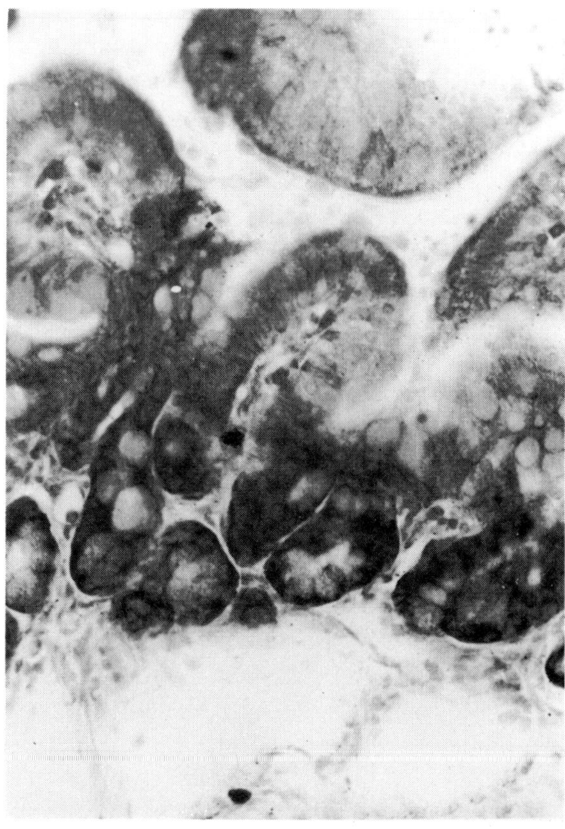

FIGURE 1.4 Autoradiograph of 'antigen-free' gut graft transplanted under kidney capsule. Note ^{3}H-thymidine labelled mesenteric lymph node cell in lamina propria. Stained methyl green pyronin. × 507. (Picture by permission of the Editor of *Immunology*)

macrophages in the lamina propria after oral feeding. The concept of *in situ* sensitization in response to intraluminal antigen does however make it very difficult to explain the presence of effector cells in completely antigen free grafts of fetal gut (Figure 1.4). Such grafts are devoid of cells at grafting but subsequently accumulate lymphocytes and plasma cells[5] and the latter have been shown to secrete IgA into the graft lumen[21]. Under these circumstances the effector cells must have migrated into the grafts from the circulating blood, and it is reasonable to conclude that this is the normal way in which the gut mucosa is populated with lymphoid cells.

Furthermore, the normal uninflamed gut of a non-primed individual does not provide the circumstances which favour the initiation of a primary response. One prerequisite of this is that there should be sufficient traffic of lymphocytes so that the limited number of cells with appropriate immunological potential can be selectively retained and so interact with antigen. Such circumstances normally only prevail in the organized lymphoid tissues. Some extravasation of lymphocyte must occur in a tissue such as the gut with extensive capillary beds but there is no indication from experiments on the traffic of labelled lymphocytes[22–24] that appreciable numbers of normal small lymphocytes enter the gut mucosa. Circumstances could, however, be radically different in an inflamed gut with the likelihood of increased extravasation of lymphocytes accompanying the increased vascular permeability comparable to that which occurs in experimentally induced inflammation in the skin[25] and, in a hyperimmune host there would be large numbers of memory cells circulating which would facilitate the induction of a further response *in situ*.

The normal mucosa is not then on *a priori* grounds a likely site for the induction of a primary response to intraluminal antigen but there is as yet no definitive evidence in favour of any other sites, although the likely alternatives are the gut associated lymphoid tissues (tonsils, Peyer's patches and appendix), the mesenteric nodes and the spleen. In assessing the rival claims of these sites the following criteria will be adopted:

1. They should be on the pathway of recirculating lymphocytes, both T and B.
2. They should receive antigen from the gut lumen and possess antigen trapping mechanisms.

3. They should contain cells which react against the priming antigen, and
4. They should contain effector cells (T and B) which will migrate to the gut mucosa.

There are many studies describing the organization of the spleen and lymph nodes (including mesenteric node) in functional terms, i.e. identifying antigen trapping mechanisms, pathways of cell traffic and production of effector cells[18,22,23,26–28] so that it is not necessary to describe them here. It should, however, be remembered that although antigen from the lumen of the gut has been traced to the portal circulation and to the mesenteric lymph[29] hard evidence that gut derived antigen in fact reaches the spleen or mesenteric nodes in its native state is difficult to come by although it is logical to deduce that this does happen.

It is necessary, however, to consider the structure and organization of Peyer's patches and appendix and their relationship in terms of lymphocyte traffic with the rest of the lymphoid system, in greater detail in order that their role in gastrointestinal immunity can be appreciated. Not only has it been disputed that these tissues are capable of responding to intraluminal antigen[20,30,31] but also many workers still regard them as mainly 'central' in function and not as 'peripheral' tissues although it is not relevant to enter into the pro's and cons of that argument here.

Functional architecture of Peyer's patches and appendix

Structure of Peyer's patches

Peyer's patches are simply aggregates of lymphocytes extended through the lamina propria and submucosa of the small intestine (Figures 1.5a and 1.5b). In the normal adult these nodules contain germinal centres. The nodular areas are, as in other lymphoid tissues, occupied by B-lymphocytes and in conventionally housed animals the T area is a narrow internodular zone which also contains post capillary venules[32,33]. Recent studies[24] revealed, however, that the open work pattern of reticulum which is characteristic of T areas (and also traffic areas) was present in the dome area (Figure 1.6) and in the zone close to the outer muscle layer. Moreover, in nude mice and axenic neonatally thymectomized mice there was an obvious depletion of lymphocytes (Figure 1.5b),

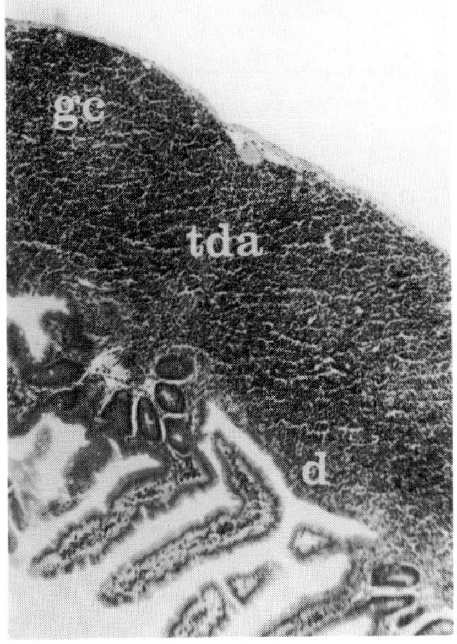

FIGURE 1.5(a) Peyer's patch from normal mouse. Stained H & E. D-dome. TDA–thymus dependent area. G.C–germinal centre. Compare with Figure 1.5(b). × 200

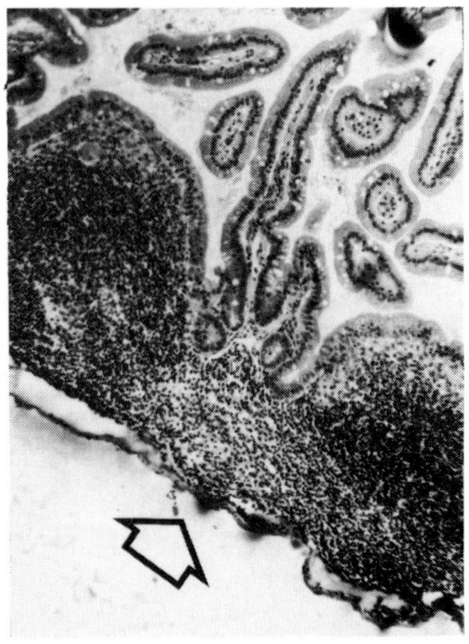

FIGURE 1.5(b) Peyer's patch from axemic neonatally thymectomized CBA mouse. Note (arrows) depleted thymus dependent (T) area between nodules and depletion in the 'dome' area. Stained H & E. ×175. (Reproduced by permission of the Editor of *Immunology*)

so that T areas are potentially much wider than was originally supposed. Peyer's patches do not have afferent lymphatics, only efferent lymphatics, which drain down to the mesenteric nodes. Interest, therefore, is centred on the dome areas as a means of access of intra-luminal antigen into Peyer's patches. The epithelium over the dome differs from that over the rest of the mucosa in being cuboidal (Figure 1.7) instead of columnar and having very few goblet cells[34]. Work on human Peyer's patches[35] has shown that there is a new type of epithelial cell (an M-cell) in the dome area which is characterized by luminal surface microfolds rather than microvilli. It is likely that there are comparable cells in Peyer's patches of other species[34,36] and also in the dome area of the appendix. There are large numbers of intraepithelial lymphocytes in dome epithelium (Figure 1.7) and interestingly they appear somewhat earlier in life (within 3 days of birth in the mouse) than intraepithelial cells elsewhere, a timing difference which equates well with the postu-

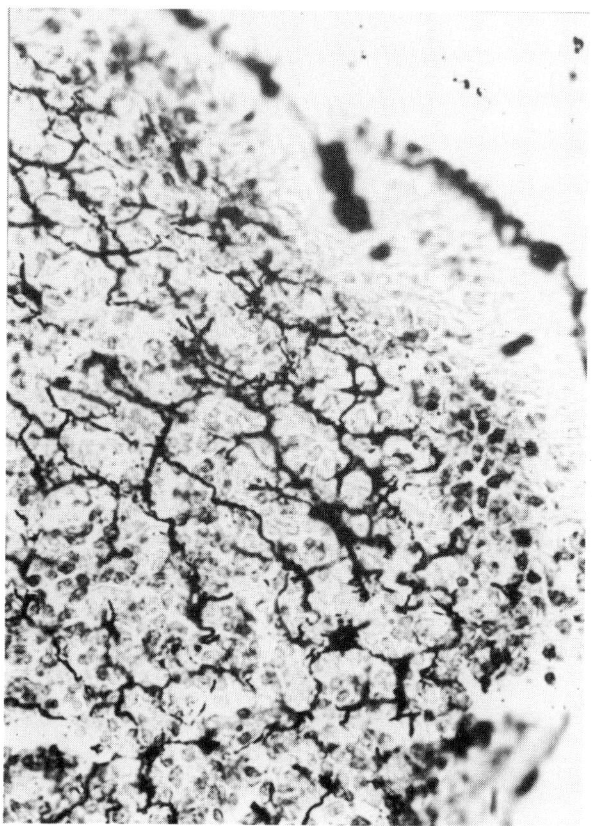

FIGURE 1.6 Peyer's patch from thymus-deprived bone marrow reconstituted CBA mouse. Note open mesh pattern of reticulum typical of traffic areas in the subepithelial layer of the dome. Stained Gordon Sweet. × 595

late that intraepithelial cells in dome epithelium are part of the affector arm of the immune response and intraepithelial lymphocytes elsewhere are part of the effector arm of the immune response. Peyer's patches can be identified before birth in the mouse and are simply composed of reticular cells, yet by 3 days after birth they are already populated by lymphocytes[5,37]. Primary nodules appear at 3–7 days, germinal centres at 4–5 weeks of age[5,38]. Peyer's patches in germ free mice do not develop germinal centres unless there is oral administration of bacteria[39], likewise, the Peyer's patches in isografts of fetal gut do not develop germinal centres and remain very small even 3–4 months after grafting[5]. There are no germinal centres in Peyer's patches in nude mice[15,35]

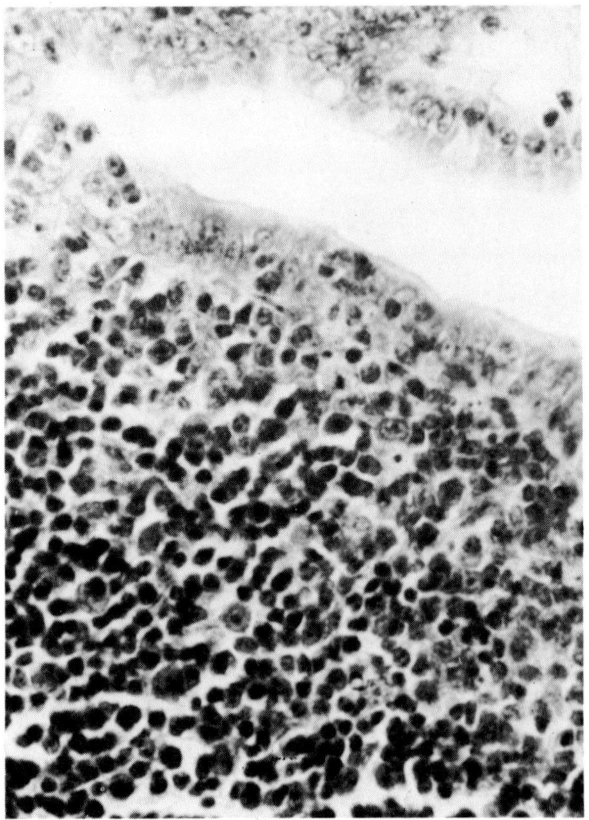

FIGURE 1.7 Peyer's patch from normal mouse. Side of dome area. Note cuboidal epithelium containing many lympocytes and large numbers of blast cells in sub-epithelial layer. × 595

whether germ free or conventionally housed but this deficiency is not peculiar to Peyer's patches since it occurs in other lymphoid tissues.

Structure of the appendix

Peyer's patches and the appendix, as well as the tonsil and sacculus rotundus, have many structural as well as functional similarities. The rabbit appendix which has been the subject of several detailed studies[41–42] is divided into segments each of which comprises a dome area with associated corona and a large nodule of lymphocytes containing a germinal centre (Figure 1.8). Most of the appendix consists of

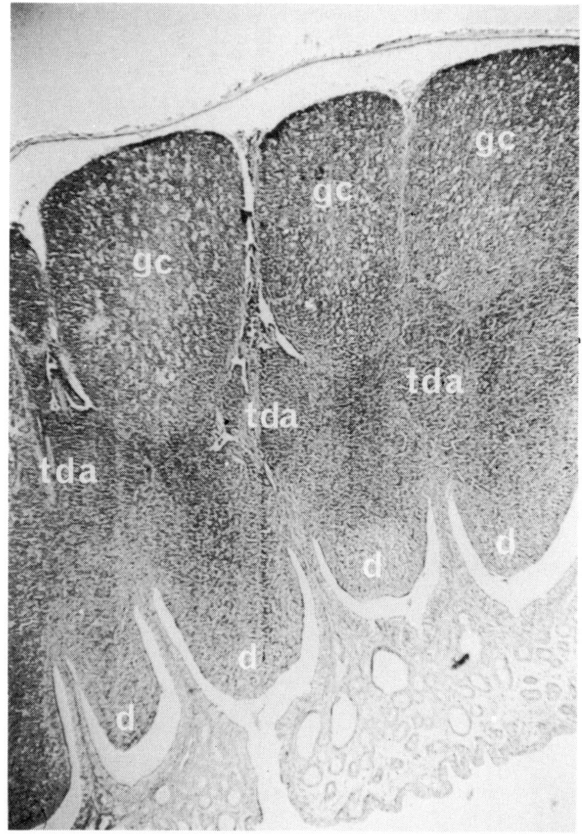

FIGURE 1.8(a) Normal appendix. TDA–thymus dependent area. D–dome. G.C.–germinal centre

B-lymphocytes although between the upper end of each nodule is a diamond shaped thymus-dependent area (TDA) with post-capillary venules. As in Peyer's patches the epithelium over the dome area is cuboidal, it lacks goblet cells and contains large numbers of intra-epithelial lymphocytes. Between each dome there is a 'mushroom' of normal gut mucosa and lamina propria attached to the dome epithelium by a narrow 'stalk'. The dome area can be identified in the latter part of gestation though it is alymphoid. Lymphocytes appear in the dome epithelium within 24 hours of birth[40] much earlier than elsewhere in mucosal epithelium. Nodules appear by 4 days after birth[40,43] and germinal centres by 7 days after birth[40].

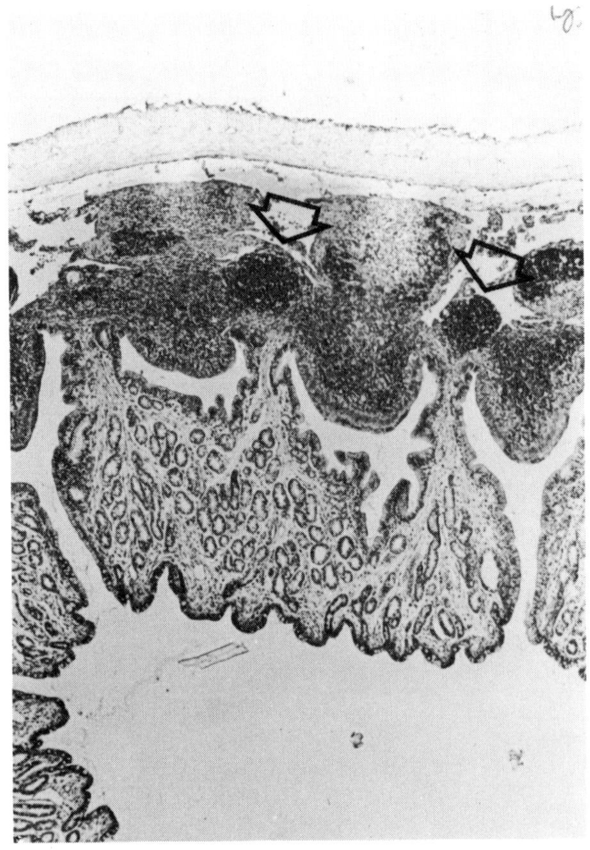

FIGURE 1.8(b) Appendix 14 days after appendicostomy and irradiation. Note depletion germinal centre and nodule but persistence of most lymphocytes in TDA and some in dome area. × 21. (Pictures by permission of Dr B. H. Waksman)

Lymphocyte traffic in Peyer's patches and appendix

Gowans and Knight[22] first demonstrated by means of autoradiography that Peyer's patches are on the route of recirculating lymphocytes. Subsequently Parrott and de Sousa[32] demonstrated that intravenously infused ^{3}H-adenosine labelled thymus cells are confined to the narrow corridor between nodules. When cell suspensions containing B-lymphocytes are injected[24,27,44], however, these are mostly found in the nodular aggregates of lymphocytes below the dome but also in the B areas stretching down and around the germinal centres (Figures 1.9a and 1.9b). Both B- and T-lymphocytes enter Peyer's patches through post-capillary venules which are very similar to those seen in lymph nodes.

In neonates the vast majority of lymphocytes (85–90%) in the Peyer's patches are θ positive[45], i.e. they are T-cells, although this reduces in adults to only 20–40%[46]. This is why the spread of labelled thymus cells appears much wider in the newborn[37] than in adults[32] although most cells are still nevertheless within the bounds of the thymus-dependent area[38]. The relative sizes of T and B areas obviously vary

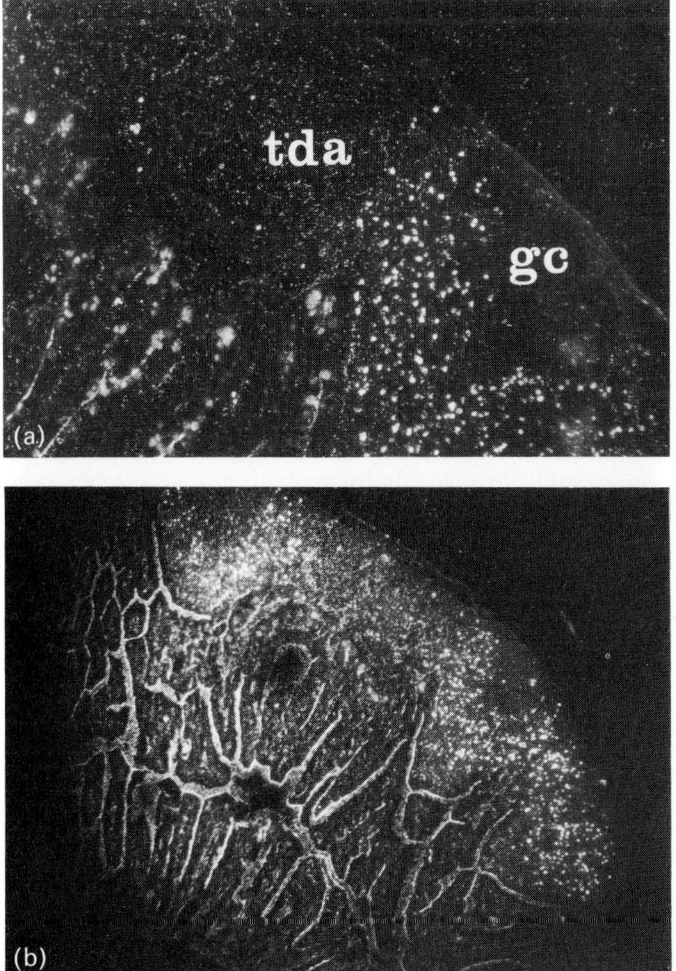

FIGURE 1.9(a) Dark ground view of [^{3}H]–adenosine labelled B-cells in normal mouse. Note preponderance of cells in nodular area below the dome in crescent formation over germinal centres. Note lack of cells in germinal centres, interfollicular T area and sub-epithelial area. × 132. (b) detail of part of (a). × 240

considerably in both Peyer's patches[24,38] and appendix according to age and extent of antigen stimulation. Joel *et al.*[37] and Waksman[38] found a few ^{3}H-thymidine labelled thymus cells in the sub-epithelial area of the dome and one or two within the epithelium itself. Thus there are T-cells as well as B-cells in close proximity to the dome epithelium.

Studies on cell migration in the appendix are restricted to rabbits which are not inbred, and this obviously limits cell transfer experiments. Nevertheless the series of observations by Keuning and his co-workers, Van den Brock[48], Veldman[41] and Nieuwenhuis[40] combining thymectomy with irradiation, irradiation with thymus shielding and the injection of ^{3}H-thymidine labelled thymocytes have clearly shown that the major area of T-cell traffic is the diamond shaped interfollicular zone. There is also some evidence of cortisone resistant cells which could be T-cells in the dome area immediately beneath the epithelium[48]. Recently it has been shown[49–51] that the appendix, like spleen and lymph node, contains both T- and B-lymphocytes which are capable of migrating to either T or B areas in other peripheral lymphoid tissues (Figure 1.10). Durkin, Caporale and Thorbecke[51] further showed that the migration of appendix cells to B areas but not T areas was inhibited by pretreatment of the appendix cells with anti-immunoglobulin, a treatment which would preferentially affect B-cells and not T-cells.

It seems reasonable to conclude that both Peyer's patches and appendix are on the route of recirculating T- and B-cells in the same way as

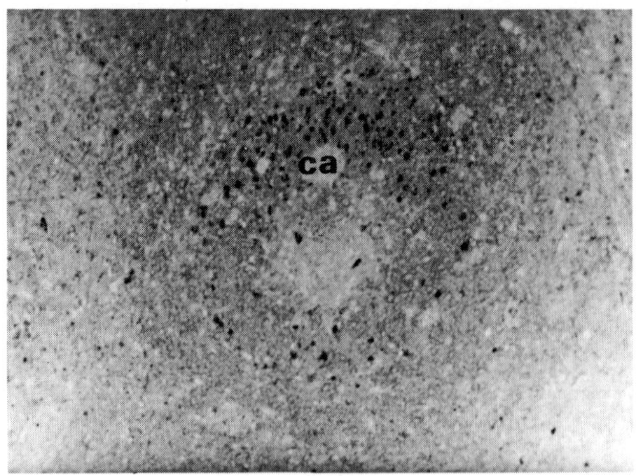

FIGURE 1.10 [^{3}H]-adenosine labelled cells separated from appendix TDA after migration to TDA of spleen. × 225. ca–central arteriole. (Picture by permission of Dr Howard Ozer)

the other lymphoid tissues, and thus are well placed to recruit from the recirculating pool, lymphocytes with the appropriate immune potential for reacting to intraluminal antigen.

Route of entry of antigen into Peyer's patches and appendix

There are no afferent lymphatics in either Peyer's patches or appendix and no organized antigen trapping mechanism similar to that in marginal sinuses of lymph nodes and the sinus in the perifollicular area of the spleen. Soluble and particulate antigens, Indian ink and even intact bacteria pass freely into the dome area of Peyer's patches of rabbits[42] and of weanling mice[36] and the dome area of the appendix in rabbits[36,52,53] presumably as a consequence of the micropinocytotic capabilities of the epithelial cells in the dome[34–36,52]. One site for antigen-lymphocyte interaction (Figures 1.7 and 1.8) would appear to be immediately below the dome, which is an area of cell traffic (Figure 1.6) and which normally contains large numbers of macrophages and frequently plasma cells as well as lymphocytes. The large numbers of lymphocytes actually within the dome epithelium should not, however, be overlooked, and it may be, as Owen and Jones[35] suggest, that some of these lymphocytes approach sufficiently close to the intestinal lumen to make direct contact with the antigen in the lumen without leaving the epithelium. The very early appearance of lymphocytes at this site certainly suggests early antigen contact.

Response of Peyer's patches and appendix to antigen challenge

It would be reasonable to expect that since both Peyer's patches and appendix receive circulating lymphocytes and antigen from the lumen of the gut oral immunization would result in the appearance of specific antibody containing cells in these tissues. There is widespread agreement, however, that such cells do not appear in either Peyer's patches[20,30] or appendix[31] although they can be detected easily in the mesenteric lymph node, lamina propria and the spleen[8,9].

Many authors have ascribed this lack of specific antibody forming cells to a deficiency in one of the three cell types (T- and B-cells and accessory macrophages) required for co-operation in antibody production. It has been shown, for example, that Peyer's patch cells are poor at inducing graft-versus-host reactions and from this it has been surmised that Peyer's patches are therefore deficient in T-cells[54] but others have reported that the response to PHA is normal[55]. In some instances the *in vitro* capacity to induce a primary response is normal[30] yet others have reported a deficiency because of the lack of adherent macrophage cells[56]. Similarly conflicting evidence has emerged from *in vitro* experiments on human tonsils[57] (normal macrophages, defective T-cells) and *in vivo* experiments on the appendix[47,58]. Many observers, in interpreting their observations, have failed to accommodate the very wide variations which can exist in these tissues particularly in the relative proportions of T- and B-cells according to the age of the individual and the size of each tissue[57]. There is, for example, a considerable change in the proportion of T-cells in mouse Peyer's patches according to age, with 80–90% in neonates[45], and 20–40% in adults[46]. T-cells in areas of Peyer's patches in normal adult rabbits vary from 10–50%[38]. Treatments such as appendicostomy, irradiation and administration of endotoxin[47] produce a very wide fluctuation in the content of both T- and B-cells and macrophages in the rabbit (Figures 1.8a and 1.8b). All these observations point to the conclusion that any deficiency in one cell is temporary and reversible and is not an inherent characteristic.

Antibody containing cells are only one facet of the immune response and their lack in Peyer's patches and appendix does not necessarily mean that these tissues cannot respond to antigen from the lumen of the gut. The failure of germinal centres to develop in Peyer's patches in germ free situations[13,39] is an obvious indicator that response to antigen can occur, as is the major change which follows when the continuity of the rabbit appendix with the gut lumen is interrupted[47]. The whole appendix shrinks, mainly because of the disappearance of the normally huge germinal centres (Figure 1.8b) and re-establishment of continuity with the bowel results in the regeneration of germinal centres. Moreover recent work of Müller-Schoop and Good[59] has clearly demonstrated that both T- and B-cells in Peyer's patches respond to intraluminal antigen. These workers measured the *in vitro* proliferation of guinea pig cells when cultured with *Clostridia*, a normal intestinal commensal, and compared the response of Peyer's patch cells to dead *Clostridia* with responses in spleen, mesenteric and inguinal lymph nodes. The responses of Peyer's patch cells were much higher than those of other cells. They also showed that after oral immunization with live BCG, Peyer's patch cells also showed a higher proliferative response to PPD *in vitro*. By contrast parenteral immunization with PPD evoked very little response in Peyer's patches. After separating B- from T-cells in Peyer's patches they demonstrated that T-cells responded very well to both antigenic stimuli but B-cells responded only to *Clostridia*, and not to PPD.

The appearance of specific antibody containing cells in tissues such as the spleen and lymph node is preceded by a sequence of cellular changes which varies greatly according to the antigen and the type of response—antibody production or cell-mediated reaction. Typically this is characterized by proliferation of T-cells and B-cells which takes place in the T and B areas of the white pulp of the spleen and the cortex of the lymph nodes. This is followed, in cell-mediated reactions, by the release of activated T-cells into the circulation and, in humoral immunity, by the production of B immunoblasts many of which go on to differentiate into plasma cells but some of which are released and migrate to other lymphoid tissues before final differentiation. It is significant that the differentiating cells evolve in the red pulp of the spleen and in the medullary cords of the lymph nodes, areas which are apart from the T and B areas where initial recognition and proliferation took place. If one examines Peyer's patches or appendix tissue there may be scattered plasma cells in the dome or interfollicular zone[4,31,42] but both tissues lack areas which are equivalent to the red pulp of the spleen or medullary cords of lymph nodes. It would appear therefore that both Peyer's patches and appendix lack the appropriate type of microenvironment for the differentiation of antibody forming cells. It should, however, be pointed out that in the abnormal circumstances of T-deprived animals there is sometimes an accumulation of plasma cells in the TDA of Peyer's patches (see below). Whether absence of the appropriate microenvironment is the sole reason for the lack of antibody producing cells or whether it is in some way related to the absence of an organized antigen processing mechanism cannot be decided on the basis of present evidence. Since, however, both the T effector cells and the IgA secretory cells in the lamina propria are 'short range' effector cells they must be distributed throughout the mucosa in order to be effective and, since the process of differentiation would limit their mobility, this does not proceed *in situ* within individual Peyer's patches or appendix, despite the fact that this renders these tissues especially vulnerable to the consequences of microbial invasion[60]. The thesis to be developed in the next section is, therefore, that the main function of the gut associated lymphoid tissues is to propagate the immune response as widely as possible by means of mobile effector precursors.

The migration pathways of T and B immunoblasts

Migration of B immunoblasts and IgA precursor cells

The one migration pathway of B immunoblasts which has been well defined is that of IgA precursor cells from the Peyer's patches to the lamina propria.

Craig and Cebra[61] transfused cell suspensions from Peyer's patches or popliteal lymph nodes (which could be identified by an allotype marker) into irradiated recipients. When the donor marker could be detected in the sera of the recipients, usually about 6 days after cell transfer, the recipients were killed. The recipients which had received Peyer's patch cells had large numbers of cells making IgA; these were found preferentially in the lamina propria and all were identified as donor allotype. In the recipients of popliteal lymph node cells most of the marked cells were making IgG rather than IgA and there were few donor cells in the lamina propria. The progress of cells from Peyer's patches to the lamina propria does, however, take some days and takes what would appear to be a somewhat circuitous route. Piecing all available evidence together it seems probable that they leave the Peyer's patches by efferent lymphatics and pass through the mesenteric node to the superior mesenteric duct which enters the thoracic duct at the cisterna chyli. The thoracic duct empties into the left subclavian vein and the cells eventually enter the lamina propria from the circulation. There are direct but limited lymphatic connections from Peyer's patches to the villi immediately surrounding them and cell traffic experiments with labelled small lymphocytes have shown that cells which have entered Peyer's patches can gain access to these villi[24] (Figure 1.11). Presumably if small lymphocytes can enter these villi from Peyer's patches then blasts could also enter. This could well be the reason for the higher accumulation of IgA producing cells in this site when compared with distant areas of the mucosa as observed by Crabbe *et al.* in their careful studies on conventional and germ free mice[4], an observation which led these workers to speculate that there was some kind of relationship between Peyer's patches and mucosal IgA producing cells. It seems likely that there are similar direct but

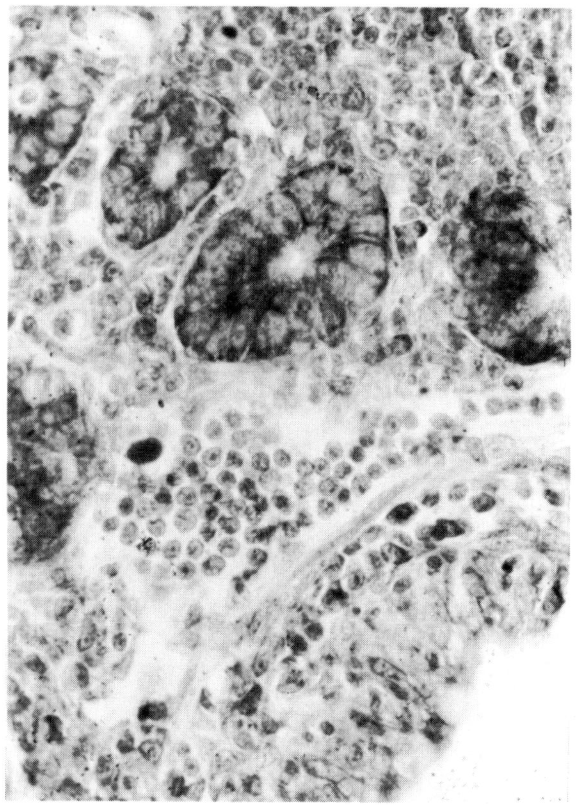

FIGURE 1.11 [^{3}H]-5-Uridine labelled spleen cells in Peyer's patch. Note labelled cell in lymphatic of villus adjacent to Peyer's patch tissue. Stained methyl green pryonin. × 525

minor pathways from the appendix to surrounding villi, e.g. in the 'mushroom' lamina propria.

The most immediate source of cells destined for the lamina propria is the thoracic duct lymph of rats and mice. Gowans and Knight[22] first demonstrated in rats that a high proportion of the large lymphocytes in thoracic duct lymph which labelled *in vitro* with a DNA precursor, in this case ^{3}H-thymidine, would within 20 hours of intravenous injection migrate preferentially to the lamina propria of the intestine, where many assumed the appearance of plasma cells. These workers also distinguished the migratory properties of these cells from those of small lymphocytes which, unlike the large lymphocytes were capable of recirculating from blood to lymph but which did not enter the lamina propria.

The propensity of large lymphocytes (immunoblasts) from thoracic duct lymph, which label *in vitro* with DNA precursors, to home to the intestine has been further classified and quantitated in a series of publications by Hall and his colleagues[62–65]. Labelled immunoblasts begin to enter the gut within 2 hours of intravenous injection and reach maximum numbers within 24 hours. Hall *et al.*[63] also demonstrated by means of electron-microautoradiographs that the final differentiation of immunoblasts to typical plasma cells with rough endoplasmic reticulum took place within the lamina propria. The B-immunoblasts, unlike some T-immunoblasts which are destined for the gut do not recirculate[22,65]. They have a short half life and it seems very unlikely that once having entered the lamina propria they could subsequently leave it. The mesenteric lymph node in both rats[66] and mice [16,24] also contains substantial numbers of immunoblasts which will migrate to the gut within 24–28 hours and there differentiate into plasma cells, but the maximum was not reached until 4 days, and the proportion is lower than in thoracic duct lymph[16]. Griscelli *et al.*[66] and Guy-Grand *et al.*[16] have also shown that a small proportion of Peyer's patch immunoblasts will migrate to the gut within 24 hours but the proportion is lower than in either mesenteric lymph node or thoracic duct. This is not because there are fewer blast-like cells in Peyer's patches than mesenteric lymph node or thoracic duct lymph; there are in fact quite large numbers[16] which accumulate preferentially in the spleen and it may be that after a longer time interval these also would arrive in the gut. There does however appear to be a direct link between the capacity to migrate to the lamina propria promptly after injection (i.e. within 24–48 hours) and the presence of intracellular IgA (i.e. cells actively secreting IgA). In the mouse very few Peyer's patch blasts contain intracellular IgA[16], although there are significant numbers with surface IgA, whereas mesenteric blasts and thoracic duct blasts have both surface and intracellular IgA[16]. In the mouse thoracic duct lymph more than 20% of all blasts contain IgA[16] and this proportion is higher in rats, sometimes over 50%[67]. Peyer's patch cells will nevertheless develop into IgA producing cells if cultured *in vitro* particularly in the presence of pokeweed mitogen[68], but it is not known whether such cultured cells would migrate to the lamina propria. The emphasis on the function of Peyer's patches as the site of IgA precursors does not preclude the possibility of other immunoglobulin precursors, e.g. IgM, multiplying there, nor that IgA precursors might also proliferate elsewhere, in particular the mesenteric nodes (since antigen from the gut lumen does drain directly to these nodes). Thus the mesenteric nodes could contain IgA producing precursors which have arisen *in situ* as well as those which have drained from the Peyer's patches. Robertson and Cooper[9] report that, after intraluminal immunization, there is an early appearance of antibody specific IgA rosettes in mesenteric nodes, as well as IgM and IgG rosettes. The spleen also responds to intraluminal immunization[9] but isotopically labelled spleen cell suspensions[24] unlike mesenteric node cell suspensions do not appear to contain cells which have an affinity for the gut. Recently, however, it has been shown that ^{3}H-thymidine labelled spleen grafts transplanted whole into the abdominal cavity do contain cells which migrate to the lamina propria[69]. These cells were at an earlier stage of differentiation than those in mesenteric nodes or thoracic duct lymph since it took about 4–5 days for the cells to reach the lamina propria.

The appendix, like Peyer's patches, lacks IgA forming cells although there are plenty in the surrounding villi and in the lamina propria in the 'mushroom' villi. It does, however, contain cells with IgA and IgM surface receptors[70] and these are mainly in the dome and corona region. Injection of antigen into the appendiceal artery or into the lumen of the appendix results in the appearance of specific antibody containing cells in the draining mesenteric lymph node and in the spleen but not the appendix itself[31,58]. Very recently Craig and Cebra[71] have obtained evidence that the appendix, like Peyer's patches, is a source of IgA precursors.

Differentiation and migration of IgA precursors is altered in circumstances in which there is a drastic reduction or an absence of T-cells. For example, in immune deficient patients T-cell deficiency is often associated with IgA deficiency and IgM producing cells often replace IgA producers in the lamina propria. A similar replacement is seen in bursectomized and thymectomized birds[72]. Athymic mice have no IgA or IgA producing cells in the lamina propria or thoracic duct lymph[16] although there are cells with surface IgA receptors in Peyer's patches[16] and the thoracic duct[73]. The picture in mice with experimentally induced T-cell deficiency is, however, somewhat contradictory, since they have normal or even raised amounts of serum IgA[74] and cells in the lamina propria of T-deprived mice secrete IgA[21] into the gut lumen. They also have normal if not increased numbers of immunoblasts in thoracic duct lymph[67,75] and often large numbers of plasma cells—a cell type not present in the lymph of normal mice. Furthermore, again unlike normal mice there are often large numbers of plasma cells in Peyer's patches of T-deprived mice, and in fact the thymus-dependent area may be partially repopulated by plasma cells[24] although it has not been demonstrated that these are making IgA.

The absence of IgA producing cells in nude mice can probably be explained on the basis of complete absence of helper T-cells to switch from IgM to IgA. The formation of excessive IgA in T-deprived mice together with the accumulation of mature antibody forming cells in Peyer's patches and thoracic duct lymph is more difficult to explain. Sufficient T-cells may still be present to initiate responses and over-production would then be the consequence of absence of suppressor T-cells, together with the stimulation by environmental pathogens. Accumulation of plasma cells could follow the slower rate of lymphocyte migration which is reported in T-deprived mice with wasting symptoms[75].

Migration pathway of T immunoblasts to the gut mucosa

Recent studies on the identity of the immunoblasts in mouse thoracic duct lymph and mesenteric lymph nodes have shown that these contain substantial numbers of T (48% in mesenteric node; 66% in thoracic duct lymph)[16] as well as B blasts. Do T blasts follow a comparable migration pattern to B immunoblasts and if so are they also primed in Peyer's patches or appendix? It was earlier shown that circulating T-cells gain access to areas in both gut associated tissues where they could be sensitized. Furthermore Müller-Schoop and Good[59] have shown that T- as well as B-cells in Peyer's patches of guinea pigs are activated by antigen in the gut lumen. Using the experimental system of injected parental strain thymocytes into F1 hybrid mice Sprent and Miller[76] obtained thoracic duct lymph cells which consisted almost entirely of ^{3}H-thymidine labelled T-lymphocytes activated against histocompatibility antigens. These cells when injected into syngeneic recipients migrated preferentially to the gut and Peyer's patches. More recently Ford and Sedgley[77] employing a similar system in rats for activated T-lymphocytes did not find any of these cells in the lamina propria, only in the TDA of Peyer's patches and other lymphoid tissues. Guy-Grand, Griscelli and Vassalli[16] however, using normal mesenteric lymph node cells and thoracic duct lymph cells, but distinguishing T blasts from B blasts by surface markers, did trace T blasts to the lamina propria and to the intraepithelial site as well as to Peyer's patches. Recently, cells have been identified in the intraepithelial site which have migrated from spleen grafts[69].

Factors which affect the migration of immunoblasts to the mucosa

In preceding sections emphasis has been placed on identifying the lymphoid cell populations in the gut mucosa as effector cells reacting to intraluminal antigen. Since the initial interaction of lymphocytes which gave rise to these effector cells takes place in the organized lymphoid tissues, the effector cell precursors must perforce migrate in what would appear to be a somewhat roundabout and potentially inefficient route to the mucosa. In fact, most of the immunoblasts in thoracic duct lymph will have drained from intestinal lymphoid tissues, and experiments (see above) have shown that a very high proportion of these do find their way to the gut, up to 50% to the small intestine and additional, though smaller, amounts to the large intestine and caecum. Such a high proportion would seem to indicate that the cells are attracted to the gut in a positive way and the most obvious attractant is the antigen against which the cells are directed. But there are several experiments demonstrating that this is not the case. Immunoblasts migrate to grafts of 'antigen free' fetal gut implanted under the skin[78] or kidney capsule[16,24] (Figure 1.4) in the same numbers as to normal gut. Immunoblasts from adult donors also migrate as well to the gut of caesarian delivered new born rats before suckling[64] as to newborn suckled or adult rats; and thus they freely enter the gut mucosa well before lymphocytes or plasma cells would normally appear. Moreover, when the number of immunoblasts in the thoracic duct is elevated by antigen applied to the flank these blasts[64,65] also accumulate in the gut wall although they are not primed to gut antigen. In a complementary experiment[16], namely injecting blasts taken from peripheral nodes, these do not migrate to the gut despite being primed against ferritin, recipients having been pretreated with ferritin by mouth in order to induce oral immunization. All the foregoing experiments will have been carried out with cell suspensions containing mixtures of both T and B immunoblasts the proportions of which will vary according to the tissue, the species, whether the animal has been maintained in a specific pathogen free or conventional environment and whether a stimulant has been used to elevate blast cell numbers. Nevertheless the overall observations are sufficiently clear to conclude that antigen does *not* attract migrating T or B blasts into the gut mucosa.

One is therefore left with the problem of what tempts immunoblasts to cross the capillaries into the gut mucosa. It need not, of course, be the same stimulus for both T and B blasts. Some authors have speculated on the role of secretory piece[16,67] produced by the epithelial cells as a positive attraction for IgA producing cells, even possibly IgM producers but not IgE or IgG producing cells and not T immunoblasts. A possible explanation may be contrived based on observations of the ready facility with which immunoblasts, particularly activated T-cells, cross blood vessels into local areas of inflammation. T blasts from lymph nodes draining the skin after application of a contact sensitizer (oxazolone) will accumulate in sites of non-specific inflammation or an inflammatory exudate induced by an unrelated contact sensitizer as easily as into the site to which the priming chemical had been applied[79,80]. Similarly the newly formed T blasts which appear in the thoracic duct during infections, e.g. with *Listeria monocytogenes*, will assemble very readily in an inflamed peritoneal cavity but in an entirely non-specific way[81]. If the normal gut is regarded by immunoblasts (particularly T blasts) as a non-specific inflammatory site then large numbers of blast cells would accumulate in the gut mucosa simply as a consequence of its large capillary network. From this argument it follows: firstly that blast cells from any source should enter the gut mucosa; secondly more blast cells should enter an inflamed gut mucosa than a normal one; thirdly immunoblasts should be readily diverted from the gut into capillary beds elsewhere; and, lastly there should be increased accumulation in the gut following removal of alternative sites to which blast cells migrate.

A variety of sources of blast cells in addition to mesenteric lymph node and thoracic duct lymph have been investigated for their capacity to migrate to the gut. These include antigenically stimulated peripheral nodes[16,66]; oxazolone stimulated blasts from peripheral nodes[24,80] which readily enter inflammatory areas of skin; and leukaemic blasts from the spleen of recipients of a transplantable cell leukaemia[83].

But none of these blast cells appear in the lamina propria or epithelium of the villi although they may be found in Peyer's patches.

There is an increase in migration of immunoblasts to the gut mucosa in parasitic worm infection[80,82] and the cells concerned do not need to be specifically activated although they were, however, taken from the mesenteric lymph node and thoracic duct lymph. A proportion of immunoblasts from mesenteric lymph node or thoracic duct lymph draining infected gut could, however, be persuaded into the peritoneal cavity following injection of casein[82] or into the site of application of a contact sensitizer[80]. In the latter case, however, the relevant proportion of immunoblasts was minor and was diverted from the spleen as much as from the gut. Lastly in recipients splenectomized before cell transfer in order to remove a major 'home' of all types of migrating lymphocytes one can detect an increase in migration to the whole gut[80] but most of this increase is diverted to Peyer's patches and not the gut mucosa.

The normal gut, therefore, does not appear to be a non-specific inflammatory site although during worm infection a small proportion of the activated cells are produced as a consequence of infection and these will subsequently accumulate in sites of non-specific inflammation as well as in the gut. It should be appreciated, however, that none of the foregoing experiments disprove the theory that all immunoblasts readily traverse capillaries regardless of source. It merely demonstrates that they do not accumulate in the gut mucosa except when derived from appropriate sources. With this reservation in mind it is relevant to return to the role of antigen in controlling the effector cell population in the gut mucosa for although it has been demonstrated that antigen does not attract immunoblasts into the gut there is equally good evidence to show that antigen determines the number of effector cells in the gut, for in 'antigen-free' conditions, epithelial (T) lymphocytes[5] and IgA forming plasma cells[4] are only 10% of the normal number. In order to resolve this apparent contradiction the following hypothesis is offered: immunoblasts cross capillaries in the gut mucosa in an entirely random fashion. Under the influence of intraluminal antigen appropriately primed effector cells are inhibited from returning to the blood stream probably as a consequence of antigen driven stimulus to final differentiation or multiplication. Such a mechanism would explain the findings of Ogra and Karzon[84] whereby local antigen preferentially stimulates local antibody production.

REFERENCES

1. Bazin, H. (1975). The secretory antibody system. Chapter 2.
2. Meader, R. D. and Landers, D. F. (1967). Electron and light microscopic observations on relationship between lymphocytes and intestinal epithelium. *Am. J. Anat.*, **121**, 763
3. Toner, P. G. and Ferguson, A. (1971). Intraepithelial cells in the human intestinal mucosa. *J. Ultrastruct. Res.*, **34**, 329
4. Crabbe, P. A., Nash, D. R., Bazin, H., Eyssen, H. and Heremans, J. F. (1970). Immunohistochemical observations on lymphoid tissues from conventional and germ-free mice. *Lab. Invest.*, **22**, 448
5. Ferguson, A. and Parrott, D. M. V. (1972). The effect of antigen deprivation on thymus-dependent and thymus-independent lymphocytes in the small intestine of the mouse. *Clin. Exp. Immunol.*, **12**, 477
6. Lascelles, A. K. and McDowell, G. H. (1974). Localized humoral immunity with particular reference to ruminants. *Transpl. Rev.*, **19**, 170
7. Tada, T. and Ishizaka, K. (1970). Distribution of γE-forming cells in lymphoid tissues of the human and monkey. *J. Immunol.*, **104**, 377
8. Crabbe, P. A., Nash, D. R., Bazin, H., Eyssen, H. and Heremans, J. F. (1969). Antibodies of the IgA type in intestinal plasma cells of germ-free mice after oral or parenteral immunization with ferritin. *J. Exp. Med.*, **130**, 723
9. Robertson, P. W. and Cooper, G. N. (1972). Immune responses in intestinal tissues to particulate antigens. Plaque-forming and rosette-forming cell responses in rats. *Aust. J. Exp. Biol. Med. Sci.*, **50**, 703
10. Murray, M., Miller, H. R. P. and Jarrett, W. F. H. (1968). The globule leukocyte and its derivation from the subepithelial mast cell. *Lab. Invest.*, **19**, 222
11. Fichtelius, K. E. (1968). The gut epithelium—a first level lymphoid organ? *Exp. Cell Res.*, **49**, 87
12. Davies, A. G. S. and Ferguson, A. (1974). Unpublished observations
13. Ferguson, A. and Parrott, D. M. V. (1972). Growth and development of 'antigen-free' grafts of foetal mouse intestine. *J. Pathol.*, **106**, 95
14. Ferguson, A. (1975). Celiac disease and gastrointestinal food allergy. In Chapter 5 this volume
15. Parrott, D. M. V. and de Sousa, M. A. B. (1974). B-cell stimulation in nude (nu/nu) mice. In *Proceeding of the First International Workshop on Nude Mice*. J. Rygaard and C. O. Povlsen (eds.) p. 61. (Stuttgart: Gustav Fischer Verlag)
16. Guy-Grand, D., Griscelli, C. and Vassalli, P. (1974). The gut-associated lymphoid system: nature and properties of the large dividing cell. *Eur. J. Immunol.*, **4**, 435
17. Sprent, J., Anderson, R. E. and Miller, J. F. A. P. (1974). Radiosensitivity of T and B lymphocytes. II. Effect of irradiation on response of T cells to alloantigens. *Eur. J. Immunol.*, **4**, 204

18. Hunter, R. L. (1972). Antigen trapping in the lamina propria and production of IgA antibody. *J. Retic. Soc.*, **11**, 245
19. Cornell, R., Walker, W. A. and Isselbacher, K. F. (1971). Small intestinal absorption of horseradish peroxidase. A cytochemical study. *Lab. Invest.*, **25**, 42
20. Bienenstock, J. and Dolezel J. (1971). Peyer's patches: lack of specific antibody-containing cells after oral and parenteral immunization. *J. Immunol.*, **106**, 938
21. Ferguson, A. (1974). Secretion of IgA into 'antigen-free' isografts of mouse small intestine. *Clin. Exp. Immunol.*, **17**, 691
22. Gowans, J. L. and Knight, E. T. (1964). The route of re-circulation of lymphocytes in the rat. *Proc. Roy. Soc. B.*, **159**, 257
23. Ford, W. L. and Gowans, J. L. (1969). The traffic of lymphocytes. *Seminars in Hematology*, **6**, 67
24. Parrott, D. M. V. and Ferguson, A. (1974). Selective migration of lymphocytes within the mouse small intestine. *Immunology*, **26**, 571
25. Smith, J. B., McIntosh, G. H. and Morris, B. (1970). The migration of cells through chronically inflamed tissues. *J. Pathol.*, **100**, 21
26. Nossal, G. J. V. and Ada, G. L. (1971). *Antigens, lymphoid cells and the immune response.* (New York and London: Academic Press)
27. Parrott, D. M. V. and de Sousa, M. A. B. (1971). Thymus-dependent and thymus-independent populations: origin, migratory patterns and life-span. *Clin. Exp. Immunol.*, **8**, 663
28. Langevoort, H. L. (1963). The histopathology of the antibody response. I. Histogenesis of the plasma cell reaction in rabbit spleen. *Lab. Invest.*, 12, 106
29. Warshaw, A. L., Walker, W. A., Cornell, R. and Isselbacher, K. J. (1971). Small intestinal permeability to macromolecules. Transmission of horseradish peroxidase into mesenteric lymph and portal blood. *Lab. Invest.*, **25**, 675
30. Henry, C., Faulk, W. P., Kuhn, L., Yoffey, J. M. and Fudenberg, H. M. (1970). Peyer's patches: immunologic studies. *J. Exp. Med.*, **131**, 1200
31. Hanaoka, M. and Waksman, B. H. (1970). Appendix and antibody formation. II. Distribution of antibody-forming cells after injection of bovine γ-globulin in irradiated, appendix shielded rabbits. *Cell. Immunol.*, **1**, 316
32. Parrott, D. M. V. and de Sousa, M. A. B. (1969). The source of cells within different areas of lymph nodes draining the site of primary stimulation with a contact sensitizing agent. In *Lymphatic tissue and germinal centres in immune responses*, L. Fiore-Donati and M. G. Hanna (eds.) p. 293 (New York: Plenum Press)
33. de Sousa, M. A. B., Parrott, D. M. V. and Pantelouris, E. M. (1969). The lymphoid tissues in mice with congenital aplasia of the thymus. *Clin. Exp. Immunol*,. **4**, 637
34. Faulk, W. P., McCormick, J. N., Goodman, J. R., Yoffey, J. M. and Fudenberg, H. H. (1971). Peyer's patches: morphologic studies. *Cell. Immunol.*, **1**, 500

35. Owen, R. L. and Jones, A. L. (1974). Epitheliae cell specialization within human Peyer's patches: an ultrastructural study of intestinal lymphoid follicles. *Gastroenterology*, **66**, 189
36. Bockman, D. E. and Cooper, M. D. (1973). Pinocytosis by epithelium associated with lymphoid follicles in the bursa of Fabricius, appendix and Peyer's patches. An electron microscopic study. *Am. J. Anat.*, **136**, 455
37. Joel, D. D., Hess, M. W. and Cottier, H. (1972). Magnitude and pattern of thymic lymphocyte migration in neonatal mice. *J. Exp. Med.*, **135**, 907
38. Waksman, B. H. (1973). The homing pattern of thymus-derived lymphocytes in calf and neonatal mouse Peyer's patches. *J. Immunol.*, **111**, 878
39. Pollard, M. and Sharon, N. (1970). Responses of Peyer's patches in germ-free mice to antigenic stimulation. *Infect. Immun.*, **2**, 96
40. Nieuwenhuis, P. (1971). *On the origin and fate of immunologically competent cells.* (Groningen: Wolters-Noordhof Publishing)
41. Veldman, J. E. (1970). *Histophysiology and electron microscopy of the immune response.* (Groningen: Wolters-Noordhof Publishing)
42. Waksman, B. H., Ozer, H. and Blythman, H. E. (1973). Appendix and M–antibody formation. VI. The functional anatomy of the rabbit appendix. *Lab. Invest.*, **28**, 614
43. Stramignoni, H., Mollo, F., Ruà, S. and Palestro, G. (1969). Development of the lymphoid tissue in the rabbit appendix isolated from the intestinal tract. *J. Pathol.*, **99**, 265
44. Howard, J. C., Hunt, S. V. and Gowans, J. L., (1972). Identification of marrow-derived and thymus-derived small lymphocytes in the lymphoid tissue and thoracic duct lymph of normal rats. *J. Exp. Med.*, **135**, 200
45. Chanana, A. D., Schaedeli, J., Hess, M. W. and Cottier, H. (1973). Predominance of theta-positive lymphocytes in gut associated and peripheral lymphoid tissues of newborn mice. *J. Immunol.*, **110**, 283
46. Raff, M. C. (1971). Surface antigenic markers for distinguishing T and B lymphocytes in mice. *Transp. Rev.*, **6**, 52
47. Blythman, H. E. and Waksman, B. H. (1973). Effect of irradiation and appendicostomy on appendix structure and responses of appendix cells to mitogens. *J. Immunol.*, **111**, 171
48. Van den Broek, A. A. (1973). Cortisone interfering with the production of T and B cells. In *Microenvironmental aspects of immunity*, B. D. Janković and K. Isaković (eds.) p. 377 (New York: Plenmun Press)
49. Durkin, H. G. and Thorbecke, G. J. (1973). Homing of B-lymphocytes to follicles: specific retention of immunologically committed cells. In *Microenvironmental aspects of immunity*, B. D. Janković and K. Isaković (eds.) p. 63 (New York: Plenum Press)
50. Ozer, H., Waksman, B. H. and Parrott, D. M. V. (1973). Unpublished observations
51. Durkin, H. G., Caporale, L. and Thorbecke, G. J. (1975). Migratory patterns of B lymphocytes. I. Fate of cells from central and peripheral

lymphoid organs in the rabbit and its selective alterations by anti-immunoglobulin. *Cell. Immunol.*, **16,** 285

52. Shimizu, Y. and Andrew W. (1967). Studies on the rabbit appendix. I. Lymphocyte–epithelial relations and the transport of bacteria from lumen to lymphoid nodule. *J. Morphol.*, **123**, 231
53. Hanaoka, M., Williams, R. M. and Waksman, B. H. (1971). Appendix and γ M–antibody formation. III. Uptake and distribution of soluble or alum-precipitated bovine γ-globulin injected into the rabbit appendix *Lab. Invest.*, **24**, 31
54. Perey, D. Y. E. and Guttman, R. D. (1972). Peyer's patch cells. Absence of graft–versus–host reactivity in mice and rats. *Lab. Invest.*, **27**, 427
55. Levin, D. M., Rosenstreich, D. L. and Reynolds, H. Y. (1973). Immunologic responses in the gastrointestinal tract of the guinea pig. I. Characterization of Peyer's patch cells. *J. Immunol.*, **111**, 980
56. Kagnoff, M. F. and Campbell, S. (1974). Functional characteristics of Peyer's patch lymphoid cells. I. Induction of humoral antibody and cell-mediated allograft reactions. *J. Exp. Med.*, **139**, 398
57. Hoffman, M. K., Schmidt, D. and Oettgen, H. F. (1973). Production of antibody to sheep red blood cells by human tonsil cells *in vitro. Nature* (*Lond.*), **243**, 408
58. Sussdorf, D. H. (1974). Plaque-forming cells in rabbits following stimulation of the appendix with sheep erythrocytes. *Immunology*, **27**, 305
59. Muller-Schoop, J. W. and Good, R. A. (1975). Functional studies of Peyer's patches: evidence for their participation in intestinal immune responses. *J. Immunol.* **114,** 1757
60. La Brec, E. H. and Formal, S. B. (1961). Experimental *Shigella* infections. IV. Fluorescent antibody studies of an infection in guinea pigs. *J. Immunol.*, **87**, 562
61. Craig, S. W. and Cebra, J. J. (1971). Peyer's patches: an enriched source of precursors for IgA producing immunocytes in the rabbit. *J. Exp. Med.*, **134**, 188
62. Hall, J. G. and Smith, M. E. (1970). Homing of lymph-borne immuno blasts to the gut. *Nature* (*Lond.*), **226**, 262
63. Hall, J. G., Parry, D. M., Smith, M. E. (1972). The distribution and differentiation of lymph-borne immunoblasts after intravenous injection into syngeneic recipients. *Cell Tissue Kinet.*, **5**, 269
64. Halstead, T. E. and Hall, J. G. (1972). The homing of lymph-borne immunoblasts to the small gut of neonatal rats. *Transplantation*, **14**, 339
65. Hall, J. G. (1974). Observations on the migration and localization of lymphoid cells. In *Progress in Immunology II*, **Vol. 3,** L. Brent and J. Holborow (eds.) p. 15. (Amsterdam: North Holland)
66. Griscelli, C., Vassalli, P. and McCluskey, R. T. (1969). The distribution of large dividing lymph node cells in syngeneic recipient rats after intravenous injection. *J. Exp. Med.*, **130**, 1427
67. Williams, A. F. and Gowans, J. L. (1975). The presence of IgA on the

surface of rat thoracic duct lymphocytes which contain internal IgA. *J. Exp. Med.*, **141**, 335

68. Cebra, J. J., Craig, S. W. and Jones, P. P. (1974). Cell types contributing to the biosynthesis of s IgA. In *The Immunoglobulin A system*, J. Nestecky, and A. R. Lawton (eds.) p. 23. (New York: Plenum Press)
69. Parrott, D. M. V., Tilney, N. L. and Sless, F. (1975). The different migratory characteristics of lymphocyte populations from a whole spleen transplant. *Clin. Exp. Immunol.*, **19**, 459
70 Calkins, C. E., Ozer, H. and Waksman, B. H. (1975). B cells in the appendix and other lymphoid organs of the rabbit: stimulation of DNA synthesis by anti-immunoglobulin. *Cell. Immunol.* **18**, 187
71. Craig, S. W. and Cebra, J. J. (1975). Rabbit Peyer's patches, appendix and popliteal lymph node B lymphocytes. A comparative analysis of their membrane immunoglobulin components and plasma cells precursor potential. *J. Immunol.*, **114**, 492
72. Perey, D. Y. E. and Bienenstock, J. (1973). Effects of bursectomy and thymectomy on ontogeny of fowl IgA, IgG and IgM. *J. Immunol.*, **111**, 633
73. Bankhurst, A. D. and Warner, N. L. (1972). Surface immunoglobulins on the thoracic duct lymphocytes of the congenitally athymic (nude) mouse. *Aust. J. Exp. Biol. Med. Sci.*, **50**, 661
74. Humphrey, J. H., Parrott, D. M. V. and East, J. (1964). Studies on globulin and antibody production in mice thymectomised at birth. *Immunology*, **7**, 419
75. Sprent, J. (1973). Circulating T and B lymphocytes of the mouse. I. Migratory properties. *Cell. Immunol.*, **7**, 10
76. Sprent, J. and Miller, J. F. A. P. (1972). Interaction of thymus lymphocytes with histo-incompatible cells. II. Recirculating lymphocytes derived from antigen-activated thymus cells. *Cell. Immunol.*, **3**, 385
77. Ford, W. L. and Sedgley, M. (1975). Personal communication
78. Moore, A. R. and Hall, J. G. (1972). Evidence for a primary association between immunoblasts and small gut. *Nature* (*Lond.*), **239**, 161
79. Asherson, G. L., Allwood, G. G. and Mayhew, B. (1973). Contact sensitivity in the mouse. XI. Movement of T blasts in the draining lymph nodes to sites of inflammation. *Immunology*, **25**, 485
80. Parrott, D. M. V., Rose, M. L., Sless, F., Freitas, A. A. and Bruce, R. G. (1975). Factors which determine the accummulation of immunoblasts in gut and skin. In *Future Trends in Inflammation II* (Basel: Burhäuse Verlag)
81. McGregor, D. D. and Logie, P. G. (1974). The mediator of cellular immunity. VII. Localization of sensitized lymphocytes in inflammatory exudates. J. Exp. Med., **139**, 1415
82. Ogilvie, B. and Love, R. (1975). Personal communication
83. Ogra, P. L. and Karzon, D. T. (1969). Distribution of polio virus antibody in serum, nasopharynx and alimentary tract following segmental immunization of lower alimentary tract with polio vaccine. *J. Immunol.*, **102**, 1423
84. Parrott, D. M. V. and de Sousa, M. A. B. (1972). Unpublished observations

CHAPTER 2

The secretory antibody system

Hervé Bazin

Introduction

In the last few years, there has been rapid progress in experimental immunology. However, gastroenterologists may find it surprising that almost all the experimental work has been carried out by using the parenteral route for administration of antigen. Although this approach allows accurate measurement of the inoculated dose, living animals are exposed to antigens at the mucous surfaces to a much greater extent than they are at the cutaneous level. Percutaneous inoculation of antigen would normally occur only by accident, whereas exposure to antigen at mucous surfaces is constant, either by food ingestion, by respiratory inhalation or by the continuous presence of commensal bacteria and viruses. The reluctance of immunologists to use the digestive or pulmonary route in antigen administration can readily be explained by the different penetration of antigen, and inconsistency of antigen absorption when administered by these routes. In the case of the oral route, the main interest in this review, antigens are subjected to gastric juice acidity, to various enzymes and to the intestinal bacterial flora. Moreover, after digestion, most of the substances absorbed by the animal via the alimentary canal have a very small molecular weight and therefore are not immunogenic. In spite of all this, the first observations of digestive immunology were made many years ago[1,2]. These early experiments were dismissed as curiosities and the fact that oral administration of antigen produced immunization was thought to be readily explained by an abnormal inflammatory state of the intestinal mucosa. A clinical example of this state was considered to be the systemic allergic reactions to foods which occur infrequently in man, usually in patients suffering from other allergic diseases. In practice, therefore, digestive immunology was ignored for many years because of the dogma that, in health, there was an intestinal barrier which was impermeable to large, immunogenic molecules.

It is now recognized that this particular field of immunology is of considerable importance, for food ingestion occurs every few hours, the intestinal flora is always present, and inhaled antigens may be coughed up and swallowed. To date most work has been carried out on the intestinal mucosal immune system, although much of the work can be criticized because the techniques used to study local immunity have been based on the spectrum of earlier work on systemic immunology, rather than being specifically designed to study the body surfaces. The possibility that local immunization would lead to secretory antibodies was probably first thoroughly investigated by Burrows[3,4]. However, it was Tomasi and his collaborators who introduced the fundamental concept of an immunological system unique to the mucosae, by their report that the relative proportions of different immunoglobulin classes were not identical in serum, extracellular fluids, and secretions.

IgA is the predominant immunoglobulin in external secretions, and the immunologists who specialized in the study of IgA directed their attention to the antibacterial and antiviral properties of antibodies of this class. However, a critical appraisal of the numerous studies of this subject leads to the conclusion that the evidence for a protective function of IgA is still not very convincing.

A new line of research has recently been opened by the demonstration that food antigens pass in small quantities through the 'intestinal barrier'. This new concept may tie in with a former observation by Sulzberger and Chase[5], on the curious phenomenon whereby tolerance could be induced by administration of antigen orally. No explanation of this Sulzberger–Chase phenomenon has yet been advanced.

At the present time many laboratories are working on digestive immunology and publications in the field are emerging in large numbers. In this review, no attempt will be made to cover all recently published papers. This chapter will be used to air current concepts in this branch of immunology, and to describe and discuss some relevant experiments.

Several excellent and exhaustive reviews are commended to the interested reader. These cover local immunity[6–9], digestive immunity[10–20], IgA immunoglobulin[21–28] and also IgE[29–34].

The intestinal immunological system

A number of observations have drawn attention to the immunological system of the digestive tract. In birds, it has been demonstrated that there are two central immunological organs. The thymus controls maturation of T-lymphocytes, mainly involved in cellular immunological reactions; and the bursa of Fabricius is responsible for the development of the B-lymphoid cells which are able to synthesize immunoglobulins. No anatomical equivalent to the bursa of Fabricius is known in mammals, but there have been many attempts to demonstrate a 'bursa equivalent' in the gut associated lymphoid tissues of mammals.

Tomasi[7] showed that the external secretions, and specifically the digestive juices, do not have the same relative proportions of the different Ig classes as serum. Moreover, the main component of the secretory Ig is IgA, which differs from its serum equivalent in that secretory

IgA has a higher molecular weight and additional antigenic determinants.

Additional pointers to the importance of an intestinal immunological system have been the studies on immune responses produced by oral antigen administration, the presence of and properties of coproantibodies, and the fact that some gastrointestinal diseases (e.g. malabsorption) are associated with immunological disturbances.

These considerations have led various groups to study immunity of the digestive tract as an entity quite different from the general immunological system, although, of course, sharing some properties with it.

Serum and secretory immunoglobulins

To date, five Ig classes have been defined in man, and equivalent Ig's are present in many laboratory animals (Table 2.1). In any animal species, the basic unit of Ig is a molecule, the molecular weight of which is around 155 000 (sedimentation coefficient 6.6S), composed of two heavy and two light chains. The heavy chains are specific to each Ig class and called α, μ, ϵ, δ and γ respectively for the IgA, IgM, IgE, IgD and IgG chains. The light chains are common to all the Ig classes but

Table 2.1 ANALOGY BETWEEN VARIOUS IMMUNOGLOBULIN CLASSES IN MAN AND IN SOME LABORATORY ANIMALS

Species	*Immunoglobulin*					*References*
Man	IgM	IgA	IgE	IgD	IgG	35
Mouse	IgM	IgA	IgE	—	IgG1 or IgF IgG2a or IgG IgG2b or IgH IgG3 or IgI	36
Rat	IgM	IgA	IgE	—	IgG1 IgG2a IgG2b IgG2c	37
Guinea pig	IgM	IgA	IgE	—	IgG1 IgG2	38
Hamster	IgM	IgA	—	—	IgG1 IgG2	39
Rabbit	IgM	IgA	IgE	—	IgG	38

may be of two different types, lambda and kappa. Each heavy or light chain is composed of a variable portion in which is found the antigen combining site and idiotypic specificity (i.e. the properties which are confined to molecules synthesized by the same clone of cell), and a constant part which defines the properties which are common to each Ig class, e.g. complement fixation, attachment to the mast cell membrane, crossing of the placental barrier, etc.

Table 2.2 SOME PHYSICAL PROPERTIES OF HUMAN IMMUNOGLOBULIN CLASSES

Property	*Immunoglobulin*				
	IgM	*IgA*	*IgE*	*IgG*	*IgD*
Sedimentation coefficient	19S	7S 9S 11S	8S	7S	7S
Molecular weight	900 000	160 000 and polymers	190 000	150 000	185 000
Heavy chains	μ	α	ϵ	γ	δ
Light chains	κ or λ	κ or λ	κ or λ	κ or λ	κ or λ
Number of basic unit (2 heavy and 2 light chains)	5	1 or 2	1	1	1
Concentration range in normal serum	0·5–2 mg/ml	1·4–4 mg/ml	0·1–0·7 ng/ml	8–16 mg/ml	0–0·4 mg/ml
Carbohydrate content (%)	12	8	12	2·4	13

The Ig prototype is the IgG molecule which is composed of two light chains (kappa or lambda), and two heavy chains (gamma). It contains about 2·4% glucid. The heaviest Ig molecule is called IgM and is composed of $(2L + 2H)5$, i.e. five basic units polymerized together. In Table 2.2 are listed some physical properties of the different Ig classes.

Two other polypeptide chains have been found in some Ig molecules, secretory piece (Secretory Component) and junction piece (J). The molecular weights of these polypeptides are 60 000 and 20 000 respectively. The secretory piece has been found in all mammals in which it has been looked for [25], and even in birds[40]. This molecule can be found free in external secretions such as saliva and milk and it can also be obtained by reduction of the secretory IgA molecules. The junction piece, discovered by Halpern and Koshland[41] has been found in secretory IgA and IgM[42]. It can be obtained by complete reduction and alkylization of the disulphide bonds of the secretory IgA or IgM molecules. This junction piece is similar in both situations and is found in the ratio of one J piece per molecule. It is synthesized by IgM and IgA plasma cells[43], and surprisingly, it seems that IgG plasma cells synthesize it also although it is not found in IgG molecules[44].

Immunoglobulins of gastrointestinal secretions

The qualitative and quantitative studies of immunoglobulins in the digestive tract are made difficult because of the presence of numerous

Table 2.3 IMMUNOGLOBULINS IN SERUM AND SECRETIONS FROM NORMAL HUMANS

	Immunoglobulin levels mg/100 ml				*References*
	IgM	*IgA*	*IgG*	*ratio IgG/IgA*	
Serum	132	328	1230	3·8	45
Whole saliva	0·55	30·38	4·86	0·16	45
Jejunal secretion	ND	27·6	34·0	1·23	46
Colonic secretion	ND	82·7	86·0	1·04	46

ND: not determined

enzymes capable of degrading Ig molecules. In addition, antigens borne by the Ig molecules are many and heterogeneous, and the problem of their quantitation is made even more complex because IgA molecules may polymerize to give proteins of various molecular weights (monomers and polymers). Finally, storage will influence the nature and types of immunoglobulins present in a sample of intestinal fluid. However, Table 2.3 gives values for immunoglobulins in the serum and secretions of normal humans.

IgA: Molecules of secretory IgA differ from the serum IgA by their high molecular weight and additional antigenic determinants. While the serum IgA is mainly monomeric (7S) in humans, the secretory IgA is mainly dimeric with a molecular weight of 380 to 400 000 (sedimentation coefficient 11S). It is composed of 2 (α_2L_2). J.SC. Light chains in a single molecule are always of the same isotype (kappa or lambda), which means that is is synthesized by only one cell and that extracellular polymerization does not occur. The secretory component is synthesized by the epithelial cells of the non-stratified mucous membranes or glands and not by the immunocytes. It is bound to the alpha chains by –S–S– bonds and covalent bonds. This piece may play a stabilizing role in the dimeric IgA molecule; it may also make this molecule more resistant to proteolytic enzymes[47]. About 90% of secretory IgA molecules possess the SC chain[48]. They also possess the J chain but this characteristic is common to all the polymeric molecules from serum or secretory immunoglobulins. The J piece seems to be necessary for SC binding on the molecules which fix it[49].

IgM: Until recently, it has been accepted that the IgM found in intestinal secretions was identical to that of the serum. Brandtzaeg[48] has demonstrated that, on the contrary, 60–70% of the IgM in secretions possesses the SC piece. The binding between SC and secretory IgM molecules seems to be different from its binding with IgA in that the SC of the secretory IgM molecule reveals antigenic determinants which are hidden in the secretory IgA molecule, and its quaternary structure is less covalently stabilized than that of secretory IgA.

Other immunoglobulins: In all the samples of intestinal secretions which have been studied, IgG and traces of IgD and IgE have been detected. These seem to be identical to their counterparts of the serum.

Secretory Ig in laboratory animals: The animals used in laboratory work have been found to have secretory immunoglobulins analogous to those in man. Thus IgA is the prevalent immunoglobulin in animals' intestinal secretions and its molecular weight is higher than in the serum (mouse[50], rat[51,52], guinea pig[53], hamster[54], rabbit[55], dog[56]). In the same way the J piece (rabbit[57], mouse[58], dog[59], guinea pig[60]) and the SC piece[61,62] have been found in the various polymeric IgAs of all the animal species studied up to now.

ORIGIN OF THE SECRETORY IMMUNOGLOBULINS

Early work by Burrow[4,63] demonstrated that guinea pig faeces contained agglutinating antibodies to *Vibrio cholerae* if the animal had been infected previously, by the intragastric route, with live or dead bacillae. The appearance of these antibodies (called coproantibodies) preceded the appearance of serum antibodies directed against the same antigen. In spite of these findings, the local origin of antibodies in the secretions was not accepted for a long time. The first studies of the gut with fluorescence microscopy, by Crabbé and his colleagues[64] revealed the incredible abundance of immunocytes in the intestinal mucosa, and especially those containing IgA. These results immediately pointed to the origin of the coproantibodies and reinforced the theory that they had a local origin and not a systemic one.

Distribution of the immunocytes in the intestinal mucosa: The digestive tract contains many cells which are part of the immunological system. Some of these are concentrated in nodules (e.g. the lymphoid tissues of the nasopharynx, Peyer's patches, appendix) and others are scattered in the intestinal mucosa where they form a lymphoid jacket or cylinder separated from the gut contents by the intestinal epithelium. A study of this lymphocytic jacket shows that most of the cells synthesizing Ig were elaborating IgA. This has been demonstrated in man[64], dog[21], rat[65], mouse[66] and chicken[67].

A study in man showed that the numbers of plasma cells making IgA, IgM and IgG were 352 000, 51 000 and 15 000 immunocytes per mm^3 respectively[68]. Some IgD immunocytes were found in man also[69] as well as IgE, these latter comprising 3–4% of the number of IgA lymphocytes[70,71]. In the context of the distribution of IgE immunocytes in the body, it is interesting that these are found mainly close to the mucosae[72] in addition to the more frequently discussed IgA immunocytes. By light or electron microscopy, IgA immunocytes cannot be distinguished from those synthesizing other Ig classes[69].

Studies using IgA producing cell lines have shown that the IgA polymers are formed at the time of their excretion from the cells, both in man and the mouse[73,74]. In most species serum IgA is polymeric, at least in part[25]. However, in man serum IgA is mainly monomeric and in the human species dimeric IgA seems to be preferentially synthesized by IgA immunocytes localized in the glandular structures[75].

The mechanism behind these different cellular aspects of synthesis of IgA is not absolutely clear. There is some evidence that the IgA immunocytes making monomeric IgA do not seem to be able to synthesize the J piece in contrast to those making polymeric IgA[76].

Peyer's patches would appear to have very few immunoglobulin synthesizing cells[77,78].

Synthesis of immunoglobulins by the intestinal mucosa: In view of the large number of plasma cells found in this organ, synthesis of Ig by the intestinal mucosa was very likely to be present and, indeed, this has been demonstrated. Aiuti *et al.*[79], Asofsky *et al.*[80] and Hurlimann *et al.*[81], have shown by radioimmunoelectrophoresis that explants from human or mouse intestinal mucosae synthesize IgA *in vitro*. In the same way Bazin *et al.*[50] showed secretion of IgA into the culture medium of mouse intestinal slices. The mean values for daily synthesis were found to be 6·55 ± 0·75 mg in 12 mouse small intestines taken from animals with serum IgA level of 1·72 ± 0·23 mg/ml, i.e. the daily intestinal production was clearly greater than the whole quantity of IgA in the rest of the animal's body. Similar results were obtained in other species[82].

It has been clearly demonstrated that the major part of IgA excreted by the mucosae or exocrine glands is not produced from the serum. In the specific case of the digestive tract, Dive[83] showed that 85% of the IgA from dog intestinal fluid was derived from local synthesis. Similarly Bazin *et al.*[84] proved that the total IgA recovered by washing mouse intestinal tract could not be increased by prior transfusion of normal mouse serum which was rich in IgA. In man, a species where the IgA is mainly monomeric, the secretory dimeric IgA molecules contain either light chains of kappa type or light chains of lambda type[85]. By using allotypic b markers, it has now been shown that the α heavy chains of the two halves of secretory IgA molecules are also identical[86]. Nevertheless, some serum immunoglobulins, including IgA do pass from serum into the intestinal secretions but the amounts are probably fairly low[87].

Mechanism of excretion of intestinal immunoglobulins: Since IgA is the predominant immunoglobulin in the intestinal fluid, its mechanism of passage into the lumen has been most extensively studied. Whether derived from serum or locally, the intestinal mucosal IgA must cross the intestinal epithelium to reach the lumen. Between the cells of this epthelium there are narrow spaces (100–150 Å), so that molecules can diffuse from the extracellular fluids towards the intestinal lumen. However, these intercellular spaces are obstructed by desmosomes and the terminal bars. Proteins do not seem to be able to cross directly into the intestine across the terminal bars [88] (Bazin and Thierry, unpublished results). Thus Ig molecules may spread up to the terminal bar[89] and at this point they must cross the cytoplasm of the epithelial cells. Selective transfer of IgA into the intestinal lumen could be explained on the one hand by a high concentration of IgA in the intestinal submucosa, merely because of the abundance of immunocytes synthesizing this Ig, but on the other hand secretory piece may be involved in the transfer mechanism. SC is synthesized by humans who have no Ig synthesis[90–92] and this molecule is produced by the serous type secretory epithelial cells[93]. SC attaches to the dimeric IgA or the pentameric IgM by means of the J piece; SC is synthesized by the epithelial cells and these seem to be responsible for the transfer of secretory IgA and IgM[93]. Therefore a simple transfer mechanism would be for the SC to be the receptor on the membranes of the epithelial cells for the Ig molecules which require to be transferred into the intestinal lumen. In the situation of a contact between SC and IgA–J or IgM–J in the extracellular fluid, another receptor should be postulated for these molecules which would allow them to cross the epithelial cells. Another possible route of secretion could be through the cell membranes themselves, the J–Ig–SC complex being capable of moving freely through the membrane and perhaps thus crossing the terminal bar in order to be transferred to the intestinal lumen without necessarily penetrating the cellular cytoplasm[94]. If such a role for SC can indeed be proven, this protein would deserve the term 'transport piece' which has been given to it[90]. A similar type of Ig excretion has also been postulated by Brandon *et al.*[95] to explain the selective transport of IgG1 through the sheep mammary epithelium. In this situation, the receptor is thought to recognize the IgG1 and transport it across the epithelial cells while it does not do so for IgG2.

Passage of Ig from the submucosa into the intestinal lumen probably occurs by at least two mechanisms. The first one is adapted to polymeric IgM and dimeric IgA, involves secretory component, and requires the presence of a J chain in the molecule. The second mechanism is applicable to IgE[72] and to IgG, immunoglobulins which do not have polymers or additional polypeptide chains in the intestinal secretions.

It is likely that most of these immunoglobulins cross the epithelial barrier through intercellular spaces and then simply diffuse through the apices of the cells. The quantitative importance of this mechanism has been demonstrated by Andersen *et al.*[96] in the dog, for most dog intestinal IgG is derived from plasma. In addition serum momeric IgA has been proved to cross the intestinal mucosa by passive diffusion. It is not unlikely that in some parts of the villi a break in the continuity of the epithelium may allow the fluid phase of gut lumen to meet the extracellular space of the villi directly. A number of factors may predispose to or increase the amount of this direct continuity, including inflammatory diseases. This subject will not be discussed further as it is outwith the remit of this chapter, which is to be confined to the physiological state.

Immunoglobulins contributed to the serum pool by the intestinal immunological system

Of the several different classes of Ig, only intestinal IgA can be considered to contribute significantly to the serum immunoglobulin pool, although other Ig classes are synthesized in the intestinal submucosa in small quantities. This feature is highlighted by comparing the absolute numbers of IgM, IgA and IgG immunocytes which are situated in the intestine and in other parts of the body. Also several recent experimental studies have demonstrated that the intestinal submucosa was an important source of IgA in dogs, guinea pigs, rats and mice. In dogs the mesenteric lymph contains 3–20 times more dimeric IgA than the quantity which could be accounted for by simple filtration through the intestinal capillary blood vessels[25]. In the same study Vaerman showed that 80% of the serum IgA is provided by the IgA immunocytes of the intestinal mucosa. In rats and guinea pigs, the situation seems to be the same[97]. A completely different approach to this problem, using irradiated mice, has led to similar conclusions. A profound and selective fall of serum IgA occurs after irradiation of mice[98,99]. This fall is observed only when the small intestine has been irradiated and not when the whole animal is irradiated with shielding of the intestine[100]. The rate of catabolism of serum IgA is unaffected by total irradiation of the mouse[101], and similarly IgA catabolism is not influenced by transfusion of additional IgA (from a BALB/c mouse plasmacytoma or normal high titre serum IgA) into axenic mice which normally possess very low serum levels of IgA[84]. Furthermore, the number of immunocytes in the intestinal lamina propria and the synthesis of IgA by mouse gut slices are not diminished by irradiation[50]. The explanation of these apparently conflicting results has been provided by histological and ultrastructural study of the intestinal mucosa after irradiation. This has shown both obstruction of the lymphatic vessels and discontinuities in the intercellular junctions of the epithelial cells. Thus, there is a massive transfer of synthesized IgA from the intestinal submucosa through an epithelium damaged by irradiation into the intestinal lumen, which therefore produces a secondary, although sudden, fall of IgA supply to the serum pool[102].

In man, studies of the concentration of IgA in mesenteric lymph have given rather different findings from those for animals[103,104]. Indeed, humans differ from most other species studied up to now by having high levels of serum IgA with a large proportion of monomeric IgA in the serum, whereas other species have mostly polymeric IgA in their serum. The supply of polymeric IgA in man may possibly be masked by relatively large amounts of monomeric IgA from other origins. Perhaps relevant to this, Hijmans *et al.*[105] demonstrated in man that the bone marrow contains a large number of IgA plasma cells and they came to the conclusion that the bone marrow may be the major source of IgA in man.

Thus, serum IgA seems to be derived from two different sources, the first one being the intestinal submucosa (and possibly other mucous surfaces) which produce polymeric IgA and the second one, other parts of the animal or man which produce monomeric IgA. Depending on the species under consideration, one or the other origin may be predominant.

Intestinal barrier

An important question to be answered is: does the intestinal epithelium represent a real and effective barrier which prevents antigenic molecules from leaving the intestinal lumen and entering the body? It is usually accepted that an inflammatory state will allow exchange of fluid in both directions across the intestinal epithelium, but opinions diverge with regard to the permeability of the intestinal barrier in normal human beings.

It is usually assumed that various substances, including bovine gammaglobulin, ovalbumin, colloidal gold (up to 175 Å), are easily absorbed by columnar epithelial cells in the jejunum and the ileum but not in the duodenum, at least in suckling rats or mice[106]. It is also accepted that this property of intestinal absorption is lost around the time of weaning[106,107]. Although many authors have worked in this field since the beginning of this century, the early studies were inconclusive because of lack of the appropriate techniques. However, a series of well conducted experiments has recently shown that, in man, as well as in experimental animals, the intestinal epithelial barrier is not completely impermeable.

The early experiments on the passage of molecules into the body from the digestive tract have been well reviewed in articles by Wells and Osborne[108], Hettwer and Kriz[109], Walzer[110], Ratner and Gruehl[111] and Alexander *et al.*[112]. These give a detailed survey of the subject up to 1935. Probably the most convincing technique used to demonstrate the passage of antigens into the body was direct or indirect anaphylaxis, in which men or experimental animals were shocked by the feeding of antigens. Ratner and Gruehl[111], in 1934, commented 'we believe that the historical survey gives sufficient evidence to warrant the conclusion that antigens enter the blood stream directly from the gastro-intestinal tract'. Indeed, between 1930 and 1935 direct passage of entire protein molecules was clearly demonstrated in man as well as in animals (guinea pig, dog, rat, rabbit). Papers later than 1930 give accurate accounts of the state of the molecules after their absorption, the factors which regulate their entry, measurements of the quantities absorbed, and the routes followed by these substances before they join the general circulation. Recent expansion of technical aspects of such research has allowed the clarification of some of these points.

Murlin *et al.*[113] showed that the absorption of insulin from Thiry–Vella loops of the jejunum of dogs, as assessed by reduction of blood sugar, was a real phenomenon. Smyth *et al.*[107] studied the absorption of proteolytic enzymes labelled with radioactive iodine, in rabbits. Similar experiments on absorption of Bromelain showed that this molecule was absorbed intact in man also[114]. Ravin *et al.* [115] found that absorption of bacterial endotoxin (*Escherichia coli* 011B_4) from the gastrointestinal tract occurred in normal rabbits. Gruskay and Cooke[116] demonstrated permeability of the intestinal tract to intact proteins (egg albumin) in healthy children. Bernstein and Ovary[117] were unable to confirm this although they showed a significant transfer of the hapten

α–ϵ– bis–DNP–L–lysine (M.W. = 478) through the intestinal mucosa. Falconer and Winborn[118] demonstrated transport of horse spleen ferritin across ligated intestinal segments in normal adult hamsters, and Cornell *et al.*[119] showed that horseradish peroxidase (M.W. = 40 000) may be taken up by a characteristic membranous subcellular system within rat small intestinal absorptive cells and that the macromolecule may be transmitted by these cells to the extracellular space of the lamina propria. This last observation was confirmed for normal rats[120] by the same team who also demonstrated[121] that the adult jejunum is the site of the most significant transfer of entire protein molecules and that the uptake mechanism is similar to the endocytosis which has been described previously in neonatal animals. These various experiments[118–120] demonstrated also that absorption of intact protein molecules by the intestine would seem to be physiological, for the organ apparently maintained its normal ultrastructure. Proteins were found to be completely absorbed in the apical surface of the cells and were found in the intracellular spaces. Absorption occurred by invagination into the cellular surface, i.e. pinocytosis.

Various authors have tried to quantitate absorption of proteins by the intestine. Only approximate values are available. Gruskay and Cooke[116] reported that 0·002% of egg albumin fed to normal children was found in their serum. Thomas and Parrott[122] found serum levels of 1–10 ng/ml. bovine serum albumin in normal rats which had been given 25 mg of protein orally. However, perhaps the most original works in this field are from Volkeimer *et al.*[123–124]. They have differentiated the resorption phenomena (diffusion, active transport and micropinocytosis) already described from the persorption phenomenon which is the entry of particulate elements into the body. They have studied transport of particles of 7–110 microns diameter (pollen powder, corn, maize, potato starch grain, lycodin spores and metallic iron particles). The tested species were rats, guinea pigs, hens, rabbits, dogs and man. In the normal digestive mucosa, they found these markers to be localized at all places where the epithelium was unstratified but mainly at the extrusion zones at the tips of villi in the jejunum. Pollen, starch grains and spores were found in the subepithelial mucosal layers as well as in the lymphatic vessels and the venous blood vessels. In normal man, 70 starch grains per 10 ml venous blood were detected after ingestion of 200 g raw oat flakes, i.e. about 20 000 starch grains for the complete blood volume. The largest persorbed particles were sand grains of 150 microns diameter. 40–70 microns diameter starch grains or spores were persorbed in predictable and constant amounts. According to these authors, the persorbed particles seem to leave the bloodstream in the urine, in pulmonary alveoli, in the cerebrospinal fluid, peritoneal cavity, milk, bile and by macrophage phagocytosis. This persorption phenomenon has been confirmed by a number of other authors, specifically Schlewinski *et al.*[125] in studies on phages and bacteria in mice, but Carter and Collins[126] found no evidence of persorption of *Salmonella* in mice.

Immunological responses induced by the oral route

Physiology of the IgA-producing system

Several supposedly fundamental properties have been attributed to the classical immunological system. These include the function of surveillance for the appearance of malignantly transformed cells, and co-operation with the reticuloendothelial system in the destruction of effete cells and molecules. In fact, such roles are still hypothetical and I would suggest that another and more relevant function of the immunological system could be the monitoring of antigens from the alimentary tract (dietary or bacterial) as well as those from other external origins. The immunological system of the mucosae seems to fit this function perfectly.

The fetus does not contain any immunoglobulin synthesizing immunocytes in the intestinal tract[69] and young germ-free animals have very few of these cells[66], in youth. The appearance of Ig secreting immunocytes in the intestine (especially those secreting IgA) is linked to the establishment of the commensal flora[128]. By using 'antigen free' fetal intestinal grafts in mice[129], Ferguson demonstrated that secretion of IgA into one segment of the small intestine is not dependent upon the presence of antigens within its lumen[130]. The same author suggested that immunoglobulins secreted in the 'antigen free' grafted intestine may have antibody activity directed against antigens present in small intestine elsewhere in the animal[130]. In a similar experiment using rats, Bazin, Beckers and Platteau (unpublished results) have demonstrated that nearly all the IgA found in an intestinal graft lumen has the allotypic marker of the host animal, and not that of the graft; they used one rat allotypic marker[131] for the host IgA and fetal intestinal grafts from (LOU/C/Iα(1a)/Wse and LOU/C/Iα(1.)/Wse) congenic strains for this experiment. These results seem to agree completely with those obtained by Guy-Grand *et al.*[132] who showed that immunoblasts from the mesenteric node (T and B) and from the thoracic duct homed not only to the lamina propria of the intestinal wall but also to the lamina propria of an intestinal graft. The contents of the alimentary tract in germ-free mice are very poor at inducing IgA immunocytes, but this is only so in young animals for old germ-free mice have large numbers of IgA immunocytes in the lamina propria (Bazin and Salomon, unpublished results).

In man, the serum level of IgA at birth is low, about 0·08 mg/ml[133], indicating the absence of transplacental passage of IgA, and a very low rate of synthesis in the newborn. IgA is found in the serum from the second month[134] but thereafter the serum level continues to rise with age[21].

At the moment, it is still impossible to define the relationship between IgA and other Ig immunocytes. It is known that IgA immunocytes are part of the B lymphoid cell pool. It is also generally assumed that the progenitors of IgA secreting cells could be the IgM immunocytes. This theory is supported by experiments of Manning[135], who found very low serum IgA levels in mice which had been treated by injection of anti-μ-chain serum. Another possibility could be a switch from IgM to IgG and then to IgA[136]. Craig and Cebra[137] have used allotypic markers to demonstrate that lymphoid cells from rabbit Peyer's patches contain precursors of the IgA immunocytes which are found in the spleen and later in the intestine. Guy-Grand *et al.*[132] confirmed these results, i.e. blast cells of the Peyer's patches home to the spleen and then to the intestine. The homing mechanism of these blasts would seem to be dependent on two factors: the necessity for the cells to synthesize dimeric IgA and the presence of free SC piece in the lamina propria.

Serum levels of IgA are influenced by the thymus. Thymectomy in birds gives a moderate decrease in serum IgA levels[138]. The use of athymic nu/nu mice has allowed a better definition of how IgA immunocytes are dependent upon the thymus. Salomon and Bazin[139] compared the serum immunoglobulins in nude mice with normal littermates and found the athymic nude animals had serum levels of 19% (IgA), 24% (IgG2a), 61% (IgG1) and 95% (IgM) of the normal mice. Nude mice have been found to have few IgA immunocytes in the intestinal wall (Bazin and Salomon, unpublished results).

Table 2.4 HALF-LIFE OF THE DIFFERENT IMMUNOGLOBULIN CLASSES (IN DAYS)

Species	*Reference*	*IgM*	*IgA*	*IgE*	*IgD*	*IgG*			
Man	140	5	6	2·3	3	24			
						IgG1	IgG2	IgG2b	IgG3
Mouse	36	0·5	0·5–1	ND		2·5–11	5·4–12	3–4	4
						IgG1	IgG2a	IgG2b	IgG2c
Rat	36	2·5	ND	0·5		ND	5·0	ND	ND

ND: not determined

The half lives of the serum immunoglobulins differ. In analysis of serum levels, the catabolic rate and the extra- and intravascular distribution must always be considered. Table 2.4 gives some values for half lives of different immunoglobulin classes. The intravascular distribution of monomeric IgA and IgG are similar, around 40%. About 80% of IgM and IgD are intravascular[141]. Animals which have a predominance of polymeric IgA in their serum probably have more than 40% of the IgA as intravascular. Although the catabolism of IgM, IgA and IgE are probably constant, the catabolism of different IgG subclasses are bound to vary according to the different serum levels[142,143].

The normal level of serum IgA in man, calculated from studies of a population of 462 normal Caucasian adults, is 2·63 ± 1·13 mg/ml[21]. In various animal species studied it has been much lower[25,37] and usually less than 1 mg/ml.

Classical immunological response

Today it is accepted that antigens from a food bolus or from the intestinal flora may enter the body. In the normal physiological condition, this entry is quite small quantitatively, but clearly demonstrable in most of the systems studied (see above). The demonstration of passage of antigen into the body through the intestinal mucosa, is corroborated by several examples of immunization by antigens given orally. This type of immunization which is completely physiological, consists of administering a substance by normal feeding or by catheter. Some experiments have also been performed by using operative models such as Thiry–Vella loops. In such conditions the observations made cannot always be accepted as being typical of antigens given by the oral route for clearly antigens could penetrate the intestinal mucosa through breaches associated with the operation such as suture lines. P. Ehrlich[1] was probably the first scientist who showed antibodies in mice which had been given ricin by the oral route. Davies[2] observed the appearance of coproantibodies (anti-*Shigella* agglutinins) in patients suffering from bacillary dysentery, one and a half days after onset of symptoms, at the time when these patients had no serum antibodies. Indeed, many publications have shown that immunization by the oral route usually leads to stimulation of the immunological system and to the appearance of specific antibodies in the intestinal secretions and serum[7,144–146]. These findings have been reanalysed in relation to the recent appreciation of the importance of a secretory immunological system, and it is best to separate results observed at cellular level from those observed at the level of the immunoglobulins.

Intestinal immunocytes after oral immunization: Levanon *et al.*[147] were apparently the first group to demonstrate the synthesis of specific antibodies at the level of the intestinal mucosa of orally immunized animals. By using the test of passive cutaneous anaphylaxis (PCA), these authors demonstrated that suspensions of cells from the lamina propria of guinea pigs who had ingested dead salmonellae, were able to sensitize normal homologous animals to the same antigenic suspension in 70% of experiments. In 1969, Crabbé *et al.*[148] provided direct evidence of a local intestinal immunological response after ingestion of an antigen. They gave germ-free C3H mice 1 mg of horse ferritin per ml of drinking water. After 30 days by means of an elegant but arduous technique (sequential immunofluorescence staining) they looked not only for the cells producing anti-horse ferritin antibodies but also for the class of immunoglobulins produced by these same cells. They found various immunocytes synthesizing antiferritin antibodies in the intestinal mucosa, and of 66 such cells, they found 58 which clearly synthesized IgA. In 1971 Dolezel and Bienenstock[149] published a very interesting article in which they reported similar results but in another species, and above all in larger numbers of cells. By using combined autoradiography and immunofluorescence, these authors were able to analyse the cells producing specific antibodies and their IgA or non-IgA immunoglobulin class. They used conventional golden hamsters to whose drinking water had been added 0·1% bovine albumin; 70–80% of the cells containing specific antibovine albumin antibodies were IgA class cells (Figure 2.1). The maximum production occurred

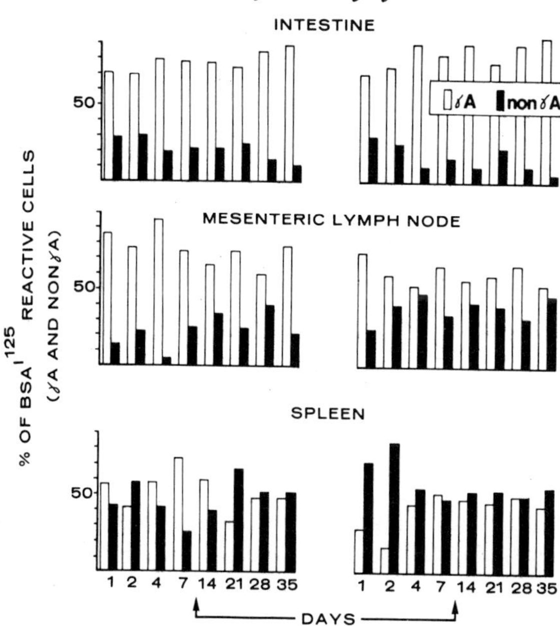

FIGURE 2.1 γA and other classes of antibody containing cells left-hand columns: oral immunization; right-hand columns footpad immunization. (With the permission of Dr J. Bienenstock (*Cell Immunol.*, 1971, **2**, 458))

on the 25th day after the beginning of oral immunization. Therefore there is clear experimental evidence that local synthesis of antibodies can occur after oral administration of an antigen. The immunological responses induced in the Peyer's patches by oral immunization are less well documented. Bienenstock and Dolezel[78] showed that the Peyer's patches in hamsters immunized by ingestion of bovine serum albumin (BSA) for 1–35 days, did not contain antibody-containing cells. Furthermore, they did not find any antigen in these lymphoid aggregates. On the other hand injection of BSA into the Peyer's patches provoked the appearance of local germinal centre formation. Pollard and Sharon[150] have reported that the intestinal infection of mice with *Salmonella paratyphi* or lymphocytic choriomeningitis virus leads to enlargement of the Peyer's patches with appearance of germinal centres. They found that this phenomenon was not observed in mice infected orally with *Streptococcus faecalis*. However, specific antibody containing cells were not searched for in these experiments.

Extraintestinal immunocytes after oral immunization: Quite a few studies have been devoted to these extraintestinal responses after oral immunization. Felsenfeld *et al.*[151] showed that the primate *Cercopithecus aethiops*, when orally immunized with *Vibrio cholerae* liposaccharides, had cells producing specific antibodies in larger numbers in the mesenteric lymph node than in the spleen. Felsenfeld and Greer[152] also demonstrated that oral immunization of gerbils with *Vibrio cholerae* antigens provoked the formation of antibody producing cells in the mesenteric lymph node and in the spleen. Robertson and Cooper[153] studied the immune response of rats after ingestion of sheep red cells. They came to the conclusion that the type of response was identical to that obtained after intravenous immunization. The technique they used did not allow more than the separation of IgM or non-IgM antibody producing cells. Rothberg *et al.*[154] studied the rabbit response to oral immunization with bovine serum albumin and concluded that local antigenic stimulation of the gastrointestinal mucosal surfaces led to a production of specific antibodies by the gut-associated lymphoid tissues. None of these studies differentiated between the classes of immunoglobulins synthesized by the specific antibody-producing cells. Crabbé *et al.*[148] also studied the immunocytes synthesizing specific antibodies in mice immunized with ferritin by the oral route, by means of the above described experimental system. Five cells only were detected in the mesenteric lymph nodes of the two mice studied, four of them being IgA class cells. No other extraintestinal cell was studied. They concluded that oral immunization led to an exclusively IgA class response. In order to allow screening of a larger number of cells from extraintestinal lymphoid organs, Bazin *et al.*[155] used a different experimental system. They added a haemolysate of 2·5% sheep red blood cells (SRBC) to the drinking water of germ-free NMRI mice. By using the direct and indirect Jerne technique, they looked for anti-SRBC antibody producing cells and the corresponding immunoglobulin class in the mesenteric lymph node and in the spleen. After a 2-week oral immunization schedule they found an increasing number of IgA class cells producing haemolytic plaques. IgM, IgG1 and IgG2 class cells were found together with IgA cells, but the latter were five times more numerous than all the other types taken together (Table 2.5). After a 10-day halt in the immunization, the anti-SRBC antibody producing cells disappeared but came back after immunization had been re-established. During primary and secondary responses, the cells synthesizing anti-SRBC antibodies appeared sooner in the mesenteric

Table 2.5 PFC PER SPLEEN IN GERM-FREE MICE ORALLY IMMUNIZED WITH SHEEP RBC

Immune response	*Primary*				*Secondary*				
Days of oral immunization	0	6	14	25	6	11	25	33	77
No of mice	7	2	6	6	2	2	3	4	4
Classes of PFC									
IgM	83	80	94	524	145	72	264	83	105
IgA	0	0	254	2967	0	310	7200	5500	3500
IgG1	0	0	0	167	0	50	230	157	235
IgG2a	0	0	0	46	0	0	230	110	10
IgG2b	0	0	0	40	0	0	10	10	10

From Bazin *et al.* (1970). *J. Immunol.*, **105**, 1049, reproduced by permission

lymph node more than in the spleen. Obviously, oral immunization was not leading to an immunological response limited to the IgA class but rather predominant in IgA, and quite different in distribution of Ig classes from the immunological response obtained by parenteral immunization. This work has also pointed to an intestinal origin for the cells synthesizing specific antibodies in the mesenteric lymph node and in the spleen. Work by Dolezel and Bienenstock[156,149] on hamsters fed orally with bovine albumin fully confirmed and extended the implications of the above discussed results. The peak time of response in the mesenteric lymph node was at 4 days, when 95% of the antibody producing cells were IgA class. In the spleen, the peak response (74% IgA) was observed on the 7th day of immunization (Figure 2.1). Andre *et al.*[157] fed BALB/c mice with sheep red blood cells by intragastric intubation and showed that, in the spleen, the immunological response occurred with predominantly IgA class cells, thus confirming the work by Bazin *et al.*[155] (Figure 2.2). An interesting finding was a discovery that a second course of antigen, given shortly after the first one, showed a state of splenic unresponsiveness. In contrast, when the second course of antigen was given three months after the first antigenic contact, this led to a response identical to the first (Figure 2.3). Indeed, all the studies performed on IgA immunological responses induced by the oral route have demonstrated that secondary responses are almost identical to primary responses[155–157].

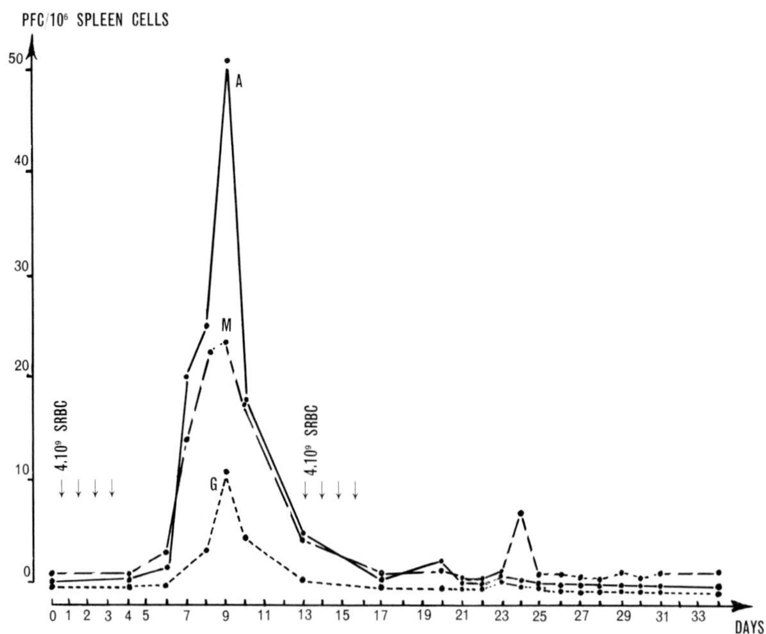

FIGURE 2.2 Antibody producing cells in the spleen of mice receiving sheep red blood cells (SRBC) by the intragastric route for two closely spaced 4-day periods. The first contact with SRBC is followed by the appearance of plaque forming cells (PFC) in the spleen, with a similar time course for PFC of M, A and G immunoglobulin classes. The contribution of PFC of the IgA class is, however, predominant. A secondary response is completely absent when a second intragastric course is initiated ten days after the end of the first (Andre, C., Bazin, H. and Heremans, J. F. (1973). *Digestion*, **9**, 166) (With the permission of the Editor of *Digestion*)

Intestinal immunocytes after parenteral immunization: In their experiments on immunization of germ-free mice with horse ferritin, Crabbé *et al.*[148] discovered after parenteral immunization a small number of specific antibody-secreting cells were present in the lamina propria of the gut, all being of the IgA class. Dolezel and Bienenstock[156] observed a predominantly IgA antibody response in the lamina propria of normal hamsters immunized parenterally with bovine serum albumin.

Specific antibodies detected in the serum and the intestinal secretions of orally immunized animals and man: Many studies were carried out in this field before the discovery of IgA and of its importance in local immunity[6, 23, 145, 158, 174].

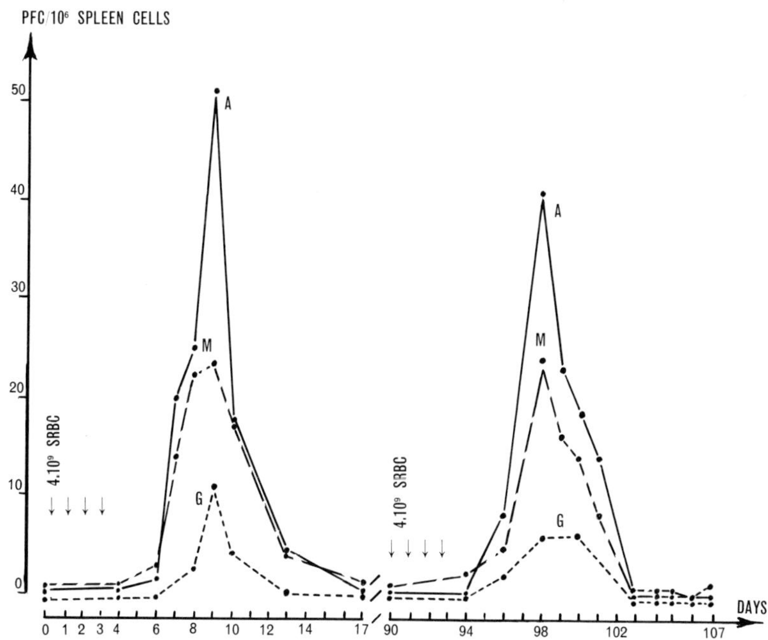

FIGURE 2.3 Antibody producing cells in the spleen of mice receiving SRBC by gastric intubation for two distant 4-day periods. Booster administration of SRBC performed three months after the first antigenic contact induced in the spleen an immunological response similar to that observed in newly primed mice (Andre, C., Bazin, H. and Heremans, J. F. (1973). *Digestion*, **9**, 166) (With the permission of the Editor of *Digestion*)

(*i*) *Secretory antibodies*

Berger *et al.*[159] as well as Ogra and Karzon[160] showed that IgA class antibodies in human intestinal secretions were able to bind poliovirus. Porter *et al.*[161,162] showed that antibodies of pig intestinal secretions directed against an *Escherichia coli* strain were mainly of the IgA class. Girard and Kalbermatten[163] discovered, after oral vaccination of children against nine strains of *E. coli*, a clearly defined opsonic activity in the intestinal secretions. This antibody activity was IgM associated in the first samples (8–10 days after oral immunization) and later IgA associated (20–44 days after immunization). Hasimoto *et al.*[164] showed that anti-adenovirus neutralizing activity in the orally infected mouse was IgA associated and appeared in the animal's intestinal contents. Eddie *et al.*[165] found specific IgG and IgA class antibodies to the orally administered antigen *Salmonella typhimurium* in rabbit intestinal fluid. Fubara and Freter[166] described the appearance of IgA class antibodies after oral immunization of mice with *Vibrio cholerae.*

(*ii*) *Serum antibodies*

In a study on circulating antibodies to milk in children, Coombs *et al.*[167] noticed that IgG class antibodies were always present in higher titres than IgA ones. Strannegard[168] observed only IgA class antibodies in rabbit orally immunized with killed toxoplasma. Ogra and Karzon[160,169] reported their discovery of IgA class anti-poliovirus specific antibody in humans orally vaccinated with inactivated virus. Crabbé *et al.*[148] reported that germ-free C3H mice synthesized only IgA class specific circulating antibodies after oral immunization with horse ferritin. On the other hand, Strannegard and Yurchison[170] pointed out that in rabbits orally immunized with sheep red blood cells, egg albumin or bovine serum albumin antigens, the serum antibodies were of the IgM, IgA and IgG classes. Girard and Kalbermatten[163] could not identify circulating antibodies in children whom they orally immunized with an extract of *E. coli* strains. Kletter *et al.*[171] showed that some new born children had circulating antibodies to cow's milk protein but in titres lower than in their mothers. Moreover, the titres of these antibodies increased at the age of a month to reach a maximum at three months and then fell. The antibodies were mainly IgG class but some IgA antibodies were also present, appearing later and increasing in amount up to the 7th month. Dolezel and Bienenstock[156], in the experiments already mentioned, found specific antibodies to bovine albumin in the serum of the orally immunized hamsters, and these antibodies were mainly of the IgM and IgG classes although sometimes also IgA. Heremans and Bazin[172] in a study of axenic mice immunized against sheep red bood cells (SRBC) found anti-SRBC antibodies in the serum, of all immunoglobulin classes but with an IgA predominance. After oral immunization of adult rats with sheep red blood cells, André and Bazin[173] detected an IgM response in the serum and IgA–IgG1 class antibody in the mesenteric lymph.

Reaginic response after oral immunization

Tada and Ishizaka[70] have reported the presence of moderate numbers of IgE immunocytes in the intestine and in the lymph nodes draining it, both in humans and monkeys. The functional correlates of these cells—anaphylactic reactions—were described a long time ago both in men and in laboratory animals after oral immunization. Richet[174] who with Portier, discovered the phenomenon of anaphylaxis, mentioned in a book on the subject written in 1923 that Rosenae and Anderson[175] were the first scientists to establish anaphylaxis induced by alimentary ingestion. These authors noticed that guinea pigs which had previously eaten horse meat could suffer an anaphylactic crisis after injection of horse serum. The chapter on alimentary anaphylaxis in Richet's book[174] is very interesting because it quotes clinical examples of alimentary allergy. One patient is mentioned who was affected after ingestion of only one shrimp (even when absolutely fresh) and yet was not upset at all by lobsters and crayfish; the second case report is probably the first clinical report in which the patient is a Nobel prizewinner, Richet himself 'in this regard I may mention my personal experience that even in very little quantity, yolk can provoke in me violent gastric pains and even vomiting'. Prausnitz and Küstner[176] reported the case of a patient who was extremely sensitive to the ingestion of cooked fish and whose serum allowed them to develop their test.

Alimentary anaphylaxis can also be induced in laboratory animals and Richet[174] reported that dogs can have anaphylactic crises after oral sensitization with 'crepitine' and subsequent ingestion of the same compound. He concluded by drawing attention to several factors: antigen (especially those of milk, egg and fish), the site of exposure (stomach or rectum), individual sensitivity, and absorption of undigested substances into the body. Another very interesting publication is that of Du Bois *et al.*[177]. These authors report cases of normal children who developed reactions of immediate hypersensitivity to foods (cows' milk: 6 of 10 tested children; egg white: 8 of 21; sheep serum: 1 of 4; almond flour: 2 of 15). Many other studies have also reported the incidence of reaginic antibodies against alimentary proteins in man.[178–185] Although this work has documented alimentary allergy, causes of the allergy are yet poorly defined. Allergy will develop in only a percentage of individuals exposed to standard antigenic stimulation.

In order to determine whether it is possible to obtain reaginic immune responses by the oral route in experimental animals, Bazin and Platteau (*Immunology*, in press) immunized LOU/M/Wsl rats with ovalbumin doses from 1 to 100 mg by the oral route together with 10^{10} *Bordetella pertussis* organisms as adjuvant. They did not obtain clear primary response in these animals when tested by passive cutaneous anaphylaxis using serum. However, after a second immunization one month later, 10, 50, or 100 mg of albumin orally, erratic responses were detected, unequivocally positive in some animals. On the other hand rats from the same strain, immunized with 1 μg of albumin parentally plus 10^{10} *Bordetella pertussis*, by the technique of Jarrett and Stewart[186], developed unequivocal reaginic responses after oral ingestion of 10–100 μg of albumin 30 days later. In these experiments titres of up to 1/512 were obtained with PCA tests. In this last experiment, the most constant responses were obtained with doses of 10 mg orally. Clearly, this experimental model provides the basis for further studies on the initiation of digestive tract allergy.

Immunological response to intestinal parasite

The immune response of the intestinal tract to intestinal parasite infection has not yet been adequately studied. In the case of many parasites the life cycle of the parasite is at first extraintestinal and later in the gastrointestinal tract. Therefore the induction of the immune response may be mostly outwith the intestine and only the final phenomenon of selfcure is localized to the gastrointestinal tract. Crandall *et al.*[187] showed that the number of IgA plasma cells were maintained at a very high level during infection of rabbits with *Trichinella*. Moreover, large numbers of IgM and IgG cells were also found in the intestine. Curtain and Anderson[188] found definite increases in the numbers of IgG synthesizing plasma cells in parasitized sheep. Bazin *et al.*[189] studied mice, Cne: NMRI germ-free and three months old, infected with *Hymenolepis nana*. This parasite of man and rodents may have a complete cycle in mice without an intermediate host and when absorbed as an egg by the mouse, it changes into the hexacanth embryo, penetrates the duodenal villi where it takes the form of cysticercoid larvae. Some 5 days later it returns to the intestinal lumen and goes down to live in the ileum. The eggs of this worm can be sterilized without killing them so that it is possible to study the specific influence of the parasite on the germ-free host animal. The lamina propria and the mesenteric lymph node from 3-month-old axenic mice contain very small numbers of IgA immunocytes (about 100 times less than conventional mice of the same age)[66]. On the 10th day of infection, the parasitized germ-free mice had numbers of IgA immunocytes approximately equal to germ-free control animals. On the 30th day of infection, however, the intestinal mucosa showed large numbers of IgA plasma cells, similar to conventional mice at the same age. Also at this 30th day of infection, the mesenteric lymph nodes of the animals contained large numbers of IgA immunocytes, clearly significantly more than the control germ-free animals. Table 2.6 summarizes the serum levels of immunoglobulins

Table 2.6 SERUM LEVELS OF IMMUNOGLOBULINS OF NMRI OUTBRED MICE INFESTED WITH *Hymenolepis nana*

	Number of mice	*Levels of serum immunoglobulins* (mg/ml)			
		IgM	*IgA*	*IgG1*	*IgG2a*
germ-free mice	3	1·21	0·04	0·19	1·03
infested germ-free mice (10th d.)	3	0·97	1·01	0·12	0·59
Infested germ-free mice (30th d.)	3	1·22	0·13	0·60	1·74
infested and infected mice* (10th d.)	3	1·17	0·28	1·03	5·50
infested and infected mice* (30th d.)	3	1·33	0·29	1·77	7·11

* Germ-free mice voluntarily contaminated with commensal micro-organisms one month before starting the experiment

in these animals. It should be noticed that IgM level, which is always normal in axenic mice, did not vary in spite of the infection either in germ-free mice or in controls which had been taken out of isolators one month before the experiment. On the other hand, IgA and IgG increased in the germ-free mice 30 days after infection with *Hymenolepis nana*.

Discussion

I. Is there a passage of antigens from the intestinal lumen in normal animals?

Intestinal permeability to macromolecules is not an important aspect of absorption of nutrients. On the other hand since relatively few molecules are required for immunological stimulation, the intestine is clearly permeable to macromolecules in sufficient quantities to affect immunity. Scientific literature now contains many examples of immunological reponses which have been orally induced, and some of the work already discussed[118,122,190–193] has shown that orally administered antigens can be detected in the intestinal mucosa as well as in the mesenteric lymphatics or blood. Passage of macromolecules through the intestinal epithelium may be modified in several ways and the limit between normal and pathological situations has not yet been defined. Walker and Isselbacher[194] analysed these various factors recently in an excellent review. One of these factors is particularly interesting, that immunization of an animal against a given antigen may lead to a modification in the absorption of this antigen through the intestine. Bockman and Winborn[118] described increase of antigenic absorption in hamsters immunized with ferritin. This might indicate local trapping of antigen by specific antibodies binding antigen in the gut wall[193]. However, the opposite result found was by Walker *et al.*[190,192,195], who reported that oral or parenteral immunization of rats with bovine serum albumin or with horseradish peroxidase led to a specific decrease of the antigen uptake by gut sacs prepared from jejunum and ileum of treated rats. Moreover, the binding of antigen to specific IgG1 and IgG2 antibodies was demonstrated by radioimmunoelectrophoretic analysis of mucosal extracts. Andre *et al.*[193] showed that rats immunized with human serum albumin had impaired absorption of antigen when this was assessed by antigen measurement in the mesenteric vein. This phenomenon was apparently related to the state of immunization of the animals and the authors suggested that the IgA class antibodies could be responsible.

These results are not necessarily contradictory if it is considered that antigenic macromolecules could be stopped, at least partially, in the lamina propria by specific binding with corresponding antibodies[20] and thus would be more readily phagocytosed if present in the lamina propria in previously immunized animals. The fact that parenteral or oral immunization could lead to the same phenomenon is not necessarily evidence against this suggestion because antibodies of local and systemic origin are present in the lamina propria. Finally, the affinity of IgA class antibodies could well be insufficient for the detection of antibody properties by radioimmunoelectrophoresis. In contrast to the report by Fahey *et al.*[196], we could not determine, even after hyperimmunization of mice, the IgA antibody properties by this technique, although it has been quite easily demonstrated in the case of other immunoglobulin classes[197].

II. Are there immunological phenomena after ingestion of antigens by the oral route in normal subjects?

There is now abundant evidence that it is relatively easy to obtain immunization by the oral route. However, in reviewing the published literature, it is important to remind oneself that negative results are seldom published. However, from the information available, it is clear that immune responses may be local or systemic or else tolerance induction may occur.

Local immunological response: Theoretically, the antigen which crosses the intestinal barrier has to pass the lamina propria to reach the lymphatic or venous vessels which will then carry it into the body. Thus the first type of response must be local and the main characteristic of the secretory immunological system of the intestine is its abundance in IgA immunocytes and relative abundance in IgE immunocytes. The study of cells synthesizing specific antibodies of the IgA class and the analysis of special secretory antibodies have clearly demonstrated the existence of immunological responses induced by the oral route and localized in the intestine.

Systemic immunological response: The existence of a lymphocyte traffic from the intestine through lymphatic vessels, mesenteric lymph nodes and blood vessels, and preferential homing back to the lamina propria has been demonstrated (Chapter 1). After antigens cross the intestinal epithelial barrier, they meet immature lymphocytes (B-lymphocytes possibly co-operating with T-cells). These cells would migrate to the general circulation and most of them will be predetermined to manufacture IgA class immunoglobulins. Some of them will stop at the mesenteric lymph node level or at the spleen where they may contribute to a systemic immune response. Others home to the lamina propria by a mechanism which may be due to the presence of secretory piece[137,198–201]. Probably not all the cells which are destined to become IgA secreting immunocytes in the lamina propria will follow this intricate route. Crabbé *et al.*[77] and Bienenstock[202] demonstrated the existence of a number of foci of IgA immunocytes adjacent to Peyer's patches and Crabbé *et al.*[77], reported that when they looked for IgA immunocytes in germ-free mice recently taken out of sterile isolators and put into an ordinary environment, the first cells of IgA class appeared around Peyer's patches. Finally, Ogra and Karson[160] showed that intestinal immunological responses could remain localized in the area of contact with the antigen. Thus, according to the species, the antigen and the localization of the antigenic stimulus, the proportion of cells evolving into IgA class antibody forming cells, may be variable and some of them may migrate a short distance, others migrating through the thoracic duct and the general circulation. These two routes of migration could explain the fact that some responses appear to stay localized and others diffuse into other mucosae to a varying degree. However, in all situations it is interesting that the circulation of IgA synthesizing cells is a very efficient mechanism which spreads these cells all along the digestive tract. A second mechanism whereby the immunological response to oral antigen may be expanded is by the contribution of the lymphoid system associated with the intestine to the serum pool of immunoglobulins. There is no doubt that in many animal species and in man, some of the antibody synthesized in the digestive tract returns to the blood vessels, and IgA represents an important part of this contribution. It must not be forgotten that the half life of antibodies varies considerably according to their immunoglobulin classes. In mice, the half life of the IgA is 0·5 days, the IgG1 is 8–11 days[101], and in man the IgA half life is about 6 days and that of IgG around 24 days[140]. It is little wonder then that the serum of orally immunized animals seems to have higher concentration of IgG class antibodies (with a long half life) than IgA antibodies[172]. A final mechanism similar to both the others above should also be mentioned. Small quantities of antigens which have not been degraded may be found in the serum of orally immunized animals[122,193]. This antigen probably has a role identical to the one which it would have had if it had been parenterally injected.

Tolerance induction by ingestion of antigen: Tolerance induction by the intestinal route has been known for many years (Suzlberger–Chase phenomenon)[5]. In the adult guinea pig, oral immunization with simple allergens such as 2.4 dinitrochlorobenzene or picryl chloride, prevents these animals from later sensitization when injected with the same substance by the parenteral route. The tolerance obtained is absolutely specific, often total, long-lasting and affecting both immediate and delayed hypersensitivity. Although tolerance is usually induced by repeated administration of antigen, Pomeranz[203] showed that a state of specific tolerance could be obtained in the guinea pig by a single administration of a high dose of picryl chloride in vegetable oil by the oral route. Silverman and Pomeranz[204] show that at least part of the ingested picryl chloride was localized in the upper gastrointestinal tract during the 12 hours after its feeding, whereas the remaining material was hydrolysed into picric acid in the gut and was eliminated in the faeces[205]. Since picryl chloride is a simple chemical sensitizer that couples rapidly to proteins, it is interesting to compare these results with those obtained by Borel and Golan[206,207] and by Lee and Sehon[208,209], who demonstrated that administration of hapten coupled with mouse IgG allowed the induction of hapten specific tolerance in mice, but also suppressed an already established response.

III. Role of the local immunological response

Many reviews and original articles have dealt with the problem of the biological role of the intestinal immunological responses. In fact, the role of this part of the immune system is still not established and it should be emphasized more often that the suggested functions of the local immune response are still a subject of research.

Of the antibodies which are present in intestinal secretions, only the IgA class ones would seem to have special properties when compared with their serum homologues. Secretory IgM, with secretory component, apparently has properties identical to those of serum IgM. On the other hand secretory IgA molecules are more resistant to digestion than the other Ig[47,210,211]. Thus, the life of IgA antibodies in the intestinal lumen is longer than that of other Igs. Secretory IgA is, as a rule, tetravalent, being a dimer of two divalent molecules. The IgA class antibodies have a very poor capacity to precipitate antigens in gel[212]. Newcome (cited by Gimsberg[17]) reported that the S-IgA from human or rabbit could precipitate albumin if it had been crosslinked by means of glutaraldehyde in a gelled medium with polyethylene glycol added. Myeloma IgA of the mouse with known antibody properties, has been studied and although it is monomeric and with high affinity constants, these molecules do not precipitate dinitrophenylized proteins (mentioned in ref. 25). IgA class antibodies do not fix complement[212,213]. Nevertheless, Adinolfi *et al.*[214] suggested that secretory IgA, in the. presence of complement and lysozyme, could lyse certain bacteria. This mechanism has not been found in other systems[165]. On the other hand, agglutinating properties of polymeric IgA seem to be good[162,212,215]. IgA antibodies may activate complement by the alternate pathway involving C3. Opsonic properties of IgA antibodies have been described[163,216,217], but at least in the mouse no specific receptors can be found on macrophage membranes for IgA molecules. Although blocking activity of IgA antibodies may be doubtful[218], it has been clearly demonstrated that they have a neutralizing capacity[104], and could be bactericidal without any help from complement[219].

The role of IgE antibodies is more difficult to understand. There is no doubt that immediate anaphylactic reactions may occur at the intestinal level but they can hardly be considered as useful. On the other hand, it has been shown recently by Capron *et al.*[220] that IgE antibodies are cytophilic for normal macrophages and may act against parasites in the rat. The role of other antibodies from the IgM, IgG and IgD classes would seem to be the same, when studed in the intestinal mucosa, as their roles in serum.

IV. Function of the immunological response

Antiviral and anti-microbial function: The first work on secretory antibodies showed that they were present in viral, microbial and parasite infections. Furthermore it has been shown in various systems that protection obtained against virus or bacterial infection correlates with the secretory antibody titres and not with the serum titre. Oral immunization against bacteria was demonstrated a long time ago to be highly effective in producing immunity against the same organisms administered orally[221]. Fubara and Freter[166,222] showed that the specific secretory IgA antibodies could protect a mouse against experimental cholera. Waldman *et al.*[223] proved the effectiveness of a killed vaccine against *Salmonella typhimurium* in the mouse, when the vaccine was given orally.

Nevertheless, the mechanism by which the coproantibodies, especially those of the IgA class, act is not clear. Intestinal bacterial infections are obviously controlled, at least in part, by interrelationships between different bacterial species as well as by local immunological phenomena[224]. A possibility that bacterial adherence may be interfered with at the level of the intestinal mucosa represents one of the best ways to study these problems[166,225,226].

Studies on the role of antibodies from intestinal secretions have been many. Lipton and Steigman[227] and Kono *et al.*[228] reported the presence in faecal extracts of neutralizing antibodies for polio virus and the Newcastle virus. Berger *et al.*[159], Ogra and Karson[229] and Keller and Dwyer[230] clearly demonstrated the existence in the intestinal secretions of IgA antibodies which neutralize polio virus. Hashimoto *et al.*[164] showed that in mice orally infected with adenovirus the neutralizing activity was bound to IgA and was found in intestinal contents of these animals *in vivo.*

Brantdzaeg[231] has separated the mechanism of intestinal immunological responses into two stages. The first line of defence, which is perhaps the normal line of defence, is composed of the synthesis and secretion of IgM, IgA and secretory piece. The second line comprises the exudation and local synthesis of IgG which is associated with chronic inflammatory phenomena. The role of intestinal IgE is little known. Even in the case of parasite infection, for example with *Nippostrongylus brasiliensis*, where the intestine is the selective site for adult parasites and also the site of their expulsion by an immunological mechanism, opinions are divergent[232]. Urquhart *et al.*[233] have integrated some of these mechanisms, postulating that a reaction of immediate hypersensitivity at the intestinal level could, through the production of a protein losing enteropathy, result in a significant transport of protective IgG class antibodies from the serum through the mucosa into the gut lumen.

Increase of the intestinal impermeability to antigens: In recent years a number of authors have suggested that one important role of the intestinal immunological responses could be to prevent alimentary, parasite or bacterial antigens from entering the body. This mechanism might be described as an ointment or dressing along the mucosa of the digestive tract. Antibodies would then be bound to the luminal surface by means of cysteine residue of mucin (Walter and Bloch, mentioned in ref. 202). By this means, non-absorbable, stable antigen–antibody complexes would be formed[234]. In man, the incidence of antibodies to bovine serum albumin has been found to decrease with age. 74% of healthy children between 4 and 5 years have such antibodies, 69% under 15 years, 30% between ages of 16 and 40 and only 7–10% of persons older than 40[180,235]. It is possible to explain this phenomenon by a reduction in the ingestion of bovine albumin, by changes in the permeability of the intestinal barrier, or by immunological hypoactivity towards chronically administered antigens[236]. Bazin *et al.*[20] proposed the hypothesis as follows: When antigens have induced an intestinal immunological response, their subsequent crossing of the intestinal barrier will result in the formation of antigen–antibody complexes and their enhanced phagocytosis by the reticuloendothelial system. Thomas and Vaes-Zadeh[237] have suggested that this antigen trapping could take place in the liver. It has also been suggested that defects in IgA synthesis could allow complement fixing reactions between gut antigens and antibodies of the IgG and IgM classes[238]. This has been studied by Eddie *et al.*[165] who showed that *Salmonella typhimurium* when agglutinated by IgA antibodies, could no longer be killed by IgM or IgG antibodies—antibodies which are normally able to kill *Salmonella* organisms by means of complement fixation. A possible role of the IgA antibodies from the digestive tract could be to stop antigens after they cross the epithelial barrier so that no Arthus reactions occur, since the complement fixing actions are inhibited.

Antigens from the lumen of the gut may well meet immunological cells in the Peyer's patches. These lymphoid cells will then leave the Peyer's patches to be distributed along the intestine, there to secrete specific antibodies, especially of the IgA class, which prevent the entry of antigens to the body or protect it against bacterial or viral infections.

Tolerance induced by the ingestion of antigen: Schulberger and Chase originally proved that an animal could be rendered refractory to cutaneous sensitization by haptens, after ingestion of this hapten. This phenomenon is still unexplained. Battisto and Miller[239] showed that adult guinea pigs could be rendered tolerant to picryl chloride or to bovine gammaglobulin by injection of these materials in minute quantities into the mesenteric veins. Pommeranz[203] has reported that a state of specific tolerance can be obtained in the adult guinea pig by a single administration of a high dose of picryl chloride orally. Cantor and Dumont[240] showed that the ingestion of dinitrochlorobenzene by adult dogs prior to parenteral immunization, suppressed the elaboration of specific antibodies to this hapten and this effect could be suppressed by previous diversion of the portal vein from the liver. Triger *et al.*[241]

extended the range of results by publishing their work on immunization with sheep red cells via the portal vein or the inferior vena cava. The humoral and cellular responses in this system were shown to be considerably reduced when antigen was administered by the portal venous route. Thomas and Parrott[122] recently published a very interesting paper in which they demonstrated that oral administration of bovine serum albumin could lead to a partial state of tolerance to this antigen. Although the mechanism involved has not been established, it is known that parenteral inoculation of an animal's own intestinal flora gives a very poor immunological response, at least in mice[242]. In man, Korenblat *et al.*[243] showed that adults in whom there were no serum antibodies to bovine albumin, were in fact in a state of immunological hyporeactivity towards this antigen. Kletter *et al.*[171] proposed that the state of non-reactivity could be due to a reduction of the digestive tract permeability to intestinal antigens which allowed only the passage of tolerogenic antigen in adults. Bazin *et al.*[20] presented the thesis that antigenic filtration could take place at the level of the epithelium or the lamina propria by classical antigen–antibody reactions which allowed passage of small tolerogenic antigen molecules. They also suggested that the passage of antigens combined with specific antibodies (mainly IgA class) into the general circulation could produce a state of tolerance. This phenomenon must be compared with the results obtained by Borel[207] and by Lee and Sehon[208,209] on the induction of tolerance to haptens attached to isogenic protein carriers. IgA antibodies would of course, be perfect candidates for such a carrier role as they do not fix complement.

V. Conclusions

To draw conclusions based on the established facts of secretory antibody system of the gastrointestinal tract is difficult. The raw fundamental data concerning the system itself are still lacking. Nevertheless, its role and its functions are certainly the subject of a considerable amount of recent work. The earlier research was directed towards antibacterial or antiviral functions, similar to the functions which have already been established in the systemic parts of the immune system. IgM and IgG antibodies are much more efficient in these properties than IgA, and the presence of a special yet functionally inferior type of immunoglobulin to perform these functions the body surfaces seems an inefficient type of specialization. A completely new research line has now opened up in relation to studies on the absorption of antigens through the intestinal epithelium, and the ways in which this absorption is altered by prior oral immunization. The function of the secretory antibody system may be a difficult aspect to measure and a difficult concept to grasp, especially if its main property turns out to be simply to be present and to be active in binding antigens, in order to prevent any other type of immune response from happening.

ACKNOWLEDGMENTS

This work has been supported by the 'Fonds Cancérologique de la C.G.E.R.' (Belgium) and the contract No 74.7.0491 by the D.G.R.S.T. (France). H. Bazin is staff member of the Euratom–Biology Division (Publication No 1127). I gratefully acknowledge Dr. A. Ferguson's help in reviewing the manuscript and I warmly thank Mrs D. Amthor for her assistance in writing the English version of this paper.

REFERENCES

1. Ehrlich, P. (1891). Experimentelle Untersuchungen über Immunität, I Uber Ricin. II Uber Aboin. *Dtsch. Med. Wschr.*, **17**, 976
2. Davies, A. (1922). Serological properties of dysentery stools. *Lancet*, **ii**, 1009
3. Burrows, W., Elliot, M. E. and Havens, I. (1947). Studies on immunity to Asiatic cholera. Excretion of coproantibody in experimental enteric cholera in guinea pig. *J. Inf. Dis.*, **81**, 261
4. Burrows, W. and Havens, I. (1948). Studies on immunity to Asiatic cholera; absorption of immune globulin from bowel and its excretion in urine and feces of experimental animals and human volunteers. *J. Infec. Dis.*, **82**, 231
5. Chase, M. W. (1946). Inhibition of experimental drug allergy by prior feeding of the sensitizing agent. *Proc. Soc. Biol. N.Y.*, **61**, 257
6. Tomasi, T. B. and Bienenstock, J. (1968). Secretory immunoglobulins. *Adv. Immunol.*, **9**, 1
7. Heremans, J. F. (1968). Immunoglobulin formation and function in different tissues. *Curr. Topics Microb. Immunol.*, **45**, 131
8. Tomasi, T. B. (1970). Structure and function of mucosal antibodies. *Ann. Rev. Med.*, **21**, 281
9. Hanson, L. A. and Brandtzaeg, P. (1973). Secretory antibody system. In *Immunologic disorders in infants and children*, E. R. Stiehm, V. A. Fulginiti and W. B. Saunders (eds.) p. 107. (Philadelphia)

10. Taylor, K. B. (1965). Role of immune responses in the gastrointestinal tract. *Fed. Proc.*, **24**, 23
11. Taylor, K. B. (1966). Immunological mechanisms of the gastrointestinal tract. *Gastroenterology*, **51**, 1058
12. Watson, D. W. (1969). Immune responses and the gut. *Gastroenterology*, **56**, 944
13. Bazin, H. (1970). L'immunité intestinale. *Path. Biol.*, **18**, 1101
14. Johnson, J. S. (1970). Section IV: Immunologic mechanisms in the gastrointestinal tract. The secretory immune system, a brief review. *J. Infect. Dis.*, **121**, 115
15. Bazin, H. (1970). L'immunité humorale au niveau de l'intestin. *Acta Gastroénterol. Belg.*, **33**, 846
16. Kraft, S. C. and Kirsner, J. B. (1971). Immunological apparatus of the gut and inflammatory bowel disease. *Gastroenterology*, **60**, 922
17. Ginsberg, A. L. (1971). Alterations in immunologic mechanisms in diseases of the gastrointestinal tract. *Amer. J. Dig. Diseases*, **16**, 61
18. Bienenstock, J. and Perey, D. Y. (1972). Immune mechanisms of mucosal resistance. *Medical Clinics of North America*, **56**, 391
19. Ferguson, A. (1972). Immunological roles of the gastrointestinal tract. *Scot. Med. J.*, **17**, 111
20. Bazin, H., André, C. and Heremans, J. F. (1973). Réponses immunologiques induites par voie orale. *Ann. Immunol. (Inst. Pasteur)*, **124 C**, 253
21. Vaerman, J. P. (1970). Studies on IgA immunoglobulins in man and animals. *Thèse Sintal Louvain*
22. Heremans, J. F. and Vaerman, J. P. (1971). Biological significance of IgA antibodies in serum and secretions. *Progr. Immunol.*, **1**, 875
23. Tomasi, T. B. and Grey, H. M. (1972). Structure and function of immunoglobulin A. *Prog. Allergy*, **16**, 81
24. Vaerman, J. P. (1973). Structure et propriétés des IgA. *Rev. franc. Mal. respiratoires*, **1**, 871
25. Vaerman, J. P. (1973). Comparative immunochemistry of IgA. *Res. Immunochem. Immunobiol.*, **3**, 91
26. Vaerman, J. P. (1973). Propriétés physiochimiques des IgA humaines, revue générale. *Ann. Immunol. (Inst. Pasteur)*. **124**, 289
27. Wang, A. C. and Fudenberg, H. H. (1974). IgA and evolution of immunoglobulins. *J. Immunogenetics*, **1**, 3
28. Heremans, J. F. (1974). Structure and function of immunoglobulin IgA. *Behring Inst. Mitt.*, **50**, 1
29. Ishizaka, K. and Ishizaka, T. (1971). Immunoglobulin E and homocytotropic properties. *Prog. Immunol. I*, **1**, 859
30. Bennich, H. and Johansson, S. G. O. (1971). Structure and function of human immunoglobulin E. *Adv. Immunol.*, **13**, 1
31. Binaghi, R. A. (1973). Les anticorps anaphylactiques des mammifères. I. Structure et propriétés physicochimiques. *Bull. Inst. Past.*, **71**, 249
32. Stanworth, D. R. (1973). *Immediate hypersensitivity*. (Amsterdam and London: North-Holland Publ. Company)

33. Bennich, H. and Von Bahr-Lindtrom, H. (1974). Structure of immunoglobulin E (IgE). *Prog. Immunol. II*, **1**, 49
34. Ishizaka, K., Ishizaka, T., Kishimoto, T. and Okudaira, H. (1974). Biosynthesis of IgE antibodies and mechanisms of sensitisation. *Prog. Immunol., II*, **4**, 7
35. An extension of the nomenclature for immunoglobulin. (1969). *Bull. O.M.S.*, **41**, 975
36. Bazin, H., Beckers, A., Platteau, B., Naze-De Mets, J. and Kints, J. P. (1973). Les immunoglobulines de la souris et du rat. *Exp. Animale*, **6**, 219
37. Bazin, H., Beckers, A. and Querinjean, P. (1974). Three classes and four (sub) classes of rat immunoglobulins: IgM, IgA, IgE and IgG1, IgG2a, IgG2b, IgG2c. *Eur. J. Immunol.*, **4**, 44
38. Binaghi, R. (1972). *Immunoglobulins. Structure des immunoglobulines en immunologie*. P. Bordet (ed.) (Paris: Flammarion Médecine–Sciences)
39. Bienenstock, J. and Bloch, K. J. (1970). Immunoglobulins of the hamster. I. Antibody activity in four immunoglobulin classes. *J. Immunol.*, **104**, 1220
40. Bienenstock, J., Perey, D. Y. E., Gauldie, J. and Underdown, B. J. (1973). Chicken, γA: Physicochemical and immunochemical characteristics. *J. Immunol.*, **110**, 524
41. Halpern, M. S. and Koshland, M. E. (1970). Novel subunit in secretory IgA. *Nature (Lond.*), **228**, 1276
42. Mestecky, J., Zikan, J. and Butler, W. T. (1971). Immunoglobulin M and secretory immunoglobulin A: presence of common polypeptide chain different from light chain. *Science*, **161**, 1163
43. Parkhouse, R. M. E. (1972). Biosynthesis of J-chain in mouse IgA and IgM. *Nature New Biology*, **236**, 9
44. Kaji, H. and Parkhouse, R. M. E. (1974). Intracellular J chain in mouse plasmocytomas secreting IgA, IgM and IgG. *Nature (Lond.*), **249**, 45
45. Brandtzaeg, P., Fjellanger, I. and Gjersuldsen, S. T. (1970). Human secretory immunoglobulins. I. salivary secretions from individuals with normal or low levels of serum immunoglobulins. *Scand. J. Haemat.*, (*suppl. 12*), **1**, 3
46. Bull, D. M., Bienenstock, J. and Tomasi, T. B. (1971). Studies on human intestinal immunoglobulin A. *Gastroenterology*, **60**, 370
47. Shuster, J. (1971). Pepsin hydrolysis of IgA. Delineation of two populations of molecules. *Immunochemistry*, **8**, 405
48. Brandtzaeg, P. (1974). Human secretory immunoglobulin M: an immunochemical and immunohistochemical study. *Immunology*, **29**, 559
49. Eskeland, T. and Brandtzaeg, P. (1974). Does J chain mediate the combination of 19 S IgM and Dimeric IgA with the secretory component rather than being necessary for their polymerization? *Immunochemistry*, **II**, 161
50. Bazin, H., Maldague, P., Schonne, E., Crabbé, P. A., Bauldon, H. and Heremans, J. F. (1971). The metabolism of different immunoglobulin

classes in irradiated mice. V. contribution of the gut to serum IgA levels in normal and irradiated mice. *Immunology*, **20**, 571

51. Bistany, T. S. and Tomasi, T. B. (1970). Serum and secretory immunoglobulins of the rat. *Immunochemistry*, **7**, 453
52. Stechschulte, D. J. and Austen, K. F. (1970). Immunoglobulins of rat colostrum. *J. Immunol.*, **104**, 1052
53. Vaerman, J. P. and Heremans, J. F. (1972). The IgA system of the guinea pig. *J. Immunol.*, **108**, 637
54. Bienenstock, J. (1970). Immunoglobulins of the hamster. II. characterization of the γA and other immunoglobulins in serum and secretions. *J. Immunol.*, **104**, 1228
55. Cebra, J. and Robbins, J. B. (1966). γA-immunoglobulin from rabbit colostrum. *J. Immunol.*, **97**, 12
56. Reynolds, H. Y. and Johnson, J. S. (1970). Quantitation of canine immunoglobulins. *J. Immunol.*, **105**, 698
57. O'Daly, J. A. and Cebra, J. J. (1971). Rabbit secretory IgA. Isolation of secretory component after selective dissociation of the immunoglobulin. *J. Immunol.*, **107**, 436
58. Rosenstein, R. W. and Jackson, P. (1973). The binding of a naphthalene dye associated with J-chain attachment in an immunoglobulin A mouse immunoglobulin. *Biochemistry*, **12**, 1659
59. Kehoe, J. M., Tomasi, T. B., Ellouz, F. and Capra, J. D. (1972). Identification of "J" chain in a homogeneous canine IgA immunoglobulin. *J. Immunol.*, **109**, 59
60. Kobayashi, K., Vaerman, J. P., Bazin, H., Lebacq-Verheyden. A. M. and Heremans, J. F. (1973). Identification of J-chain in polymeric immunoglobulins from a variety of species by cross-reaction with rabbit antisera to human J-chain. *J. Immunol.*, **111**, 1590
61. Benveniste, J., Lespinats, G. and Salomon, J. C. (1971). Serum and secretory IgA in axenic and holoxenic mice. *J. Immunol.*, **107**, 1656
62. Vaerman, J. P., Heremans, J. F., Bazin, H. and Beckers, A. (1975). Identification and some properties of rat secretory component. *J. Immunol.*, **114**, 265
63. Burrows, W. E. and Ware, L. L. (1953). Studies on immunity to Asiatic cholera. VII. prophylatic immunity to experimental enteric cholera. *J. Infect. Dis.*, **92**, 164
64. Crabbé, P. A., Carbonara, A. O. and Heremans, J. F. (1965). The normal human intestinal mucosa as a major source of plasma cells containing γA-immunoglobulin. *Lab. Invest.*, **14**, 235
65. Nash. D. R., Vaerman, J. P., Bazin, H. and Heremans, J. F. (1969). Identification of IgA in rat serum and secretions. *J. Immunol.*, **103**, 145
66. Crabbé, P. A., Bazin, H., Eyssen, H. and Heremans, J. F. (1968). The normal microbial flora as a major stimulus for proliferation of plasma cells synthesizing IgA in the gut. The germ-free intestinal tract. *Int. Arch. Allergy*, **34**, 362
67. Lebacq-Verheyden, A. M., Vaerman, J. P. and Heremans, J. F. (1972).

Immunohistologic distribution of the chicken immunoglobulins. *J. Immun.*, **109**, 652
68. Crabbé, P. A. and Heremans, J. F. (1966). Etude immunohistochimique des plasmocytes de la muqueuse intestinale humaine normale. *Revue Franc. Etud. clin. biol.*, **II**, 484
69. Crabbé, P. A. (1967). Signification du tissu lymphoïde des muqueuses digestives. *Thésis* (Bruxelles: Arscia)
70. Tada, T. and Ishizaka, K. (1970). Distribution of γE-forming cells in lymphoid tissues of the human and monkey. *J. Immunol.*, **104**, 377
71. Ishizaka, K. and Ishizaka, T. (1971). IgE and reaginic hypersensitivity. *Ann. N.Y. Acad. Sci.*, **190**, 443
72. Ishizaka, K., Ishizaka, T., Tada, T. and Newcomb, R. W. (1969). Site of synthesis and function of gamma-E. In *Secretory immunologic system*, D. H. Dayton, P. A. Small, R. M. Chanock, H. E. Kaufman and T. B. Tomasi (eds.) p.71. (Washington DC: US Govt. Printing Office)
73. Abel, C. A. and Grey, H. M. (1968). Studies on the structure of mouse γA myeloma proteins. *Biochemistry*, **7**, 2682
74. Matsuoka, Y., Yagi, Y., Moore, G. E. and Pressman, D. (1970). Isolation and characterization of IgA produced by an established human lymphocytoid cell line. *J. Immunol.*, **104**, 1
75. Brandtzaeg, P. (1973). Two types of IgA immunocytes in man. *Nature New Biology*, **243**, 142
76. Brandtzaeg, P. (1974). Human immunocytes may contain J-chain along with IgD, IgM, IgG or dimeric IgA, but not along with pure monomeric IgA. Personal communication
77. Crabbé, P. A., Nash, D. R., Bazin, H., Eyssen, H. and Heremans, J. F. (1970). Immunohistochemical observations on lymphoid tissues from conventional and germfree mice. *Lab. Invest.*, **22**, 448
78. Bienenstock, J. and Dolezel, J. (1971). Peyer's patches: lack of specific antibody containing cells after oral and parenteral immunization. *J. Immunol.*, **106**, 938
79. Aiuti, F., Turbessi, G. and Ugolini, A. (1969). Synthesis *in vitro* of immunoglobulins produced by different human mucous membranes. *Experientia*, **25**, 1089
80. Asofsky, R. and Thorbecke, G. I. (1961). Site of formation of immunoglobulins and of a component of C′3. II. Production of immunoelectro phoretically identified serum proteins by human and monkey tissues *in vitro*. *J. Exp. Med.*, **114**, 471
81. Hurlimann, J. and Darling, H. (1971). *In vitro* synthesis of Immunoglobulin -A by salivary glands from animals of different species. *Immunology*, **21**, 101
82. Kagnoff, M. F., Serfilippi, D. and Donalson, R. M. (1973). *In vitro* kinetics of intestinal secretory IgA secretion. *J. Immunol.*, **110**, 297
83. Dive, C. (1971). *Les protéines de la bile. Leur composition et leur origine.* (Bruxelles: Arscia)

84. Bazin, H., Levi, G. and Heremans, J. F. (1971). The metabolism of different immunoglobulin classes in irradiated mice. IV. Fate of circulating IgA of tumour or transfusion origin. *Immunology*, **20**, 563
85. Bienenstock, J. and Strauss, H. (1970). Evidence for synthesis of human colostral γA as 11 S dimer. *J. Immunol.*, **105**, 274
86. Lawton, A. R. and Mage, R. G. (1969). The synthesis of secretory IgA in the rabbit. I. Evidence for synthesis as an 11S dimer. *J. Immunol.*, **102**, 693
87. Butler, W. T., Rossen, R. D. and Waldmann, T. A. (1967). The mechanism of appearance of immunoglobulin A in nasal secretions in man. *J. Clin. Invest.*, **46**, 1883
88. Orzalesi, N., Riva, A. and Testa, F. (1971) Fine structure of human lacrimal gland. I. The normal gland. *J. Submicr. Cytology*, **3**, 283
89. Brandtzaeg, P., Fjellanger, I. and Gjeruldsen, S. T. (1967). Localization of immunoglobulins in human nasal mucosa. *Immunochemistry*, **4**, 57
90. South, M. A., Cooper, M. D., Wollheim, F. A., Hong, R. and Good, R. A. (1966). The IgA system. I. Studies of the transport and immunochemistry of IgA in the saliva. *J. Exp. Med.*, **123**, 615
91. Tourville, D. R., Adler, R. H., Bienenstock, J. and Tomasi, T. B. (1969). The human secretory immunoglobulin system: immunohistological localization of γA, secretory 'piece', and lactoferrin in normal human tissues. *J. Exp. Med.*, **129**, 411
92. Brandtzaeg, P. (1971). Human secretory immunoglobulins. 4. Quantitation of free secretory piece. *Acta Pathol. Microb. Scand.*, **79 B**, 189
93. Brandtzaeg, P. (1974). Mucosal and glandular distribution of immunoglobulin components: Immunohistochemistry with a cold ethanol-fixation technique. *Immunology*, **26**, 1101
94. Brandtzaeg, P. (1974). Mucosal and glandular distribution of immunoglobulin components: differential localization of free and bound SC in secretory epithelial cells. *J. Immunol.*, **112**, 1553
95. Brandon, M. R., Watson, D. L. and Lascelles, A. K. (1971). The mechanism of transfer of immunoglobulin into mammary secretion of cows. *Austr. J. Exp. Biol. Med. Sci*, **49**, 613
96. Andersen, S. B., Glenert, J. and Wallevik, K. (1963). Gammaglobulin turnover and intestinal degradation of gamma globulin in the dog. *J. Clin. Invest.*, **42**, 1873
97. Vaerman, J. P., Andre, C., Bazin, H. and Heremans, J. F. (1973). Mesenteric lymph as a major source of serum IgA in guinea pigs and rats. *Eur. J. Immunol.*, **3**, 580
98. Micklem, H. S. and Bazin, H. (1967). Concentration of immunoglobulins in lethally X-irradiated mice. *Nature (Lond.)*, **215**, 742
99. Bazin, H. and Doria, G. (1970). The metabolism of different immunoglobulin classes in irradiated mice. III. Effects of supralethal doses of X-rays. *Int. J. Radiat. Biol.*, **17**, 359
100. Bazin, H., Maldague, P. and Heremans, J. F. (1970). The metabolism of

different immunoglobulin classes in irradiated mice. II. Role of the gut. *Immunology*, **18**, 361

101. Bazin, H. and Malet, F. (1969). The metabolism of different immunoglobulin classes in irradiated mice. I. Catabolism. *Immunology*, **17**, 345

102. Bazin, H. (1971). Etude du métabolisme des différentes classes d'immunoglobulines chez la souris normale et irradiée. *Thesis*–Faculté des Sciences de Paris

103. Cruchaud, A., Laperrouza, C. and Megevand, R. (1968). Agammaglobulinemia in monozygous twins: therepautic prospects. *Birth Defects Original Article*, **series IV**, 315

104. Tomasi, T. B. and Grey, H. M. (1972). Structure and function of immunoglobulin. *A. Prog. Allergy*, **16**, 81

105. Hijmans, W., Schuit, H. R. and Hulsing-Hesseling, E. (1971). An immunofluoresence study on intracellular immunoglobulins in human bone marrows cells. *Ann. N.Y. Acad. Sci.*, **177**, 290

106. Clark, S. L. (1959). The ingestion of proteins and colloidal materials by columnar absorptive cells of the small intestine in suckling rats and mice. *J. Biophys. Biochem. Cytol.*, **5**, 41

107. Smyth, R. D., Brennan, R. and Martin, G. J. (1964). Studies establishing the absorption of the bromelains (proteolytic enzymes) from the gastrointestinal tract. *Exp. Med. Surg.*, **22**, 46

108. Wells, H. G. and Osborne, T. B. (1911). The biological reactions of the vegetable proteins. I. Anaphylaxis. *J. Infec. Dis.*, **8**, 66

109. Hettwer, J. P. and Kriz, R. A. (1925). Absorption of undigested protein from the alimentary tract as determined by the direct anaphylaxis test. *Am. J. Physiol.*, **73**, 539

110. Walzer, M. (1927). Studies in absorption of undigested proteins in human beings; simple direct method of studying absorption of undigested protein. *J. Immunol.*, **14**, 143

111. Ratner, B. and Gruehl, H. L. (1934). Passage of native proteins through the normal gastrointestinal wall. *J. Clin. Invest.*, **13**, 517

112. Alexander, H. L., Shirley, K. and Allen, D. (1936). The route of ingested egg white to the systemic circulation. *J. Clin. Invest.*, **15**, 163

113. Murlin, J. R., Tomboulian, R. L., and Pierce, H. B. (1937). Absorption of insulin from Thiry–Vella loops of the intestine in normal and depancreatized dogs. *Am. J. Physiol.*, **120**, 733

114. Miller, J. H. and Opher, A. W. (1964). The increased proteolytic activity of human blood serum after the oral administration of bromelain. *Exp. Med. Surg.*, **22**, 277

115. Ravin, H. A., Rowley, D., Jenkins, C. and Fine, J. (1960). On the absorption of bacterial endotoxin from the gastrointestinal tract of the normal and shocked animal. *J. Exp. Med.*, **112**, 783

116. Gruskay, F. L. and Cooke, R. E. (1955). Gastrointestinal absorption of unaltered protein in normal infants and in infants recovering from diarrhea. *Pediatrics*, **16**, 763

117. Bernstein, I. D. and Ovary, Z. (1968). Absorption of antigens from the gastrointestinal tract. *Int. Arch. Allerg.*, **33**, 521
118. Bockman, D. E. and Winborn, W. B. (1966). Light and electron microscopy of intestinal ferritin absorption. Observations in sensitized and non-sensitized hamsters (*Mesocricetus auratus*). *Anat. Rec.*, **155**, 603
119. Cornell, R., Walker, W. A. and Isselbacher, K. J. (1971). Small intestinal absorption of horse radish peroxidase. A cytochemical study. *Lab. Invest.*, **25**, 42
120. Warshaw, A. L., Walker, W. A., Cornell, R. and Isselbacher, K. J. (1971). Small intestinal permability to macromolecules. Transmission of horse radish peroxidase into mesenteric lymph and portal blood. *Lab. Invest.*, **25**, 675
121. Walker, W. A., Cornell, R., Davenport, L. M. and Isselbacher, K. J. (1972). Macromolecular absorption. Mechanism of horse radish peroxidase uptake and transport in adult and neonatal rat intestine. *J. Cell. Biol.*, **54**, 195
122. Thomas, H. C. and Parrott, D. M. V. (1974). The induction of tolerance to a soluble protein antigen by oral administration. *Immunology*, **27**, 631
123. Volkheimer, G., Schulz, F. H., Wendland, H. and Hausdorf, E. D. (1967). Le phénomène de la persorption et son importance en allergologie. *Maroc médical*, **47**, 626
124. Volkeimer, G., Schulz, F. H., Lindenau, A. and Beitz, U. (1969). Persorption of metallic iron particles. *Gut*, **10**, 32
125. Volkeimer, G., Schultz, F. H., Lehman, H., Aurich, I., Hübner, R., Hübner, M., Hallmayer, A., Münch, H., Oppermann, H. and Strauch, S. (1968). Primary portal transport of persorbed starch granules from the intestinal wall. *Med. Exp.*, **18**, 103
126. Schlewinski, E., Graben, N., Funk, J., Sahm, E. and Raettig, H. (1971). Oral immunization with non-living micro-organisms or their antigens. *Zbl. Bakt. Hyg. I. Abt. Orig. A.*, **218**, 93
127. Carter, P. B. and Collins, F. M. (1974). The route of enteric infection in normal mice. *J. Exp. Med.*, **139**, 1189
128. Dolezel, J., Strauss, H. and Bienenstock, J. (1971). Antigen in feed as cause of antibody in unimmunized animals. *Int. Arch. Allergy*, **40**, 749
129. Ferguson, A. and Parrott, D. M. V. (1972). Growth and development of 'antigen free' grafts of foetal mouse intestine. *J. Path.*, **106**, 95
130. Ferguson, A. (1974). Secretion of IgA into 'antigen free' isografts of mouse small intestine. *Clin. Exp. Immunol.*, **17**, 691
131. Bazin, H., Beckers, A., Vaerman, J. P. and Heremans, J. F. (1974). Allotypes of rat immunoglobulins. I. An allotype at the α-chain locus. *J. Immunol.*, **112**, 1035
132. Guy-Grand, D., Griscelli, C. and Vassali, P. (1974). The gut-associated lymphoid system: nature and properties of the large dividing cells. *Eur. J. Immunol.*, **4**, 435
133. Faulkner, W. and Borella, L. (1970). Measurement of IgA levels in human cord serum by a new radioimmunoassay. *J. Immunol.*, **105**, 786

134. McKay, E. and Thom, H. (1969). Observations on neonatal tears. *J. Pediat.*, **75**, 1245
135. Manning, D. D. (1972). Induction of temporary IgA deficiency in mice injected with heterologous anti-immunoglobulin heavy chain antisera. *J. Immunol.*, **109**, 1152
136. Cooper, M. D., Lawton, A. R. and Kincade, P. W. (1972). A two-stage model for development of antibody-producing cell. *Clin. Exp. Immun.*, **11**, 143
137. Craig, S. W. and Cebra, J. J. (1971). Peyer's patches: an enriched source of precursors for IgA-producing immunocytes in the rabbit. *J. Exp. Med.*, **134**, 188
138. Perey, D. Y. E. and Bienenstock, J. (1973). Effects of bursectomy and thymectomy on ontogeny of fowl IgA, IgG, and IgM. *J. Immunol.*, **111**, 633
139. Salomon, J. C. and Bazin, H. (1972). Low levels of some serum immunoglobulin classes in nude mice. *Rev. Europ. études clin. et biol.*, **17**, 880
140. Daguet, G. L. (1972). *Elements d'immunologie médicale.* p. 62 (Paris: Flammarion)
141. Seligman, M. and Klein, M. (1971). Structure et activité biologique des immunoglobulines. *Rev. Prat.*, **21**, 883
142. Fahey, J. L. and Sell, S. (1965). The immunoglobulins of mice. V. The metabolic (catabolic) properties of five immunoglobulin classes. *J. Exp. Med.*, **122**, 41
143. Tada, T., Okumura, K., Platteau, B., Beckers, A. and Bazin, H. (1975). Half-lives of two types of rat homocytotropic antibodies in circulation and in the skin. *Int. Arch. Allergy*, **48**, 116
144. Ross, V. (1932). The role of the soluble specific substance in oral immunization against pneumococcus types II and III. *J. Exp. Med.*, **55**, 1
145. Pierce, A. E. (1959). Specific antibodies at mucous surfaces. *Vet. Rev. Annot.*, **5**, 17
146. Freter, R. (1962). Detection of coproantibody and its formation after parenteral and oral immunization of human volunteers. *J. Infec. Dis.*, **111**, 37
147. Levanon, Y., Raettig, H. and Rossetini, S. M. O. (1968). Positive immunological reaction of gut cells from orally immunized animals demonstrated by passive cutaneous anaphylaxis. *Experientia*, **24**, 600
148. Crabbé, P. A., Nash, D. R., Bazin, H., Eyssen, H. and Heremans, J. F. (1969). Antibodies of the IgA type in intestinal plasma cells of germfree mice after oral or parenteral immunization with ferritin. *J. Exp. Med.*, **130**, 723
149. Dolezel, J. and Bienenstock, J. (1971). γA and non-γA immune response after oral and parenteral immunization of the hamster. *Cell. Immunol.*, **2**, 458
150. Pollard, M., and Sharon, N. (1970). Responses of the Peyer's patches in germ-free mice to antigenic stimulation. *Infection and Immunity*, **2**, 96

151. Felsenfeld, O., Greer, W. E. and Felsenfeld, A. D. (1967). Cholera toxin neutralization and some cellular sites of immune globulin formation in *Cercopithecus aethiops*. *Nature (Lond.)*, **213**, 1249
152. Felsenfeld, O. and Greer, W. E. (1968). Vibriocidal activity, immune globulin producing cells and immune globulin levels in *Theropithecus gelada* after administration of a *Vibrio cholerae* antigen. *Immunology*, **14**, 319
153. Robertson, P. W. and Cooper, G. N. (1972). Immune responses in intestinal tissues to particulate antigens. Plaque-forming and rosette-forming cell responses in rats. *Austr. J. Exp. Biol. Med. Sci.*, **50**, 703
154. Rothberg, R. M., Kraft, S. C. and Michalek, S. M. (1973). Systemic immunity after local antigenic stimulation of the lymphoid tissue of the gastrointestinal tract. *J. Immunol.*, **111**, 1906
155. Bazin, H., Levi, G. and Doria, G. (1970). Predominant contribution of IgA antibody-forming cells to an immune response detected in extra-intestinal lymphoid tissues of germ-free mice exposed to antigen by the oral route. *J. Immunol.*, **105**, 1049
156. Dolezel, J. and Bienenstock, J. (1971). Immune response of the hamster to oral and parenteral immunization. *Cell. Immunol.*, **2**, 326
157. André, C., Bazin, H. and Heremans, J. F. (1973). Influence of repeated administration of antigen by the oral route on specific antibody-producing cells in the mouse spleen. *Digestion*, **9**, 166
158. Anderson, A. F., Schloss, O. M. and Myers, C. (1925). The intestinal absorption of antigenic protein by normal infants. *Proc. Soc. Exp. Biol. Med.*, **23**, 180
159. Berger, R., Ainbender, E., Hodes, H. L., Zepp, H. D. and Hevizy, M. M. (1967). Demonstration of IgA polioantibody in saliva, duodenal fluid and urine. *Nature (Lond.)*, **214**, 420
160. Ogra, P. L. and Karzon, D. T. (1969). Distribution of poliovirus antibody in serum, nasopharynx and alimentary tract following segmental immunization of lower alimentary tract with poliovaccine. *J. Immunol.*, **102**, 1423
161. Porter, P., Kenworthy, R., Noakes, D. E. and Allen, W. D. (1974). Intestinal antibody secretion in the young pig in response to oral immunization with *Escherichia coli*. *Immunology*, **27**, 841
162. Porter, P., Noakes, D. E. and Allen, W. D. (1970). Intestinal secretion of immunoglobulins and antibodies to *Escherichia coli* in the pig. *Immunology*, **18**, 909
163. Girard, J. P. and de Kalbermatten, A. (1970). Antibody activity in human duodenal fluid. *Eur. J. Clin. Invest.*, **1**, 188
164. Hashimoto, K., Yoshikawa, M., Sugihara, Y. and Sasaki, S. (1971). Intestinal resistance in the experimental enteric infection of mice with a mouse adenovirus. II. Determination of the neutralizing substance in the intestinal tract as an IgA antibody. *Jap. J. Microb.*, **15**, 499
165. Eddie, D. S., Schulkind, M. L. and Robbins, J. B. (1971). The isolation and biologic activities of purified secretory IgA and IgG anti-*Salmonella*

typhimurium 'O' antibodies from rabbit intestinal fluid and colostrum. *J. Immunol.*, **106**, 181

166. Fubara, E. S. and Freter, R. (1973). Protection against enteric bacterial infection by secretory IgA antibodies. *J. Immunol.*, **111**, 395
167. Coombs, R. R. A., Jonas, W. E., Lachmann, P. J. and Feinstein, A. (1965). Detection of IgA antibodies by the red cell linked antigen-antiglobulin reaction; antibodies in the sera of infants to milk proteins. *Int. Arch. Allergy*, **27**, 321
168. Strannegard, O. (1967). The formation of toxoplasma antibodies in rabbits. *Acta Path. Microb. Scand.*, **71**, 439
169. Ogra, P. L., Karzon, D. T., Righthand, F. and MacGillivray, M. (1968). Immunoglobulin response in serum and secretions after immunization with live and inactivated poliovaccine and natural infection. *New Engl. J. Med.*, **279**, 893
170. Strannegard, O. and Yurchision, A. (1969). Formation of agglutinating and reaginic antibodies in rabbits following oral administration of soluble and particulate antigens. *Int. Arch. Allergy*, **35**, 579
171. Kletter, B., Gery, I., Freier, S. and Davies, A. M. (1971). Immune responses of normal infants to cow milk. *Int. Arch. Allergy*, **40**, 556
172. Heremans, J. F. and Bazin, H. (1971). Antibodies induced by local antigenic stimulation of mucosal surfaces. *Ann. N.Y. Acad. Sci.*, **190**, 268
173. André, C. and Bazin, H. (1972). Variation du taux des anticorps spécifiques appartenant aux différentes classes d'immunoglobulines dans le sérum et la lymphe mésentérique du rat après ingestion de globules rouges hétérologues. *Biologie et Gastro-entérologie*, **5**, 281
174. Richet, C. (1923). *L'anaphylaxie.* (Paris: Félix Alcan)
175. Rosenau, M. J. and Anderson, J. F. (1906). A study of the cause of sudden death following the injection of horse serum. *Hyg. Lab Bul.*, **29**, 95
176. Prausnitz, C. and Küstner, H. (1921). Studies on supersensitivity. *Centralbl. f. Backteriol. 1. Abt. Orig.*, **86**, 160
177. Du Bois, R. O., Schloss, O. M. and Anderson, A. F. (1925). The development of cutaneous hypersensitiveness following the intestinal absorption of antigenic protein. *Proc. Soc. Exp. Biol. Med.*, **23**, 176
178. Peterson, R. D. A. and Good, R. A. (1963). Antibodies to cow's milk proteins. Their presence and significance. *Pediatrics*, **31**, 209
179. Saperstein, S., Anderson, D. W., Goldman, A. S. and Kniker, W. T. (1963). Milk allergy. III. Immunological studies with sera from allergic and normal children. *Pediatrics*, **32**, 580
180. Barrick, R. H. and Farr, R. S. (1965). The increased incidence of circulating anti-beef albumin in the sera of allergic persons and some comments regarding the possible significance of this occurrence. *J. Allergy*, **36**, 374
181. Bleumink, E. and Young, E. (1968). Identification of the atopic allergen in cow's milk. *Int. Arch. Allergy*, **34**, 521

182. Kletter, B., Gery, I., Freier, S., Moah, Z. and Davies, M. A. (1971). Immunoglobulin E antibodies to milk proteins. *Clin. Allergy*, **1**, 249
183. Parish, W. E. (1971). Detection of reaginic and short-term sensitizing anaphylactic or anaphylactoid antibodies to milk in sera of allergic and normal persons. *Clin. Allergy*, **1**, 369
184. Haddad, Z. H. and Korotzer, J. L. (1972). Immediate hypersensitivity reactions to food antigens. *J. Allergy Clin. Immunol.*, **49**, 210
185. Hoffman, D. R. and Haddad, Z. H. (1974). Diagnosis of IgE mediated reactions to food antigens by radioimmunoassay. *J. Allergy Clin. Immunol.*, **54**, 165
186. Jarrett, E. E. E. and Stewart, D. C. (1974). Rat IgE production. I. Effect of dose of antigen on primary and secondary reaginic antibody response. *Immunology*, **27**, 365
187. Crandall, R. B., Cebra, J. J. and Crandall, C. A. (1967). The relative proportions of IgG-, IgA- and IgM- containing cells in rabbit tissues during experimental trichonosis. *Immunology*, **12**, 147
188. Curtain, C. C. and Anderson, N. (1971). Immunocytochemical localization of the ovine immunoglobulins IgA, IgG1, IgG1a and IgG2: effects of gastrointestinal parasitism in the sheep. *Clin. Exp. Immunol.*, **8**, 151
189. Bazin, H., Ferretti, G., Jelo, E. and Levi, G. (1973). Reazioni immunitarie elle infestazioni da *Hymenolepnis nana*. *Parrassitologia*, **15**, 3
190. Walker, W. A., Isselbacher, K. J. and Bloch, K. J. (1972). Intestinal uptake of macromolecules. I. Effect of oral immunization. *Science*, **177**, 608
191. Walker, W. A., Cornell, R., Davenport, L. M. and Isselbacher, K. J. (1972). Macromolecular absorption mechanism of horseradish peroxidase uptake and transport in adult and neonatal rat intestine. *J. Cell. Biol.*, **54**, 195
192. Walker, W. A., Isselbacher, K. J. and Bloch, K. J. (1973). Intestinal uptake of macromolecules. II. Effect of parenteral immunization. *J. Immunol.*, **111**, 221
193. André, C., Lambert, R., Bazin, H. and Heremans, J. F. (1974). Interference of oral immunization with the intestinal absorption of heterologous albumin. *Eur. J. Immunol.*, **4**, 701
194. Walker, W. A. and Isselbacher, K. J. (1974). Uptake and transport of macromolecules by the intestine: possible role in clinical disorder. *Gastroenterology*, **67**, 531
195. Walker, W. A., Wu, M., Isselbacher, K. J. and Bloch, K. J. (1975) Intestinal uptake of macromolecules. III. Studies on the mechanism by which immunization interferes with antigen uptake. *J. Immunol.*, **115**, 854
196. Fahey, J. L., Wunderlich, J. and Mishell, R. (1964). The immunoglobulins of mice. I. Four major classes of immunoglobulins: 7S γ2-, 7Sγ1-, γ1a(β2a)- and 18S γ1M- globulins. *J. Exp. Med.*, **120**, 223
197. Bazin, H. (1967). Less immunoglobulines de la souris. II. Etude des

anticorps synthétisés dans les différentes classes d'immunoglobulines en réponse à l'injection de deux antigènes protéiques solubles. *Ann. Inst. Pasteur* (*Paris*), **112**, 162

198. Moore, A. R. and Hall, J. G. (1972). Evidence for a primary association between immunoblasts and small gut. *Nature* (*Lond.*), **239**, 161
199. Jensenius, J. C. and Williams, A. F. (1974). Total immunoglobulin of rat thymocytes and thoracic duct lymphocytes. *Eur. J. Immunol.*, **4**, 98
200. Bienenstock, J., Rudzik, O., Clancy, R., Day, R. and Perey, D. (1974). Rabbit IgA: reconstitution experiments with bronchus associated lymphoid tissue (BALT) and Peyer's patches (GALT). *Fed. Proc.*, **33**, 594
201. Heremans, J. F. (1974). Immunoglobulin IgA. New perspectives. *La Ricerca Clin. Lab.*, **4**, 275
202. Bienenstock, J. (1974). The physiology of the local immune response and the gastrointestinal tract. *Prog. Immunol. II*, **4**, 197
203. Pomeranz, J. R. (1970). Immunologic unresponsiveness following a single feeding of picryl chloride. *J. Immunol.*, **104**, 1486
204. Silverman, A. S. and Pomeranz, J. R. (1972). Studies on the localization of hapten in guinea pigs fed picryl chloride. *Int. Arch. Allergy*, **42**, 1
205. Chase, M. W., Battisto, J. R. and Ritts, R. E. (1963). The acquisition of immunologic tolerance via simple allergenic chemicals. In *Conceptual advances in immunology and oncology* p. 396 (New York: Harper and Row)
206. Golan, D. T. and Borel, Y. (1971). Nonantigenicity and immunologic tolerance: the role of the carrier in the induction of tolerance to the hapten. *J. Exp. Med.*, **134**, 1046
207. Borel, Y. (1971). Induction of immunological tolerance by a hapten (DNP) bound to a non-immunogenic protein carrier. *Nature* New Biology, **230**, 180
208. Lee, W. Y. and Sehon, A. H. (1975). Suppression of reaginic antibody formation. I. induction of hapten-specific tolerance. *J. Immunol.*, **114**, 829
209. Lee, W. Y. and Sehon, A. H. (1975). Suppression of reaginic antibody formation. II. The use of adoptive transfer system for the study of immunological unresponsiveness. *J. Immunol.*, **114**, 837
210. Tomasi, T. and Calvanico, N. (1968). Human secretory γA. *Fed. Proc.*, **27**, 617
211. Brown, W. R., Newcomb, R. W. and Ishizaka, K. (1970). Proteolytic degradation of exocrine and serum immunoglobulin. *J. Clin. Invest.*, **49**, 1374
212. Ishizaka, K., Ishizaka, T., Lee, E. H. and Fudenberg, H. (1965). Immunochemical properties of human γA isohemagglutinin. I. Comparisons with γG and γM-globulin antibodies. *J. Immunol.*, **95**, 197
213. Frommhagen, L. H. and Fudenberg, H. (1962). The role of aggregated γ-globulins in the anticomplementary activity of human and animal sera. *J. Immunol.*, **89**, 336

214. Adinolfi, M., Glynn, A. A., Lindsay, M. and Milne, C. M. (1966). Serological properties of γA antibodies to *Escherichia coli* present in human colostrum. *Immunology*, **10**, 517
215. McClelland, D. B. L., Samson, R. R., Parkin, D. M. and Sharman, D. J. C. (1972). Bacterial agglutination studies with secretory IgA prepared from human gastrointestinal secretions and colostrum. *Gut*, **13**, 450
216. Knop, J., Breu, H., Wernet, P. and Rowley, D. (1971). The relative anti-bacterial efficiency of IgM, IgG and IgA from pig colostrum. *Aust. J. Exp. Biol. Med. Sci.*, **49**, 405
217. Brandtzaeg, P., Fjellanger, I. and Gjeruldsen, S. T. (1968). Adsorption of immunoglobulin A onto oral bacteria *in vivo*. *J. Bacteriol.*, **96**, 242
218. Turk, A., Lichtenstein, L. M. and Norman, P. S. (1970). Nasal secretory antibody to inhalant allergens in allergic and non-allergic patients. *Immunology*, **19**, 85
219. Burdon, D. W. (1973). The bactericidal action of immunoglobulin A. *J. Med. Microbiol.*, **6**, 131
220. Capron, A., Dessaint, J. P., Capron, M. and Bazin, H. (1975). Specific IgE antibodies in immune adherence of normal macrophages to *Schistosoma mansoni* schistosomules. *Nature* (*Lond.*), **253**, 474
221. Ross, V. (1930). Oral immunization against pneumococcus. Use of bile salt dissolved organisms, etc., time of appearance of immunity and dosage. *J. Exp. Med.*, **51**, 585
222. Fubara, E. S. and Freter, R. (1972). Source and protective function of coproantibodies in intestinal disease. *Am. J. Clin. Nutrition*, **25**, 137
223. Waldman, R. H., Grunspan, R. and Ganguly, R. (1972). Oral immunization of mice with killed *Salmonella typhimuriam* vaccine. *Infection and immunity*, **6**, 58
224. Shedlofsky, S. and Freter, R. (1974). Synergism between ecologic and immunologic control mechanisms of intestinal flora. *J. Infec. Dis.*, **129**, 296
225. Williams, R. C. and Gibbons, R. J. (1972). Inhibition of bacterial adherence by secretory immunoglobulin A; a mechanism of antigen disposal. *Science*, **177**, 697
226. Freter, R. (1969). Intestinal immunity. Studies of the mechanism of action of intestinal antibody in experimental cholera. *Texas Rep. Biol. Med.*, **27**, suppl. 299
227. Lipton, M. M. and Steigman, A. J. (1963). Human coproantibody against polioviruses. *J. Infec. Dis.*, **112**, 57
228. Kono, R., Akao, Y., Sasagawa, A. and Nomura, Y. (1969). Studies on the local immunity of intestinal tract of chickens after oral administration of Newcastle disease virus. *Japan J. Med. Sci. Biol.*, **22**, 235
229. Ogra, P. L. and Karzon, D. T. (1971). Formation and functions of poliovirus antibody in different tissues. *Prog. Med. Virology*, **13**, 156
230. Keller, R. and Dwyer, J. E. (1968). Neutralization of poliovirus by IgA coproantibodies. *J. Immunol.*, **101**, 192

231. Brandtzaeg, P. (1973). Structure, synthesis and external transfer of mucosal immunoglobulins. *Ann. Immunol.* (*Inst. Pasteur*), **124C**, 417

232. Jarret, E. E. E. (1973). Reaginic anti-bodies and helminth infection. *Vet. Rec.*, **93**, 480

233. Urquhart, G. M., Mulligan, W., Eadie, R. M. and Jennings, F. W. (1965). Immunological studies on *Nippostrongylus brasiliensis* infection in the rat: The role of local anaphylaxis. *Exp. Parasitol.*, **17**, 210

234. Heremans, J. F. (1969). In *The secretory immunologic system*, D. H. Dayton *et al.* (eds.), p. 309. (Washington DC: US Govt. Printing Office)

235. Rothberg, R. M. and Farr, R. S. (1965). Anti-bovine serum albumin and anti-alpha lactalbumin in the serum of children and adults. *Pediatrics*, **35**, 571

236. Korenblat, P. E., Rothberg, R. M., Minden, P. and Farr, R. S. (1968). Immune responses of human adults after oral and parenteral exposure to bovine serum albumin. *J. Allergy*, **41**, 226

237. Thomas, H. C. and Vaez-Zadeh, F. (1974). An homeostatic mechanism for the removal of antigen from the portal circulation. *Immunology*, **26**, 375

238. Beale, A. J., Parish, W. E., Douglas, A. P. and Hobbs, J. R. (1971). Impaired IgA responses in coeliac disease. *Lancet*, **i**, 1198

239. Battisto, J. R. and Miller, J. (1962). Immunological unresponsiveness produced in adult guinea pigs by parenteral introduction of minute quantities of hapten or protein antigen. *Proc. Soc. Exp. Biol.*, (*N.Y.*), **111**, 111

240. Cantor, H. M. and Dumont, A. E. (1967). Hepatic suppression of sensitization to antigen absorbed into the portal system. *Nature* (*Lond.*), **215**, 744

241. Triger, D. R., Cynamon, M. H. and Wright, R. (1973). Studies on hepatic uptake of antigen. I. Comparison of inferior vena cava and portal vein routes of immunization. *Immunology*, **25**, 941

242. Foo, M. C. and Lee, A. (1972). Immunological response of mice to members of autochthonous intestinal microflora. *Infection and Immunity*, **6**, 525

243. Korenblat, P. E., Rothberg, R. M., Minden, P. and Farr, R. S. (1968). Immune responses of human adults after oral and parenteral exposure to bovine serum albumin. *J. Allergy*, **41**, 104

CHAPTER 3

Gastrointestinal tract and immunodeficiency

HANS D. OCHS AND MARVIN E. AMENT

Introduction

The embryonic gut plays an important role in the development of both the cellular and the humoral immune systems. The thymus and the avian bursa of Fabricius, both central lymphoid structures responsible for the development of normal immunity, are derivatives of the primitive gut. Experimental evidence suggests that multipotential stem cells, originating in the bone marrow, are induced by the thymus to differentiate into T-lymphocytes and, in the avian example by the bursa of Fabricius into B-lymphocytes and antibody secreting plasma cells[1,2]. Removal of the appendix, sacculus rotundus and Peyer's patches in young rabbits results in an antibody deficiency syndrome similar to that observed in the bursectomized chicken[3]. A human analogue to the avian bursa has not been defined unequivocally but it has been postulated that gut associated lymphoid tissues may represent a bursa equivalent[4]. Owen, Cooper and Raff[5] have recently shown that immunoglobulin bearing lymphocytes can develop from stem cells which migrated from the yolk sac to the liver. Liver fragments obtained from 12–15-day-old mice were grown in culture. B-cells, initially absent, could be detected immunohistochemically after 1 week of culture, suggesting that the liver may be the B-cell induction site in mammals. During postnatal life, the human gut develops the histological characteristics of a secondary lymphoid organ[6]. Lymphoid follicles, germinal centres, small lymphocytes and plasma cells are abundant, and the intimate proximity of lymphoid tissue with the surface of the gastrointestinal tract assures a close contact with a multitude of microbial and alimentary antigens. Coproantibodies can readily be detected in stool eluates. It has been shown that secretory IgA is quantitatively the most important gamma globulin in the intestinal secretions[7,8]. This 11-S gamma globulin has unique physical and biological properties which are discussed in a separate chapter. It is not surprising that IgA producing plasma cells are numerous in the lamina propria of the entire gut including the rectal mucosa[7] and outnumber IgM and IgG secreting plasma cells by ratios of 20:3:1. In addition, IgE containing plasma cells are regularly found in the mucosa of the normal gastrointestinal tract[9]. Large numbers of small lymphocytes, probably T-lymphocytes, are distributed diffusely or in aggregates throughout the intestinal tract.

The close relationship between gut and immune system is suggested by:

(i) An increased incidence of gastrointestinal disease has been observed in patients with immunodeficiency syndromes demonstrating the importance of an intact immune system for the integrity of the gut.

(ii) The development of both humoral and cellular immune deficiency in intestinal lymphangiectasia demonstrates the importance of the anatomical structure of the gastrointestinal tract for normal function of the immune system. In this condition, the continuous loss of gammaglobulin and long-lived lymphocytes (T-cells) results in hypogammaglobulinaemia, delayed homograft rejection and decreased lymphocyte transformation in response to mitogens[10].

(iii) It has been suggested that a number of gastrointestinal diseases represent an abnormal immune reaction in which the gut is the target organ: examples are Crohn's disease, ulcerative colitis, gluten intolerance and graft–versus–host disease.

Classification of primary immunodeficiency syndromes and incidence of gastrointestinal disease

Primary immunodeficiency syndromes are a heterogenous group of diseases which are characterized by impairment of the B-cell system (humoral immunity), the T-cell system (cell-mediated immunity) or both. Impairment of the normal development of functioning B-cells will lead to deficiency in immunoglobulin synthesis. Failure to generate an effective T-cell system will result in defective cell-mediated immunity. On the basis of these observations, a working party of the World Health Organization[11] recently developed a classification of the primary immunodeficiency syndromes (Table 3.1).

Table 3.1 CLASSIFICATION OF PRIMARY IMMUNODEFICIENCY SYNDROMES AND INCIDENCE OF GASTROINTESTINAL (GI) DISEASE

Type of immunodeficiency	*Incidence of GI disease*	*Characteristic GI symptoms, findings and morphologic abnormalities*
1. B-cell defects:		
infantile X-linked agammaglobulinaemia	(+)	*Giardia lamblia* (rare)[82], absence of plasma cells in mucosa, early crypt abscesses[14]
X-linked immunodeficiency with hyper-IgM	—	—
selective IgA deficiency	++	celiac sprue[36,46], NLH, *Giardia lamblia*[28], malignancy[123]
transient hypogammaglobulinaemia of infancy	—	—
immunodeficiency syndrome with normal serum immunoglobulin levels	(+)	diarrhea, malabsorption[20]

variable immunodeficiency (acquired hypogamma-globulinaemia)	+++	NLH[27], celiac sprue, severe B_{12} malabsorption[32], *Giardia lamblia*, colitis[14], malig-nancy[27]
2. T.-cell defect		
DiGeorge syndrome (thymic hypoplasia)	(+)	recurrent diarrhea, failure to thrive[112]
3. B- and T-cell defects:		
immunodeficiency with ataxia-telangiectasia	(+)	Vitamin B_{12} malabsorption[14], carcinoma of stomach[122],
immunodeficiency with thrombocytopenia and eczema (Wiskott-Aldrich syndrome)	+++	severe recurrent bloody diarrhea[19], malabsorption[14]
immunodeficiency with short-limbed dwarfism	+	diarrhea, crypt abscesses[134]
cartilage hair hypoplasia	+	recurrent diarrhea, failure to thrive, steatorrhea, vacuo-lated, lipid laden macro-phages[113],
immunodeficiency with thymoma	(+)	frequently diarrhea[123]
severe combined immuno-deficiency (a) autosomal recessive (with or without red blood cell adenosine deami-nase deficiency; with reticuloendo-theliosis) (b) X-linked (c) sporadic	+++	severe diarrhea, malabsorp-tion, absence of plasma cells, vacuolated and lipid containing macro-phages[107,108,113]

Repeated bacterial or severe viral or fungal infections are the most common findings in primary immunodeficiency syndromes[12].

However, shortly after the recognition of immunodeficiency disease it became apparent that gastrointestinal illnesses were frequently associated with immunodeficiency. Bruton, who described the first case of immunodeficiency syndrome, recorded that his patient had several episodes of vomiting and 'violent gastrointestinal upset' before treatment with gammaglobulin injections was started. Since then, numerous cases presenting with severe gastrointestinal symptoms of acute or chronic diarrhea, vomiting, steatorrhea, malabsorption, weight loss or failure to thrive have been recorded. It became apparent that gastrointestinal disease develops frequently in some primary immunodeficiency syndromes and less frequently in others (Table 3.1). Twenty to 50% of the patients with adult-onset immunodeficiency syndromes (variable immunodeficiency syndromes) develop chronic diarrhea and malabsorption[12,13]. Symptoms of acute colitis, including diarrhea and tenesmus have been reported in a number of patients[14–18]. In contrast, congenital antibody deficiency syndromes (e.g., infantile X-linked agammaglobulinaemia, X-linked immunodeficiency with hyper-IgM) rarely develop chronic gastrointestinal disease[12,14]. Most infants with severe combined immunodeficiency disease develop intractable diarrhea and malabsorption. Chronic bloody diarrhea starting in early infancy is almost always present in the Wiskott–Aldrich syndrome[19]. Esophageal strictures developed in two siblings with chronic mucosal candidiasis causing severe dysphagia[20].

Gastrointestinal abnormalities associated with B-cell deficiencies

Gastric abnormalities in immunodeficiency

The association of pernicious anaemia and immunodeficiency disease has been reported by many investigators[21–34]. Twomey *et al.*[32] found gastric atrophy in seven of 10 individuals with this syndrome. Gastric mucosa was infiltrated with lymphocytes but void of plasma cells. Intrinsic factor was absent in the gastric secretions of all patients studied. Nine patients had histamine-fast achlorhydria and the tenth showed minimal gastric acid secretion. None of the patients with pernicious anaemia and immune deficiency had demonstrable serum antibodies against parietal cell antigens or against intrinsic factor; in contrast, immunologically normal patients with pernicious anaemia frequently develop autoantibodies[32]. All patients in this study with immunodeficiency syndrome showed severe Vitamin B_{12} malabsorption.

Small bowel disease in immunodeficiency

Malabsorption: Damage to the small bowel mucosa may result in malabsorption Steatorrhea represents the most severe degree of malabsorption and is frequently reported in patients with acquired immunodeficiency; they often develop a sprue-like syndrome with severe villus damage[35,36]. Steatorrhea has also been associated with *Giardia lamblia* infections[14,37]. Six patients with immunodeficiency and *Giardia lamblia* infection had moderate to severe steatorrhea. Fat absorption became normal in every individual after eradication of the organisms[14].

Normal absorption of vitamin B_{12} requires the secretion of intrinsic factor from the chief cells in the stomach, normal absorptive function of the small intestine, and the presence of a specific vitamin B_{12} binding protein in the serum[38,39]. Malabsorption of vitamin B_{12} in patients with immunodeficiency may be due to: (1) Lack of intrinsic factor because of atrophy of the gastric mucosa (described earlier); (2) malabsorption of the vitamin B_{12}-intrinsic factor complex in the small bowel due to mucosal abnormalities; or (3) adverse intraluminal factors.

A significant defect in the absorption of vitamin B_{12} in spite of added intrinsic factor has been reported frequently[14,16,28,32,37,40–42]. The majority of these patients were infected with *Giardia lamblia*[14,16,28,32,37,40].

Vitamin B_{12} absorption was evaluated in one study of 10 patients with Giardiasis[14]. Four patients had severe and five had mild to moderate vitamin B_{12} malabsorption. After eradication of the parasite, two patients failed to show any improvement in vitamin B_{12} absorption and the addition of intrinsic factor in one case was ineffective. This latter patient required parenteral vitamin B_{12} injections for treatment of megaloblastic anaemia. Most of these patients had other findings of malabsorption and their biopsies showed moderate to severe damage to the villi. The significance of *Giardia lamblia* in these patients will be discussed later. Mild to moderate vitamin B_{12} malabsorption was also seen in patients who did not have Giardiasis[14,33,40,42]. Six of eight asymptomatic patients with variable immunodeficiency syndromes and three of six patients with ataxia telangiectasia showed abnormal vitamin B_{12} absorption that did not improve with added intrinsic factor[14]. Some of these individuals had mild abnormalities of their villus architecture, others had normal small bowel mucosa; none were infected with *Giardia lamblia*. The mechanism of vitamin B_{12} malabsorption in these patients is unclear.

Hypocalcaemia was found in a patient with hypogammaglobulinaemia and tetany[43]. Calcium and vitamin D supplement promptly corrected the signs and symptoms of hypocalcaemia.

Disaccharidase deficiency associated with immunodeficiency: A high incidence of disaccharidase deficiency was found in a group of patients with a variety of immunodeficiency syndromes[44]. Three of six patients with 'congenital X-linked hypogammaglobulinaemia' had isolated lactase deficiency. Seven of eight patients with a T-cell defect were found to have decreased lactase, sucrase and maltase. All but one of these patients had significant diarrhea. The possibility of a secondary disaccharidase deficiency due to gastrointestinal disease of long duration cannot be excluded. Of our patients only one of seven individuals with infantile X-linked agammaglobulinaemia had an abnormal lactose tolerance test and low lactase activity in small bowel tissue, and none had gastrointestinal symptoms during the study. Normal disaccharidase activity was present in patients with selective IgA deficiency, X-linked immunodeficiency with hyper-IgM, and ataxia telangiectasia. Three asymptomatic patients with variable immunodeficiency syndrome (acquired hypogammaglobulinaemia) had abnormal lactose tolerance; intestinal disaccharidase determinations were performed on the biopsies of one patient and showed selective lactase deficiency. All four patients with lactase deficiency developed watery diarrhea within 4 hours of drinking the lactose solution (2g/kg)[14].

Histological abnormalities of small bowel biopsies in patients with immunodeficiency: The development of peroral biopsy techniques has facilitated the study of the structure of the intestinal mucosa by providing biopsy material at minimal risk. Particularly useful is the hydraulic biopsy tube[45], which is designed to take any number of biopsies desired from different sites of the small intestine. Using this technique it has been shown that lesions of the intestinal mucosa are often patchy and might be missed if only single biopsies were taken. The following mucosal abnormalities may be present in patients with immunodeficiency syndromes: (i) decreased number or absence of plasma cells; (ii) large lymphoid follicles within the lamina propria, causing protrusion of the overlaying mucosa, described by Heremans[27] as nodular lymphoid hyperplasia; (iii) a flat mucosa with absence of villi, similar to celiac disease[41,46], but lacking plasma cells.

(i) Plasma cells are absent in the small bowel mucosa of patients with infantile X-linked agammaglobulinaemia and in most individuals with variable (acquired) immunodeficiency syndromes[14]. Patients with selective IgA deficiency often have normal numbers of plasma cells, but the predominant cell type is the IgM containing one[36,46]. Similarly, patients with ataxia telangiectasia have predominantly IgM-containing plasma cells in their rectal biopsies[47].

(ii) Nodular lymphoid hyperplasia (NLH). In 1966 Hermans[27] and colleagues described eight patients with a syndrome characterized by (1) hypogammaglobulinaemia involving all three major immunoglobulin classes; (2) unusual susceptibility to infections, especially of the respiratory tract; (3) gastrointestinal disturbances, in particular diarrhea and occasionally malabsorption; (4) the presence of *Giardia lamblia* in the stools; (5) the histological findings of nodular lymphoid hyperplasia of the small intestine. Earlier, two isolated cases of NLH were described, one case at autopsy[48] and another radiologically and histologically[49]. The clinical presentation, histologic abnormalities and immunologic findings of this syndrome have been studied extensively in recent years by a number of investigators[14,16,21,43,44,50–59,61].

Nodular lymphoid hyperplasia is most often seen in adult patients with late onset antibody deficiency syndromes. In the paediatric age group only one infant, a 2-year-old girl with diarrhea, thrombocytopenia, decreased IgG and elevated serum IgM, and four teenage children have been found with NLH. In most instances the susceptibility to infections precedes gastrointestinal symptoms by several years.

The classical symptoms of NLH are recurrent sinopulmonary infections and diarrhea with or without steatorrhea. However, a few patients without respiratory infections[27,52,59,60] and a few others without diarrhea[14,61] have been described. *Giardia lamblia* has been recovered from the stool or seen in small bowel biopsies in the majority of the patients with this syndrome. Treatment with quinacrine or metronidazole eradicated *Giardia* and reversed the symptoms in most patients[14,16,21,37,56,57].

The lymphoid nodules, however, do not disappear after eradication of the parasite. Additional evidence that *Giardia lamblia* causes gastrointestinal symptoms is provided by the observation that an asymptomatic patient with NLH suddenly developed diarrhea simultaneously with the appearance of *Giardia lamblia* in the stool[53]. In some instances, however, treatment of *Giardia* did not result in improvement of the gastrointestinal symptoms[16,27,43,60]. It is not clear why eradication of the parasite causes improvement of gastrointestinal symptoms in some patients and apparently not in others; some of these nonresponding patients may have received inadequate treatment; others may have intestinal disturbances not related to *Giardia lamblia*[14,37].

Upper gastrointestinal and small bowel series of patients with NLH show multiple small filling defects along the length of the small bowel which are uniform in size, smooth in contour, and only a few millimetres in diameter (Figure 3.1A). Similar lesions could be demonstrated

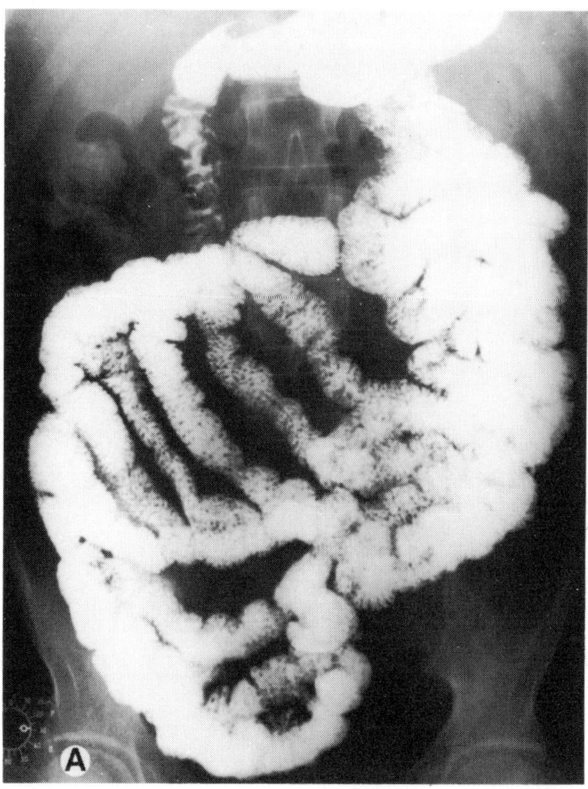

FIGURE 3.1A Small bowel series from a patient with nodular lymphoid hyperplasia of the small intestine showing multiple small filling defects which are uniform in size and only a few millimetres in diameter

radiologically in the right colon[55] and in the rectosigmoid area[50]. Microscopic examination (Figure 3.1B) of these lesions reveal large lymphoid follicles within the lamina propria, causing protrusion of the overlying mucosa, resulting in a nodular or polypoid appearance. There are germinal centres within the follicles. Epithelium over the enlarged follicles is generally normal. Characteristically, plasma cells

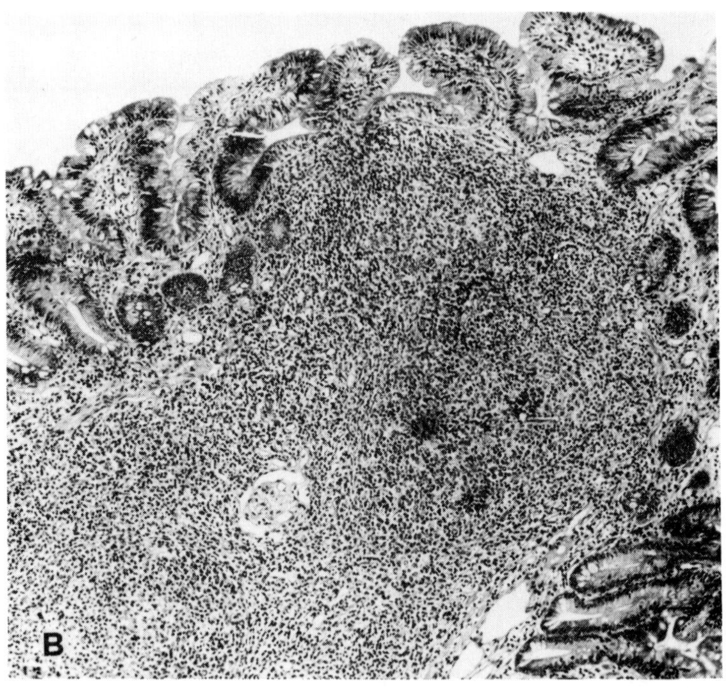

FIGURE 3.1B Typical biopsy of a patient with nodular lymphoid hyperplasia of the small intestine. The hyperplastic lymphoid follicle is prominent and has short distorted villi over its surface (H & E × 84)

are absent or markedly decreased in number[27]. The lymphoid cells of these follicles contain no detectable immunoglobulin[56] when immunofluoresecent techniques are used. In the majority, but not in all of these patients, the villi and epithelial cells of the small intestine are normal, distinguishing NLH from the sprue-like syndrome associated with 'acquired' hypogammaglobulinaemia.

Other manifestations associated with nodular lymphoid hyperplasia are splenomegaly, large tonsils, eczema, achlorhydria, pernicious anaemia, carcinoma of the stomach or colon and acute pancreatitis[62], sarcoidosis[63], ring chromosome 18[57] and tetany secondary to severe steatorrhea[43].

The immunological defect found most often in NLH consists of decreased IgG, with very low or absent IgM and IgA. The association of nodular lymphoid hyperplasia with selective IgA deficiency has been observed in a few patients[27,60]; serum IgA of these patients is low or absent and respiratory infections are usually not reported. Antibody responses in NLH are absent or very low to a number of protein antigens[14,16,57,61]. In one study four individuals with NLH were repeatedly immunized with bacteriophage ϕX 174, a potent protein antigen[14]. A very low antibody response consisting of IgM antibody only was observed in two patients. One responded with low antibody titres consisting mainly of IgM, and the fourth individual responded with a normal titre but only a small fraction of the specific antibody was of the IgG class. In contrast, normal individuals make mainly IgG antibody after repeated immunization with this antigen[64]. Cellular immunity is not affected in NLH, and it has been speculated[56] that the development of lymphoid nodules may depend on an intact cell-mediated immune system.

No distinctive immunologic characteristics separate hypogammaglobulinaemic patients with NLH from those without NLH[14,59]. It appears that NLH represents a particular reaction of the alimentary tract to late onset immunodeficiency that involves impairment of the B-cell system and requires functioning T-cells.

A number of hypotheses to explain the pathophysiology of NLH have been proposed[51,57,62]. An increased number of lymphoid cells in the lamina propria without the formation of nodules has been observed in some patients with hypogammaglobulinaemia[42,65,66], indicating that different degrees of lymphoid hyperplasia may exist, NLH being the most proliferative form. Marked follicular lymphoid hyperplasia with few or no plasma cells[51,63] was found in lymph node biopsies from patients with NLH of the intestine and hypogammaglobulinaemia. Patients with this form of immunodeficiency frequently have B-lymphocytes in the peripheral blood[20,51,67]. It has been suggested that B-lymphocytes of these patients have surface recognition antibodies and respond to antigens by proliferation. Because of a block in further differentiation, these antigen-stimulated B-lymphocytes are prevented from becoming mature plasma cells and do not secrete the antibodies needed to modulate and restrict the proliferative response of specific clones[51]. The lymphoid nodules might then be the end result of a 'piling up of plasma cell precursors'[57]. Since IgG antibodies are most effective in this feedback control[68], it is not surprising that many patients with NLH who often are able to make IgM antibodies but have impaired production of IgG and IgA antibodies and show a striking overgrowth of germinal centres, resulting in the formation of lymphoid nodules.

(iii) Celiac sprue (celiac disease). A sprue-like syndrome with response to gluten withdrawal from the diet has frequently been associated with selective IgA deficiency[36,46,69–72]. The incidence of celiac sprue in selective IgA deficiency is believed to be 12 times as high as in individuals with normal serum immunoglobulins[72]. Symptoms may first appear in childhood or in adult life and respond almost always to the removal of gluten from the diet. Patients with celiac sprue and IgA deficiency have similar abnormalities of absorption and mucosal damage as found in celiac patients with normal serum IgA levels. However, most mucosal plasma cells of patients with selective IgA deficiency and celiac sprue stain immunohistochemically for IgM[36], and those of celiac patients with normal immunoglobulins stain predominantly for IgA. Furthermore, serum IgM levels are decreased and IgA levels are increased in immunologically normal patients with celiac disease[71,73], whereas patients with absent serum IgA tend to have elevated serum IgM levels.

Clinical and laboratory findings of a malabsorption syndrome have been found in patients with 'acquired' hypogammaglobulinaemia involving all immunoglobulin classes[14,16,18,28,35,37,40–42,66,74–78]. The diagnosis of mucosal damage has been confirmed in many patients by small bowel biopsies. Severity of malabsorption and steatorrhea appeared to correlate best with intestinal mucosal changes, particularly villus damage which was most pronounced in patients with steatorrhea[14,16]. The patchy nature of the lesions, which became apparent when multiple biopsies were taken simultaneously[14,37] might explain why steatorrhea was present in some individuals who reportedly had only one normal small intestinal biopsy[40,58,79]. Most patients with hypogammaglobulinaemia and malabsorption syndrome do not respond to gluten-free diet[14,28,37,76,77]. A few individuals, however, seem to improve if gluten is eliminated from their diet[41,80,81]. *Giardia lamblia* and bacterial overgrowth of the proximal intestine with enteropathogens have been implicated in the pathogenesis of this syndrome. The clinical, laboratory and histologic abnormalities of celiac sprue associated with general hypogammaglobulinaemia are the same as in that associated with selective IgA deficiency. The same pathophysiologic mechanisms seem responsible for both entities.

The role of micro-organisms in gastrointestinal disease associated with immunodeficiency: The intestinal parasite *Giardia lamblia* has often been found in patients with humoral immune deficiency and gastrointestinal disease[14,16,21,27,28,35,37,41,43,50,51,53,54,56–58,79,82,83]. Most patients affected with *Giardia lamblia* had late-onset immunodeficiency of the variable type, involving the humoral immune system only. Markedly decreased serum IgG and low or absent serum IgA and IgM were common findings. *Giardia lamblia* has also been described in a few individuals with selective IgA deficiency[28,60]. Lack of serum IgE was observed by a few investigators[20,84]. In contrast, *Giardia lamblia* has not been reported in patients with T-cell deficiency, severe combined immune deficiency, and in only one patient with infantile X-linked agammaglobulinaemia[82].

The symptomatology of patients with immunodeficiency and *Giardia lamblia* ranges from mild diarrhea and abdominal discomfort to severe watery diarrhea, extreme weight loss, malabsorption and complete loss of villus structure[14]. To determine the incidence and pathologic significance of *Giardia lamblia* infection, we recently studied the gastrointestinal tract of 39 patients[14] with a variety of immunodeficiency syndromes (Table 3.2). The nature of the immune defect

Table 3.2 GASTROINTESTINAL (GI) SYMPTOMS AND FINDINGS IN PATIENTS* WITH IMMUNODEFICIENCY AND *Giardia lamblia* INFECTION[7]

GI symptoms (diarrhea and/or vomiting)	8/11†
Steatorrhea	5/10
B_{12} malabsorption	10/10
Lactose intolerance	4/9
Generalized disaccharidase deficiency	2/4
Villus abnormalities	7/11

* Variable immunodeficiency: 10 patients
Infantile X-linked Agammaglobulinaemia: 1 patient
† Numbers of patients affected/number of patients studied

had been determined using standard procedures and patients were classified according to the World Health Organization recommendations. *Giardia lamblia* was found in eight of nine patients with gastrointestinal symptoms such as diarrhea, weight loss, vomiting and anorexia, but the parasite could be demonstrated in only three of 30 patients free of gastrointestinal symptoms. Pathologic findings associated with giardiasis in our patients included: malabsorption of folate and vitamin B_{12}, steatorrhea, lactose intolerance, generalized disaccharidase deficiency, protein losing enteropathy and mild to severe abnormalities of villus architecture. After eradication of the parasites with metronidazole, gastrointestinal symptoms disappeared and serum carotene and folate levels became normal. Six patients who originally had steatorrhea showed significant weight gain, and fat absorption became normal. Protein losing enteropathy which was present in one individual disappeared following treatment with metronidazole. Serum immunoglobulin levels, however, did not change in any of the treated individuals. Lactose intolerance was present in four of the six symptomatic patients tested before treatment, and it disappeared in all four after treatment. Intestinal disaccharidase levels were abnormal in two of four patients tested; the enzyme activity returned to normal after eradication of the parasite. Vitamin B_{12} absorption was studied in 10 patients with giardiasis. Four patients had severe (less than 5% urinary excretion in 24 hours) and five had mild to moderate (greater than 5% but less than 10% excretion in 24 hours) vitamin B_{12} malabsorption. Two of these patients had achlorhydria. After eradication of the parasite, normal vitamin B_{12} absorption (greater than 10% excretion in 24 hours) was observed in all but two patients.

An average of five small bowel biopsies was taken from each patient before and after treatment for giardiasis (Figure 3.2). The patterns of mucosal architecture observed ranged from normal or mildly abnormal biopsies to 'flat' lesions characteristic of 'hypogammaglobulinaemic sprue' (Figure 3.2A); lymphoid nodules were frequently seen. The severity of villus abnormalities correlated with gastrointestinal symptoms and steatorrhea. Eradicaton of giardiasis was followed by significant improvement of the abnormalities in villus architecture in all patients (Figure 3.2B). Some mild to moderate histological changes, however, remained in most patients. In contrast, neither the size nor the number of lymphoid follicles were affected by eradication of the parasites.

The following case report illustrates further the significance of *Giardia lamblia* as a cause of severe gastrointestinal disease in a patient with variable immunodeficiency syndrome: a male patient, born in 1925, was referred to the University Hospital in 1961 because of increasing weight loss and diarrhea. He was hospitalized with pneumonia in 1944 and 1947, and otitis media occurred frequently during childhood and later during adult life. Steatorrhea (15–25 g of fat in his stools per day) was found consistently and vitamin B_{12} absorption was severely impaired

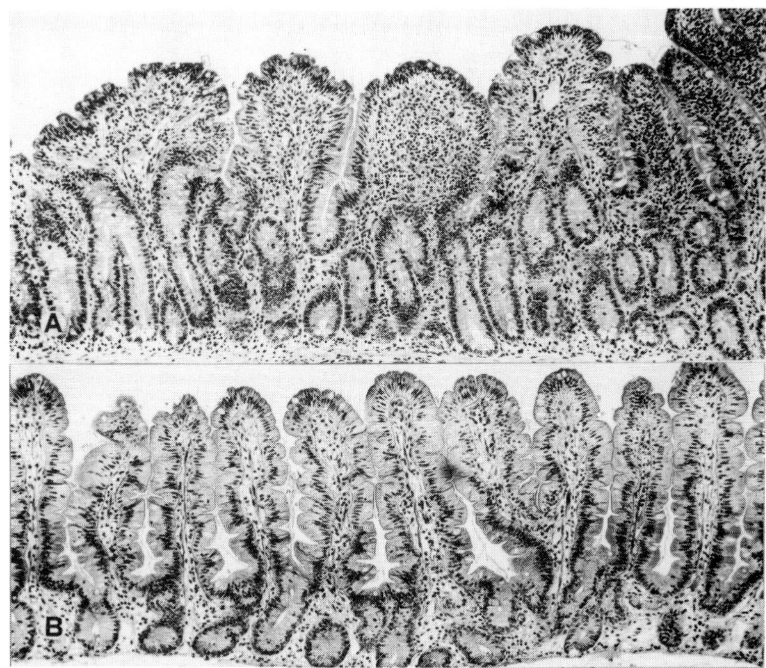

FIGURE 3.2A Shows a representative peroral biopsy taken near the duodeno–jejunal junction of a patient with variable immunodeficiency, severe gastrointestinal symptoms and malabsorption due to *Giardia lamblia* infestation. The villus architecture is severely abnormal (H & E × 72)

FIGURE 3.2B Represents a biopsy taken 5 weeks after completion of treatment to eradicate giardiasis; the villus architecture is normal (H & E × 72)

(less than 1% vitamin B_{12} was excreted in 24 hours). Small bowel biopsies revealed moderate to severe damage; no disaccharidase activity could be demonstrated in small bowel tissue and the diagnosis of celiac sprue was made. Clinical improvement was not observed. The patient was started on a strict gluten-free diet, and no significant changes of the histological appearance of the small bowel mucosa were noticed. Conversely, exposure to gluten was not followed by worsening of the symptoms. Repeated sigmoidoscopic examinations were negative. Neither lactose-free diet nor a trial to eliminate other proteins than gluten was successful in improving the gastrointestinal symptoms. Because of uncontrollable diarrhea and continuous weight loss, the patient was started on prednisone in 1963 at a dose of 15 mg/day, later reduced to 10 mg/day. Significant clinical improvement was observed, but small bowel biopsies remained abnormal. Further attempts to reduce the steroid dose resulted in prompt exacerbation of the gastrointestinal symptoms.

Immunologic studies were initiated in 1965, demonstrating hypogammaglobulinaemia (IgG 400–660 mg%, IgA 7 mg%, IgM 9 mg%). A Schick test remained positive after repeated immunizations with diphtheria toxoid. Antibody response to typhoid vaccine was low. Repeated immunization with bacteriophage ϕX 174 resulted in an increased antibody response, indicating adequate immunologic memory; however, the antibody after the third phage injection consisted mainly of IgM and less than 10% was of the IgG class; normal controls make predominantly IgG antibody[64]. Plasma cells were not detected in small bowel biopsies. Intramuscular injection of gamma globulin and intravenous infusion of plasma was followed by a rise of temperature, sweating, low blood pressure and chest pain. No further gammaglobulin was given.

Small bowel biopsies obtained in April 1970 again showed absence of villi. Smears of mucus and sections of the biopsies revealed large numbers of *Giardia* trophozoites. A review of previous biopsies obtained during a 9-year period showed that *Giardia* were present in each biopsy. The patient was treated with metronidazole (Flagyl) and began to feel subjectively better after 2 days. The number of stools diminished as did stool volume. He gained 4·6 kg in 2 weeks. Steroids were tapered and discontinued 3 months later. The elimination of steroids resulted in generalized myalgia, stiffness and pain in the ankle joints, wrists and proximal interphalangeal joints. Aspirin and ACTH did not improve these complaints, but treatment with indomethacin relieved the arthralgia. Small bowel biopsies obtained after eradication of *Giardia* showed only mild mucosal lesions; steatorrhea had disappeared and vitamin B_{12} absorption was markedly improved (7% of administered B_{12} was excreted in 24 hours). Diarrhea and abdominal pain disappeared, and the patient gained a total of 12 kg.

This and other reports[14,28,37,82] demonstrate dramatic improvement following eradication of *Giardia lamblia*. The findings of our study suggest that giardiasis was the main cause of gastrointestinal complaints in eight of the nine symptomatic patients. However, mild abnormalities of structure and function of the intestinal tract remained after the eradication of the parasite. The cause of malabsorption was not established in the ninth patient[14].

In spite of careful examination of stool specimens in an experienced laboratory, *Giardia* was present in the stool in only one-third of the infected patients[14]. Histologic examinations of serial sections of small intestinal biopsies (Figure 3.3A, 3.3B) detected *Gairdia lamblia* in every case. This method, however, is often time consuming and requires considerable skill. Examination of Giemsa-stained smears (Figure 3.3C) of mucus from the biopsies is an easier and more rapid method of

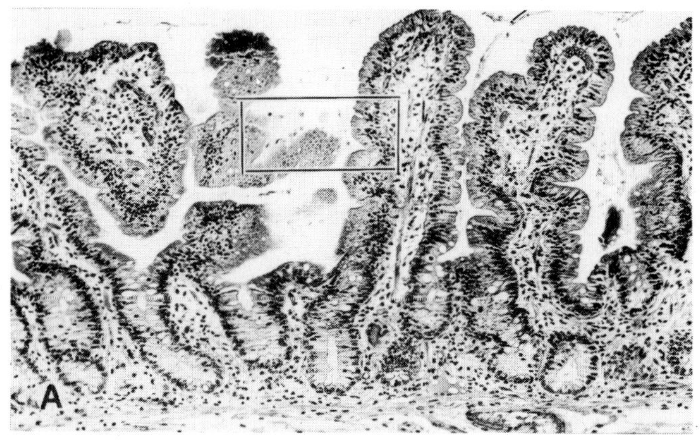

FIGURE 3.3A Small intestinal biopsy from a 12-year-old girl with variable immunodeficiency syndrome who was free of gastrointestinal symptoms; malabsorption of vitamin B_{12} was demonstrated. The villus architecture is mildly abnormal, trophozoites are present in the lumen (H & E × 84)

establishing the diagnosis; the parasite could be demonstrated in all but one case. Other investigators[28] agree that stool examination is unreliable for the diagnosis of giardiasis. Furthermore, if several biopsies were taken simultaneously, not every one demonstrated the trophozoites. The evaluation of multiple biopsies from patients with giardiasis suggests the patchy nature of the small intestinal lesions. The villus architecture often varied from normal to severely abnormal in different biopsies obtained at the same time from the same individual. If only a single small bowel biopsy is obtained, one should not be surprised to find little correlation among morphologic abnormalities, gastrointestinal symptoms and tests of absorptive function.

There has been considerable difference of opinion regarding the pathogenicity of *Giardia lamblia* in normal individuals. The incidence of positive stool examinations for *Giardia* cysts in the United States ranges between 1·5% and 20% depending on the socio-economic status of the population examined[85]. Some studies seem to indicate that

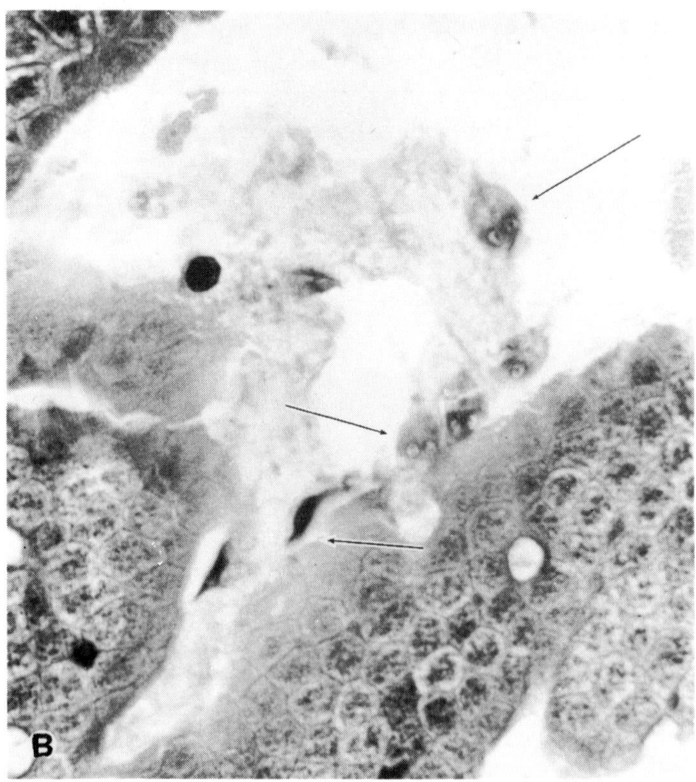

FIGURE 3.3B High power view of A shows trophozoites both in sagittal and full face projections (↑). Some trophozoites appear attached to the surface epithelium (H & E × 308)

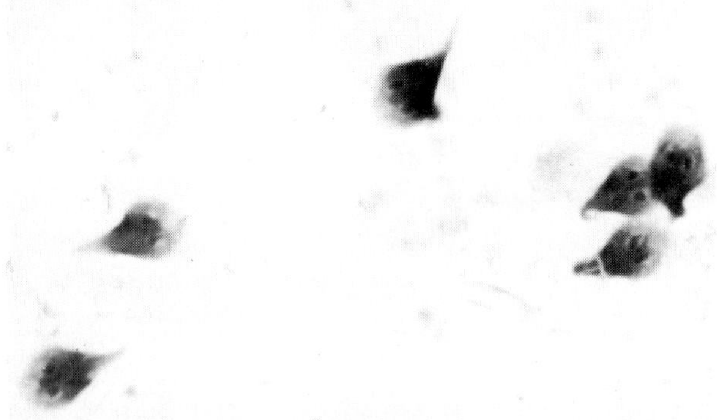

FIGURE 3.3C This preparation of trophozoites has been obtained by touching a glass slide with the mucosal surface of a small bowel biopsy obtained from a patient with humoral immunodeficiency and gastrointestinal symptoms (Giemsa × 352)

Giardia lamblia does not cause significant gastrointestinal disease and that its presence is a coincidental finding[86–88]. However, during the past years, convincing evidence has been accumulated indicating that in some individuals *Giardia lamblia* can cause intestinal disease, ranging from mild diarrhea and abdominal pain to severe malabsorption and weight loss[85,89–97]. Many of these patients were healthy individuals before travelling outside the United States. Treatment with quinacrine hydrochloride or metronidazole eradicated the parasites in most instances, and the patients became asymptomatic[85,90,93,95,98]. Histological abnormalities of the small bowel mucosa returned to normal shortly after treatment was completed[89,99]. Further evidence of the pathogenicity of *Giardia lamblia* for man has been provided by the demonstration of tissue invasion using special staining techniques[100] or electronmicroscopy[99].

Bacterial overgrowth in the duodenum and jejunum with aerobic organisms (*Streptococcus*, *Staphylococcus*, *Haemophilus*, *Diphtheroides*, coliforms, yeast) and anaerobic organisms (*Bacteroides*, *Lactobacillus*, *Clostridia*) have been reported in many patients with hypogammaglobulinaemia[9,14,16,21,37,43,54,58,66,79] but not in patients with selective IgA deficiency or in immunologically normal controls[9,14]. An aetiologic relationship between proximal bacterial overgrowth and intestinal lesions has been suggested but never proven. In a recent study[14] bacterial overgrowth of the proximal jejunum with colonic types of micro-organisms could be demonstrated in 12 of 24 patients with immunodeficiency syndromes. The presence or absence of colonic types of micro-organisms in the proximal jejunum of these patients did not correlate either with gastrointestinal symptoms, steatorrhea, lactose intolerance, vitamin B_{12} malabsorption, or the presence of *Giardia lamblia*. No significant changes in proximal intestinal bacterial flora, except for the elimination of *Giardia*, were observed in five patients after treatment with metronidazole was completed. However, all five patients showed marked clinical improvement. Furthermore, treatment with chloramphenicol did eliminate bacterial overgrowth but did not improve gastrointestinal symptoms and malabsorption, and did not alter the abnormalities of the villus architecture in a patient with variable immunodeficiency who was free of *Giardia lamblia*, indicating that bacterial overgrowth is not a major cause of gastrointestinal disease[14]. Further evidence of the insignificance of bacterial overgrowth in causing intestinal pathology comes from the observation that in spite of the presence of bacterial colonization in the upper small intestine in patients with pernicious anaemia, no intestinal symptoms were reported[58].

Patients with immunodeficiency seem to have a tendency to develop chronic salmonellosis and shigellosis, often resistant to therapy[15,33,34,66,79,101–103]. Waldmann[34] described chronic infections with *Salmonella* or *Shigella* in five of 12 hypogammaglobulinaemic patients with symptoms of diarrhea and steatorrhea. Chronic salmonellosis which did not respond to gammaglobulin treatment, plasma infusions and antibiotics has been observed repeatedly[102,103].

Disease of the colon in immunodeficiency

Symptoms of colitis have developed in a few patients with humoral immunodeficiency[14–18]. Colitis was associated in some patients with malabsorption indicating that both the small and large bowels were involved[16,18]. The absence of malabsorption in other patients[15,16] suggests that bowel disease was restricted to the colon.

Only two of 39 patients with immunodeficiency syndromes who were observed for several years developed symptoms of colitis such as watery diarrhea and tenesmus[14]. Both individuals had 'acquired' hypogammaglobulinaemia (variable immunodeficiency syndrome) and received adequate gammaglobulin therapy at the time when the symptoms developed. No malabsorption could be demonstrated, and small bowel biopsies showed normal villus architecture. A careful search for *Giardia lamblia* was negative. Sigmoidoscopic examination revealed an edematous mucosa which was friable and developed petechial haemorrhages when touched with a cotton swab. Rectal biopsies in both patients showed marked edema, haemorrhage and polymorphonuclear leukocytes in the lamina propria. Plasma cells were lacking and no crypt abscesses were found. Surface epithelium was absent in many areas. Short-term treatment with prednisone was followed by clinical remission and reversal of the abnormalities previously seen at sigmoidoscopy. Seventeen additional individuals from the same patient population were examined by sigmoidoscopy. One young adult showed multiple sessile polyps of the rectum, and a barium enema showed polyps throughout the entire colon. She also had nodular lymphoid hyperplasia of the small intestine. Histologically, the colonic polpys were of the juvenile type. We recently observed a patient with late onset immunodeficiency syndrome and malabsorption. She did not have giardiasis and did not respond to a gluten-free diet. Her small bowel biopsies showed a moderate to severe mucosal lesion. Initially proctosigmoidoscopic examination was normal, but rectal biopsy showed polymorphonuclear leukocytes in lamina propria. One year after onset of symptoms, diarrhea and malabsorption became intractable. Proctosigmoidoscopy showed a diffusely friable rectal mucosa and rectal biopsy revealed diffuse crypt abscesses and severe acute inflammation of the lamina propria. Symptoms and proctosigmoidoscopic changes did not respond to systemic corticosteroids or salicylazosulphapyridine[65].

The absence of plasma cells from the rectal mucosa of patients with agammaglobulinaemia was recognized early in the study of immune defects[104]. No plasma cells were found in rectal biopsies from eight patients with infantile X-linked agammaglobulinaemia and in those obtained from 19 patients with variable immunodeficiency syndrome[14]. In contrast, patients with ataxia telangiectasia have numerous plasma cells in their rectal mucosa; immunofluorescent studies have shown that the majority of their plasma cells produced IgM and not IgA as in normal individuals[47].

Multiple early crypt abscesses and polymorphonuclear leukocytes in the lamina propria were seen in the rectal biopsies (Figures 3.4A, 3.4B) of six of the eight patients with infantile X-linked agammaglobulinaemia[14]. None of them had gastrointestinal symptoms. The rectal mucosa was macroscopically normal at sigmoidoscopy. These microscopic abnormalities may represent an attempt to compensate for the defect of the humoral immune system.

Gastrointestinal abnormalities associated with T-cell deficiency

Abnormalities of the small bowel

Almost all children with severe combined immunodeficiency have chronic watery diarrhea and malabsorption[20,105–109]. Diarrhea and malabsorption usually are intractable, and a characteristic wasting syndrome becomes apparent in most of these infants[107,108] who gradually become unable to absorb any nutrients. Hitzig[107] reviewed the clinical and immunological characteristics of 70 infants with combined immune deficiency. Severe diarrhea was present in 86% and contributed significantly to the rapid deterioration of these infants. *Candida* infec-

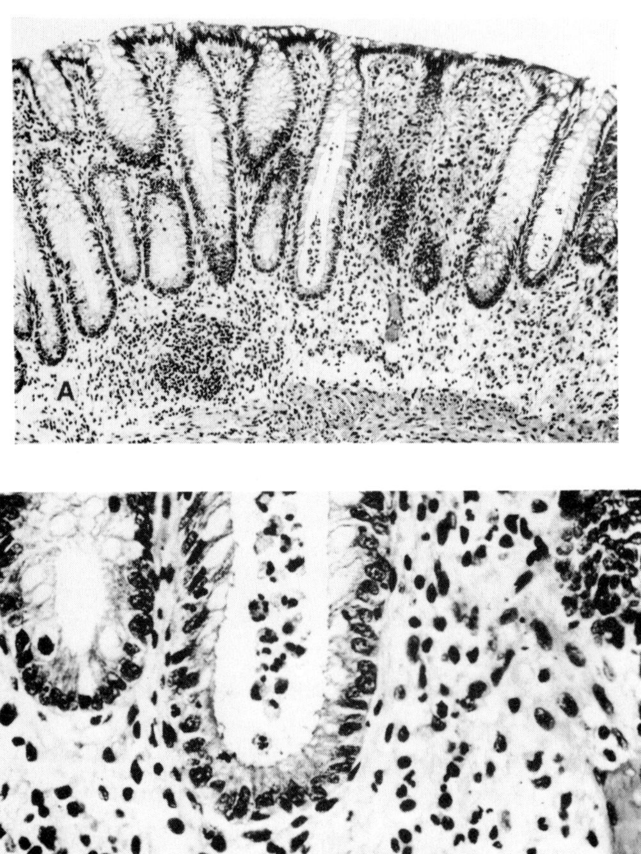

FIGURE 3.4 Rectal biopsy from a patient with infantile X-linked agammaglobulinemia who was free of gastrointestinal symptoms and did not have microscopic changes at rectosigmoidoscopy. A shows edema of the lamina propria and the presence of leukocytes in the lumen and wall of the rectal glands (H & E × 72). B is a high-power view demonstrating neutrophils in the lumen and wall of the rectal glands. Plasma cells are absent (H & E × 264)

tion was found in 79%, frequently involving the entire gastrointestinal tract. However, treatment of this infection has not resulted in reversal of diarrhea and malabsorption[65]. A high incidence of intestinal symptoms has been observed in combined immune deficiency with absence of red blood cell adenosine deaminase as well as in those without this enzyme defect[110]. Diarrhea and generalized malabsorption are also common symptoms of patients with defects of T-cell function alone[44,111–115].

Patients with ataxia telangiectasia have combined immune deficiency with some B-and T-cell function remaining. Although gastrointestinal symptoms are not of major concern, mild vitamin B_{12} malabsorption was recently described[14] in three of six patients with this syndrome. No *Giardia lamblia* was present and the addition of intrinsic factor did not improve vitamin B_{12} absorption. All three showed mild abnormalities of proximal small intestinal biopsies.

A primary symptom of Wiskott-Aldrich syndrome is early onset of severe bloody diarrhea[19,116]. One of three patients recently studied has mild steatorrhea. Vitamin B_{12} absorption was slightly abnormal in two and moderately decreased in one patient[14]. Because of the risk of intestinal haemorrhage, small bowel biopsies have not been obtained and adequate histological studies of the intestinal mucosa have not been done.

Alterations of the small bowel epithelium and the presence of large vacuolated macrophages in the lamina propria were recently described[112] in children with impaired cell-mediated immunity, chronic diarrhea and malabsorption. Electronmicroscopy revealed abnormalities of the absorptive cells and lipid droplets within the smooth endoplasmic reticulum, the Golgi apparatus and the basal portion of epithelial cells. These findings are non-specific and indicate absorptive cell damage. Many macrophages of the lamina propria showed lipid accumulation and dense inclusions. One of the four patients studied had isolated T-cell deficiency; the other three patients had combined immune deficiency.

Rectal biopsies obtained from patients with combined immune deficiency show complete absence of plasma cells[107,108]. Patients with isolated T-cell defects or with combined immune deficiency with only partial impairment of the B-cell system have plasma cells in the rectal mucosa. Immunohistochemical studies suggest that many of these patients have predominantly IgM producing plasma cells in their rectal mucosa[47].

Esophageal strictures secondary to chronic candidiasis

Esophageal strictures have recently been observed[20] in two adult siblings with chronic mucosal candidiasis and possibly a mild T-cell defect. Both required intravenous therapy with amphotericin B and repeated esophageal dilatation.

A 28-year-old white male was in good general health until 1966 when he developed whitish plaques on his tongue and oral mucosa causing discomfort and pain during eating. His 25-year-old sister developed oral thrush at 3 years of age and since that time has had almost continuously white plaques on her tongue and oral mucosa. She had urinary tract infection several times and severe vulvo-urethrovaginitis due to *Candida albicans* during her last pregnancy. Neither one has

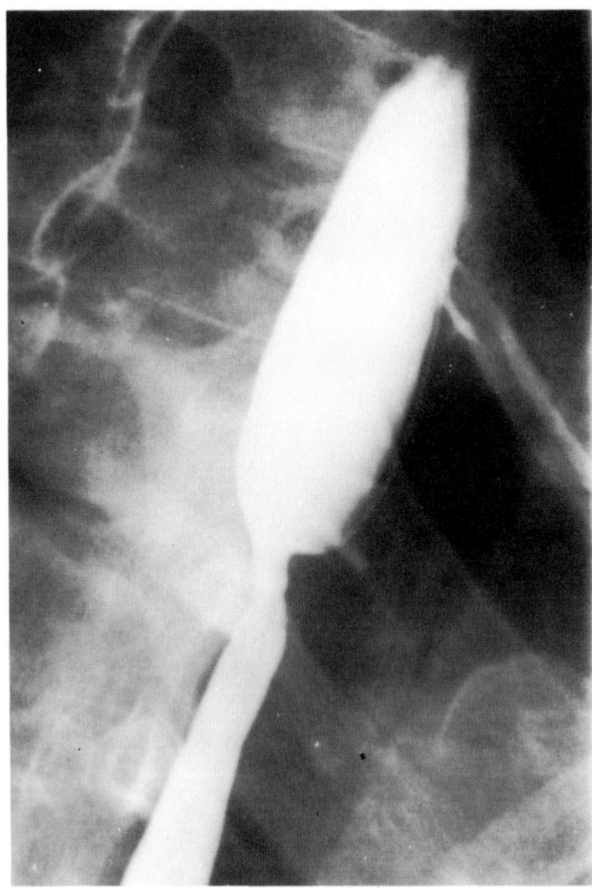

FIGURE 3.5 Esophragram of a patient with candidiasis confined to the oral cavity and esophagus demonstrating an esophageal stricture.

cutaneous candidiasis, and no history of susceptibility to bacterial or viral infections was reported. Serum calcium and phosphorus were repeatedly normal. No endocrinopathy was present. A tongue biopsy obtained from both patients in 1973 showed 'monilial granuloma'. Treatment with nystatin brought some local improvement but did not eliminate the problem. The young woman had noticed dysphagia in the past 5 years and had to chew her food very carefully. Her brother noticed difficulty in swallowing solids during the past year and by 1974 was unable to swallow solid food. He lost a considerable amount of weight prior to his admission to the University Hospital. X-ray examinations revealed focal esophageal strictures, in the man at T3, measuring 6 mm in diameter and extending for 1 cm, and in the women in the mid-esophagus (Figure 3.5). Esophagoscopy showed that the strictures were symmetrical and that the mucosa was inflamed and covered with white exudate. The endoscope could not be passed through the strictures. The tongues of both patients were coated with a moist, whitish film extending to the buccal mucosa, tonsils and pharynx. Cultures revealed *Candida albicans*. Treatment with oral amphotericin B showed only minimal improvement. Intravenous amphotericin B at a dose of 15 mg/day cleared the mouth lesions, and mechanical dilatation improved the dysphagia. Both therapeutic measurements had to be repeated two months later.

Immunological evaluation revealed possible hypergammaglobulinaemia (IgG 1500–1600 mg%, IgA 330–410 mg%, IgM 125–220 mg%). Schick tests were negative, and both patients had adequate isohaemagglutinin titres. Skin test reactivity was minimal in both patients; the brother had a 3 mm reaction to streptokinase/streptodornase (SK/SD) and negative reactions to PPD, mumps and dermatophytin O. The sister showed a slight reaction to SK/SD, a 4 × 4 mm reaction to mumps, and a 3 × 3 mm reaction to dermatophytin O. Both patients had normal *in vitro* lymphocyte transformation when stimulated with phytohaemagglutinin, Concavallin A, pokeweed mitogen, and allogeneic cells. Absolute lymphocyte counts and granulocyte counts were normal. Granulocytes showed a normal nitroblue tetrazolium reduction and had adequate amounts of myeloperoxidase.

This peculiar susceptibility to candidiasis, limited to the mucous membranes, seems to be due to an inherited abnormality. The minimal skin reactivity to a number of antigens, tested before amphotericin B therapy, might be significant and indicate a mild T-cell defect.

Malignancy of the gastrointestinal tract associated with immunodeficiency

The increased incidence of malignancies in patients with immunodeficiency syndromes is now well documented and has recently been summarized[117]. Lymphomas and other malignancies of the lymphoid system are the most common ones; neoplasms involving the gastrointestinal tract are less common. Carcinoma of the stomach has been reported by a number of investigators[32,54,118–120]. Hermans[120] summarized the clinical and immunological data of five cases with gastric carcinoma who had the characteristic findings of late-onset immunodeficiency syndrome, frequent respiratory infections (five patients), atrophic gastritis (three patients), pernicious anaemia (two patients), malabsorption (five patients), nodular lymphoid hyperplasia (two patients), hypothyroidism (one patient), and *Giardia lamblia* (three patients). Two of these patients developed carcinoma of the stomach at an unusually early age, at 27 years and 31 years respectively. Histologically, two were adenocarcinoma, two scirrhous adenocarcinoma, and in one case the malignancy was not specified.

Creagan *et al.*[118] studied a family in which eight males and four females from four generations developed carcinoma of the stomach. In addition, two members of that kindred died of cancer of the colon and three developed colitis. Several asymptomatic members of this family and one patient with carcinoma had evidence of cell-mediated immunodeficiency, manifested by impaired lymphocyte transformation *in vitro*, skin test anergy and lymphopenia. In addition, a high prevalence of autoantibodies to parietal cells was noticed in this family. The association of ataxia telangiectasia and adenocarcinoma of the stomach[121] has been observed in two sisters who both developed a rapidly spreading gastric carcinoma during the second decade of life. Other malignancies of the gastrointestinal tract associated with immunodeficiency syndromes are carcinoma of the colon and of the rectum[27,62]. Several patients with isolated IgA deficiency and carcinoma of the digestive tract have been reported involving the esophagus[122], stomach[123] and colon[124].

Gastrointestinal manifestations in chronic granulomatous disease

Chronic granulomatous disease (CGD) of childhood is an inherited illness manifested by repeated bacterial infections[125-127]. The phagocytic cells of these patients can ingest but not kill certain microorganisms[128]. The most frequent pathological findings are lymphadenopathy, hepatosplenomegaly, chronic lung disease and skin and liver abscesses. Persistent, unexplained diarrhea and perianal abscesses have been observed in approximately 20% of these patients[129].

In a recent study[130], we evaluated the structure and function of the gastrointestinal tract in nine patients with CGD (Table 3.3). Three

Table 3.3 GASTROINTESTINAL (GI) SYMPTOMS, FINDINGS AND MORPHOLOGICAL ABNORMALITIES IN NINE PATIENTS WITH CHRONIC GRANULOMATOUS DISEASE

GI symptoms (diarrhea and/or vomiting)	4/9*
Steatorrhea	2/9
B_{12} malabsorption	6/9
Lactose intolerance	none/9
Lipid-filled pigmented histiocytes	
small bowel mucosa	7/8
rectal mucosa	8/8
Granuloma and giant cells	
small bowel mucosa	none/8
rectal mucosa	5/8

* Numbers of patients affected/number of patients studied

individuals had diarrhea and one or more nontender ventral or perianal fistulas; one boy reported intermittent vomiting of undigested food. One of the symptomatic patients had a history of frequent unexplained fever, nausea, anorexia and abdominal pain of 16 months' duration. His stool frequency gradually increased from two to five per day, and intermittent diarrhea developed. Physical and sigmoidoscopic findings, X-ray changes in small bowel series and morphologic changes in rectal biopsies were undistinguishable from those seen in Crohn's disease of the small intestine and colon. Steatorrhea was demonstrated in this and one other patient. Mild to moderate vitamin B_{12} malabsorption was found in six patients; intrinsic factor did not significantly improve vitamin B_{12} absorption in four individuals tested. Those patients with steatorrhea had vitamin B_{12} malabsorption. None of the patients had lactose intolerance.

Small bowel biopsies were taken from eight patients. The biopsies were normal in every way, except for PAS-positive brownish yellow

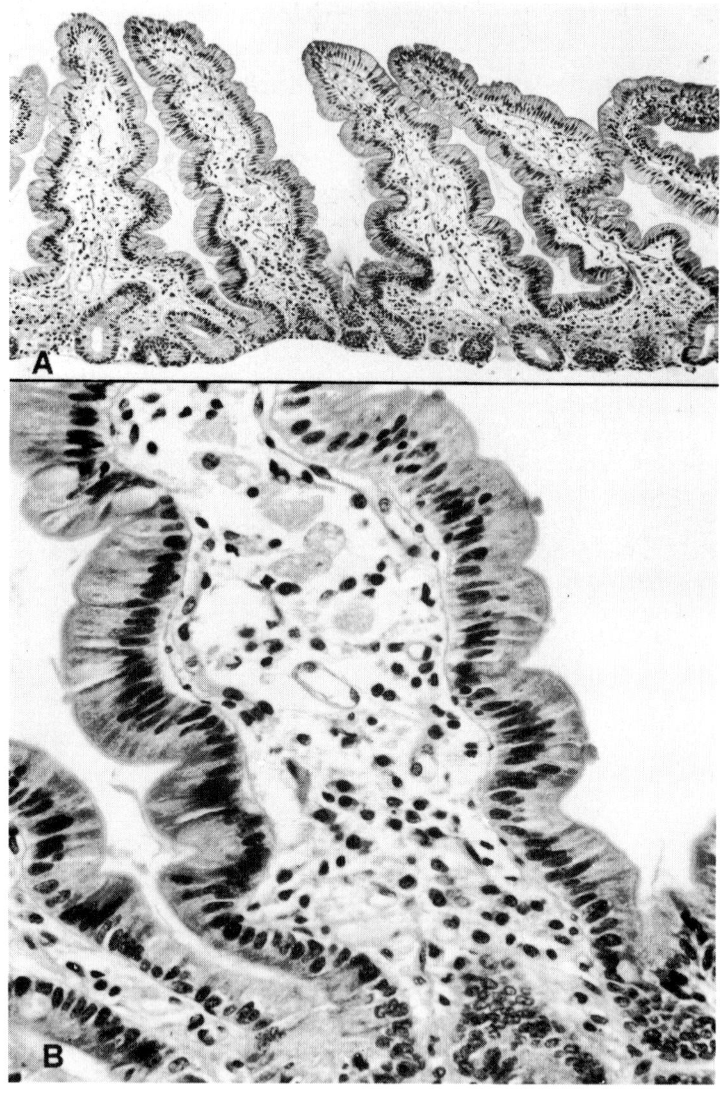

FIGURE 3.6 A shows a small intestinal biopsy from a patient with CGD. The villus architecture is normal. The lamina propria contains large numbers of histiocytes with fine granular cytoplasm (H & E × 72). B is a high-power view (× 264) showing the pigmented histiocytes

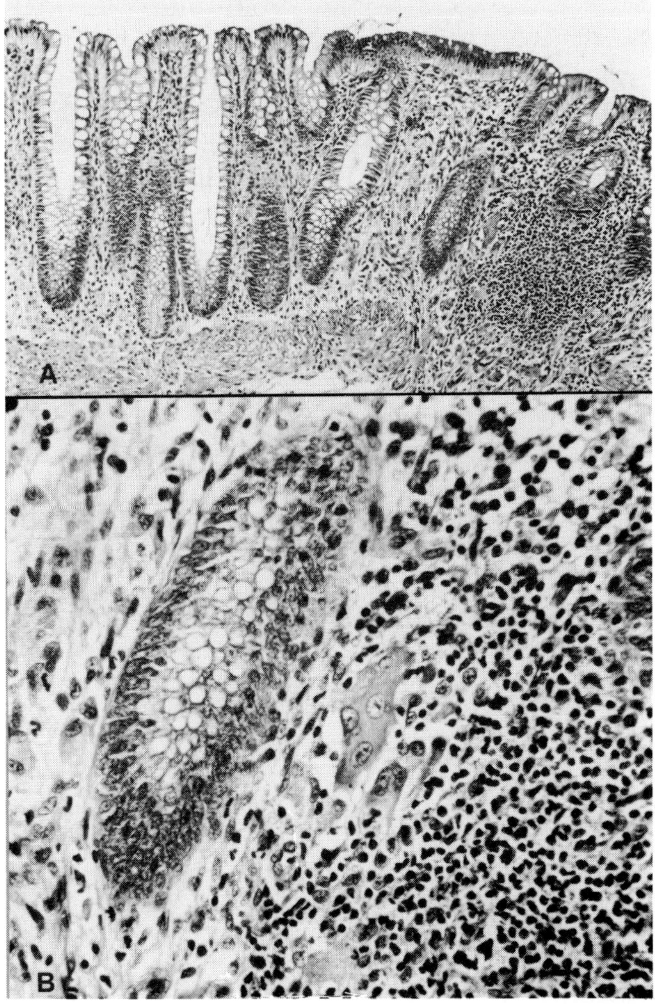

FIGURE 3.7A Rectal biopsy from a patient with CGD. The surface epithelium is intact, and the glandular architecture is normal. A giant cell is seen adjacent to a lymph nodule (H & E × 72)
FIGURE 3.7B High-power view (× 264) demonstrating the giant cell in detail

vacuolated histiocytes wtihin the lamina propria of seven of the eight patients (Figures 3.6A, 3.6B). They were variable in size and ranged from 50 to 100 μm in diameter. Most histiocytes were round but irregular in shape and had vacuoles. Giant cells or granulomas were not found in any of the small bowel biopsies. Every rectal biopsy contained abnormal histiocytes similar to those seen in the small bowel biopsies. Most of these cells were in the lamina propria, but occasionally they were found in the submucosa. Five of the eight patients had granulomas and giant cells in rectal biopsies (Figures 3.7A, 3.7B). One patient with abnormal findings at sigmoidoscopy showed disorganized architecture of the rectal glands but no crypt abscesses were seen.

The presence of 'foamy' histiocytes in the intestinal mucosa has been described in CGD, in patients with T-cell deficiency[113] and in patients with Whipple's disease. It is of interest that a persistent defect in T-cell function manifested by skin test anergy, diminished PHA responsiveness and prolonged survival of skin allografts has recently been demonstrated in patients with Whipple's disease[131,132]. The common abnormality in these three entities seems to be a defective local defence mechanism involving macrophages and/or T-lymphocytes.

REFERENCES

1. Warner, N. L., Szenberg, A. and Burnet, F. M. (1962). The immunological role of different lymphoid organs in the chicken. I. Dissociation of immunological responsiveness. *Aust. J. Exp. Biol. Med. Sci.*, **40**, 373
2. Cooper, M. D., Perey, D. Y., Peterson, R. D. A., Gabrielsen, A. E. and Good, R. A. (1968). The two-component concept of the lymphoid system. In *Immunologic deficiency diseases in man.* R. A. Good and D. Bergsma (eds.) *Birth Defects Original Article Series, NY*, **Vol. IV, No. 1**, 7
3. Cooper, M. D., Perey, D. Y., Gabrielsen, A. E., Sutherland, D. E. R., McKneally, M. F. and Good, R. A. (1968). Production of an antibody deficiency syndrome in rabbits by neonatal removal of organized intestinal lymphoid tissues. *Int. Arch. Allergy*, **33**, 65
4. Cooper, M. D., Perey, D. Y., McKneally, M. F., Gabrielsen, A. E., Sutherland, D. E. R. and Good, R. A. (1966). A mammalian equivalent of the avian bursa of Fabricus. *Lancet*, **i**, 1388
5. Owen, J. J. T., Cooper, M. D. and Raff, M. C. (1974). *In vitro* generation of B-lymphocytes in mouse foetal liver, a mammalian 'bursa equivalent'. *Nature*, **249**, 361
6. Watson, D. W. (1969). Immune responses and the gut. *Gastroenterology*, **56**, 944
7. Crabbé, P. A. and Heremans, J. F. (1966). The distribution of immunoglobulin-containing cells along the human gastrointestinal tract. *Gastroenterology*, **51**, 305
8. Crabbé. P. A. and Heremans, J. F. (1969). The significance of local IgA in the physiology of the intestinal mucosa. *Folia Med. Neerl.*, **12**, 100

9. Brown, W. R., Butterfield, D., Savage, D. and Tada, T. (1972). Clinical, microbiological and immunological studies in patients with immunoglobulin deficiencies and gastrointestinal disorders. *Gut*, **13**, 441
10. Weiden, P. L., Blaese, R. M., Strober, W., Block, J. B. and Waldmann, T. A. (1972). Impaired lymphocyte transformation in intestinal lymphangiectasia; evidence for at least two functionally distinct lymphocyte populations in man. *J. Clin. Invest.*, **51**, 1319
11. Fudenberg, H. H., Good, R. A., Goodman, H. C., Hitzig, W., Kunkel, H. G., Roitt, I. M., Rosen, F. S., Rowe, D. S., Seligmann, M. and Soothill, J. R. (1971). Primary immunodeficiencies. Report of a World Health Organization Committee. *Pediatrics*, **47**, 927
12. Rosen, F. S. and Janeway, C. A. (1966). The gammaglobulins. III. The antibody deficiency syndromes. *New Engl. J. Med.*, **275**, 709
13. Gitlin, D., Gross, P. A. M. and Janeway, C. A. (1959). The gamma globulins and their clinical significance. II. Hypogammaglobulinemia. *New Engl. J. Med.*, **260**, 72
14. Ament, M. E., Ochs, H. D. and Davis, S. D. (1973). Structure and function of the gastrointestinal tract in primary immunodeficiency syndromes: a study of 39 patients. *Medicine*, **52**, 227
15. Conn, H. O. and Quintiliani, R. (1966). Severe diarrhea controlled by gamma globulin in a patient with agammaglobulinemia, amyloidosis and thymoma. *Ann. Intern. Med.*, **65**, 528
16. Hughes, W. S., Cerda, J. J., Holtzapple, P. and Brooks, F. P. (1971). Primary hypogammaglobulinemia and malabsorption. *Ann. Intern. Med.*, **74**, 903
17. Rosecan, M., Trobaugh, F. E. and Danforth, W. H. (1955). Agammaglobulinemia in the adult. *Am. J. Med.*, **19**, 303
18. Zelman, S. and Lewin, H. (1958). Adult agammaglobulinemia associated with multiple congenital anomalies. *Am. J. Med.*, **25**, 150
19. Wiskott, A. (1937). Familiärer, angeborener Morbus Werlhoffii. *Monatsschr. Kinderh.*, **68**, 212
20. Ochs, H. D. Unpublished observations
21. Ajdukiewicz, A. B., Youngs, G. R. and Bouchier, I. A. D. (1972). Nodular lymphoid hyperplasia with hypogammaglobulinaemia. *Gut*, **13**, 589
22. Clark, R., Tornyos, K., Herbert, V. and Twomey, J. J. (1967). Studies on two patients with concomitant pernicious anemia and immunoglobulin deficiency. *Ann. Intern. Med.*, **67**, 403
23. Conn, H. O., Binder, H. and Burns, B. (1968). Pernicious anemia and immunologic deficiency. *Ann. Intern. Med.*, **68**, 603
24. Crowder, R. V., Thompson, W. T. and Kupfer, H. G. (1959). Acquired agammaglobulinemia with multiple allergies and pernicious anemia. *Arch. Int. Med.*, **103**, 445
25. Gibbs, D. D. and Pryor, J. S. (1961). Hypogammaglobulinaemia ('acquired' adult form) and pernicious anaemia. *Proc. Roy. Soc. Med.*, **54**, 590

26. Goodman, D. H., Smith, R. S. and Northey, W. T. (1967). Hypogammaglobulinemia, allergy and absence of intrinsic factor. *J. Allergy*, **40**, 131
27. Hermans, P. E., Huizenga, K. A., Hoffman, H. N., Brown, A. L. and Markowitz, H. (1966). Dysgammaglobulinemia associated with nodular lymphoid hyperplasia of the small intestine. *Am. J. Med.*, **40**, 78
28. Hoskins, L. C., Winawer, S. J., Broitman, S. A., Gottlieb, L. S. and Zamcheck, N. (1967). Clinical giardiasis and intestinal malabsorption. *Gastroenterology*, **53**, 265
29. Larsson, S. O., Hagelquist, E. and Coster, C. (1961). Hypogammaglobulinaemia and pernicious anaemia. *Acta Haemat.*, **26**, 50
30. Lee, F. I., Jenkins, G. C., Hughes, D. T. D. and Kazantzis, G. (1964). Pernicious anaemia, myxoedema and hypogammaglobulinaemia—a family study. *Br. Med. J.*, **1**, 598
31. Lewis, E. C. and Brown, H. E. (1957). Agammaglobulinemia associated with pernicious anemia and diabetes mellitus. *Arch. Int. Med.*, **100**, 296
32. Twomey, J. J., Jordan, P. H., Jarrold, T., Trubowitz, S., Ritz, N. D. and Conn, H. O. (1969). The syndrome of immunoglobulin deficiency and pernicious anemia. *Am. J. Med.*, **47**, 340
33. Twomey, J. J., Jordan, P. H., Laughter, A. H., Meuwissen, H. J. and Good, R. A. (1970). The gastric disorder in immunoglobulin-deficient patients. *Ann. Int. Med.*, **72**, 499
34. Waldmann, T. A. and Laster, L. (1964). Abnormalities of albumin metabolism in patients with hypogammaglobulinemia. *J. Clin. Invest.*, **43**, 1025
35. Cohen, N., Paley, D. and Janowitz, H. D. (1961). Acquired hypogammaglobulinemia and sprue: Report of a case and review of the literature. *J. Mount Sinai Hosp. NY.*, **28**, 421
36. Crabbé, P. A. and Heremans, J. F. (1966). Lack of gamma A-immunoglobulin in serum of patients with steatorrhoea. *Gut*, **7**, 119
37. Ament, M. E. and Rubin, C. E. (1972). Relation of giardiasis to abnormal intestinal structure and function in gastrointestinal immunodeficiency syndromes. *Gastroenterology*, **62**, 216
38. Hakami, N., Neiman, P. E., Canellos, G. P. and Lazerson, J. (1971). Neonatal megaloblastic anemia due to inherited transcobalamin II deficiency in two siblings. *New. Engl. J. Med.*, **285**, 1163
39. Hitzig, W. H., Dohmann, U., Pluss, H. J. and Vischer, D. (1974). Hereditary transcobalamin II deficiency: Clinical findings in a new family. *J. Pediat.*, **85**, 622
40. Gerson, C. D., Janowitz, H. D. and Paronetto, F. (1972). Hypogammaglobulinemia and malabsorption: immunofluorescent localization of immunoglobulins in the jejunal mucosa. *Mount Sinai J. Med. NY*, **39**, 158
41. Huizenga, K. A., Wollaeger, E. E., Green, P. A. and McKenzie, B. F. (1961). Serum globulin deficiencies in non-tropical sprue, with

report of two cases of acquired agammaglobulinemia. *Am. J. Med.*, **31**, 572

42. Pelkonen, R., Siurala, M. and Vuopio, P. (1963). Inherited agammaglobulinemia with malabsorption and marked alterations in the gastrointestinal mucosa. *Acta. Med. Scand.*, **173**, 549
43. Anderson, F. L., Pellegrino, E. D. and Schaefer, J. W. (1970). Dysgammaglobulinemia associated with malabsorption and tetany. *Am. J. Dig. Dis.*, **15**, 279
44. Dubois, R. S., Roy, C. C., Fulginiti, V. A., Merrill, D. A. and Murray, R. L. (1970). Disaccharidase deficiency in children with immunologic deficits. *J. Pediat.*, **76**, 377
45. Quinton, W. E., Flick, A. L. and Rubin, C. E. (1962). The design of a hydraulic suction tube for peroral biopsy of the human gastrointestinal tract. *Gastroenterology*, **42**, 281
46. Crabbé, P. A. and Heremans, J. F. (1967). Selective IgA deficiency with steatorrhea. A new syndrome. *Am. J. Med.*, **42**, 319
47. Eidelman, S. and Davis, S. D. (1968). Immunoglobulin content of intestinal mucosal plasma-cells in ataxia telangiectasia. *Lancet*, **i**, 884
48. Firkin, B. G. and Blackburn, C. R. B. (1958). Congenital and acquired agammaglobulinemia. A report of four cases. *Quart. J. Med.*, **27**, 187
49. Frik, W., Heinkel, K. and Zeitler, G. (1963). Vermehrung und Hyperplasie von Lymphfollikeln als Ursache granulärer Füllungsdefekte im Röntgenbild des gesamten Dünndarms. *Fortschr. Roentgenstr.*, **99**, 65
50. Bird, D. C., Jacobs, J. B., Silbiger, M. and Wolff, S. M. (1969). Hypogammaglobulinemia with nodular lymphoid hyperplasia of the intestine: report of a case with rectosigmoid involvement. *Radiology*, **92**, 1535
51. Cooper, M. D., Lawton, A. R. and Bockman, D. E. (1971). Agammaglobulinaemia with B lymphocytes. *Lancet*, **ii**, 791
52. Goldstein, G. W., Krivit, W. J. and Hong, R. (1969). Hypoimmunoglobulin G, hyperimmunoglobulin M, intestinal nodular hyperplasia and thrombocytopenia: An unusual association. *Arch. Dis. Child.*, **44**, 621
53. Grise, J. W. (1968). Dysgammaglobulinemia with nodular lymphoid hyperplasia of the small intestine. *Radiology*, **90**, 579
54. Hersh, T., Floch, M. H., Binder, H. J., Conn, H. O., Prizont, R. and Spiro, H. M. (1970). Disturbance of the jejunal and colonic bacterial flora in immunoglobulin deficiencies. *Am. J. Clin. Nutrition*, **23**, 1595
55. Hodgson, J. R., Hoffman, H. N., and Huizenga, K. A. (1967). Roentgenologic features of lymphoid hyperplasia of the small intestine associated with dysgammaglobulinemia. *Radiology*, **88**, 883
56. Johnson, B. L., Goldberg, L. S., Pops, M. A. and Weiner, M. (1971). Clinical and immunological studies in a case of nodular lymphoid hyperplasia of the small bowel. *Gastroenterology*, **61**, 369
57. Michaels, D. L., Go, S., Humbert, J. R., Dubois, R. S., Stewart, J. M. and Ellis, E. F. (1971). Intestinal nodular lymphoid hyperplasia, hypogammaglobulinemia, and hematologic abnormalities in a child with a ring 18 chromosome. *J. Pediat.*, **79**, 80

58. Parkin, D. M., McClelland, D. B. L., O'Moore, R. R., Percy-Robb, I. W., Grant, I. W. B. and Shearman, D. J. C. (1972). Intestinal bacterial flora and bile salt studies in hypogammaglobulinaemia. *Gut*, **13**, 182
59. Penny, R. (1969). Nodular lymphoid hyperplasia of the small intestine and hypogammaglobulinemia. *Gastroenterology*, **56**, 982
60. Gryboski, J. D., Self, T. W., Clemett, A. and Herskovic, T. (1968). Selective immunoglobulin A deficiency and intestinal nodular lymphoid hyperplasia. Correction of diarrhea with antibiotics and plasma. *Pediatrics*, **42**, 833
61. Kirkpatrick, C. H., Waxman, D., Smith, O. D. and Schimke, R. N. (1968). Hypogammaglobulinemia with nodular lymphoid hyperplasia of the small bowel. *Arch. Int. Med.*, **121**, 273
62. Hermans, P. E. (1967). Nodular lymphoid hyperplasia of the small intestine and hypogammaglobulinemia: Theoretical and practical considerations. *Fed. Proc.*, **26**, 1606
63. Davis, S. D., Eidelman, S. and Loop, J. W. (1970). Nodular lymphoid hyperplasia of the small intestine and sarcoidosis. *Arch. Int. Med.*, **126**, 668.
64. Ochs, H. D., Davis, S. D. and Wedgwood, R. J. (1971). Immunologic responses to bacteriphage ϕX 174 in immunodeficiency diseases. *J. Clin. Invest.*, **50**, 2559
65. Ament, M. E. Unpublished observations
66. Collins, J. R. and Ellis, D. S. (1965). Agammaglobulinemia, malabsorption and rheumatoid-like arthritis. *Am. J. Med.*, **39**, 476
67. Siegal, F. P., Pernis, B. and Kunkel, H. G. (1971). Lymphocytes in human immunodeficiency states: A study of membrane-associated immunoglobulins. *Eur. J. Immunol.*, **1**, 482
68. Uhr, J. W. and Möller, G. (1968). Regulatory effect of antibody on the immune response. *Adv. Immunol.*, **8**, 81
69. Bjernulf, A., Johansson, S. G. O. and Parrow, A. (1971). Immunoglobulin studies in gastrointestinal dysfunction with special reference to IgA deficiency. *Acta Med. Scand.*, **190**, 71
70. Claman, H. N., Merrill, D. A., Peakman, D. and Robinson, A. (1970). Isolated severe gamma A deficiency: immunoglobulin levels, clinical disorders, and chromosome studies. *J. Lab. Clin. Med.*, **75**, 307
71. Mann, J. G., Brown, W. R. and Kern, F. (1970). The subtle and variable clinical expressions of gluten-induced enteropathy (adult celiac disease, nontropical sprue). An analysis of 21 consecutive cases. *Am. J. Med.*, **48**, 357
72. Savilahti, E., Pelkonen, P. and Visakorpi, J. K. (1971). IgA deficiency in children. A clinical study with special reference to intestinal findings. *Arch. Dis. Child.*, **46**, 665
73. Hobbs, J. R. and Hepner, G. W. (1968). Deficiency of γ M-globulin in coeliac disease. *Lancet*, **i**, 217
74. Allen, G. E. and Hadden, D. R. (1964). Congenital hypogamma-

globulinaemia with steatorrhea in two adult brothers. *Br. Med. J.*, **2**, 486

75. Cooke, W. T., Weiner, W. and Shinton, N. K. (1957). Agammaglobulinaemia—report of two adult cases. *Br. Med. J.*, **1**, 1151
76. Johnson, R. L., VanArsdel, P. P., Tobe, A. D. and Ching, Y. (1967). Adult hypogammaglobulinemia with malabsorption and iron deficiency anemia. *Am. J. Med.*, **43**, 935
77. Kabler, J. D. (1960). Rare malabsorption syndromes. *Ann. Int. Med.*, **52**, 1221
78. Sanford, J. P., Favour, C. B. and Tribeman, M. S. (1954). Absence of serum gamma globulins in an adult. *New Eng. J. Med.*, **250**, 1027
79. McCarthy, C. F., Austad, W. I. and Read, A. E. A. (1965). Hypogammaglobulinemia and steatorrhea. *Am. J. Dig. Dis.*, **10**, 945
80. Green, I. and Sperber, R. J. (1962). Hypogammaglobulinemia, arthritis, sprue and megaloblastic anemia. *New York J. Med.*, **62**, 1679
81. Swift, P. N. (1962). Hypogammaglobulinaemia, steatorrhoea and megaloblastic anaemia. Response to gluten-free diet and folic acid. *Postgrad. Med. J.*, **38**, 633
82. Ochs, H. D., Ament, M. E. and Davis, S. D. (1972). Giardiasis with malabsorption in X-linked agammaglobulinemia. *New Eng. J. Med.*, **287**, 341
83. Zamcheck, N., Hoskins, L. C., Winawer, S. J., Broitman, S. A. and Gottlieb, L. S. (1963). Histology and ultrastructure of the parasite and the intestinal mucosa in human giardiasis: effects of Atabrine therapy (abstract). *Gastroenterology*, **44**, 860
84. Brown, W. R., Lansford, C. L. and Hornbrook, M. (1973). Serum immunoglobulin E(IgE) concentrations in patients with gastrointestinal disorders. *Am. J. Dig. Dis.*, **18**, 641
85. Moore, G. T., Cross, W. M., McGuire, D., Mollohan, C. S., Gleason, N. N., Healy, G. R. and Newton, L. H. (1969). Epidemic giardiasis at a ski resort. *New Engl. J. Med.*, **281**, 402
86. Cantor, D., Biempica, L., Toccalino, H. and O'Donnell, J. C. (1967). Small intestine studies in giardiasis. *Am. J. Gastroent.*, **47**, 134
87. Monat, H. A. and McKinney, W. L. (1946). Giardiasis: Question of pathogenicity. *US Naval. Med. Bull.*, **46**, 1204
88. Palumbo, P. J., Scudamore, H. H. and Thompson, J. H. (1962). Relationship of infestation with *Giardia lamblia* to intestinal-malabsorption syndromes. *Proc. Staff Meetings Mayo Clinic*, **37**, 589
89. Alp, M. H. and Hislop, I. G. (1969). The effect of *Giardia lamblia* infestation on the gastro-intestinal tract. *Aust. Ann. Med.*, **18**, 232
90. Babb, R. R., Peck, O. C. and Vescia, F. G. (1971). Giardiasis. *JAMA*, **217**, 1359
91. Cortner, J. A. (1959). Giardiasis, a cause of celiac syndrome. *Am. J. Dis. Child.*, **98**, 311
92. Court, J. M. and Stanton, C. (1959). The incidence of *Giardia lamblia* infestation of children in Victoria. *Med. J. Aust.*, **2**, 438

93. Powell, E. D. U. (1956). Giardiasis. *Irish J. Med. Sci.*, **371**, 509
94. Rendtorff, R. C. (1954). The experimental transmission of human intestinal protozoan parasites. *Am. J. Epidem.*, **59**, 209
95. Véghelyi, P. (1939). Celiac disease imitated by giardiasis. *Am. J. Dis. Child*, **57**, 894
96. Yardley, J. H. (1967). Giardiasis. *Gastroenterology*, **52**, 301
97. Yardley, J. H., Takano, J. and Hendrix, T. R. (1964). Epithelial and other mucosal lesions of the jejunum in giardiasis. Jejunal biopsy studies. *Bull. Johns Hopkins Hosp.*, **115**, 389
98. Bassily, S., Farid, Z., Mikhail, J. W., Kent, D. C. and Lehman, J. S. (1970). The treatment of *Giardia lamblia* infection with mepacrine, metronidazole and furazolidone. *J. Trop. Med. Hyg.*, **73**, 15
99. Morecki, R. and Parker, J. G. (1967). Ultrastructural studies of the human *Giardia lamblia* and subjacent jejunal mucosa in a subject with steatorrhea. *Gastroenterology*, **52**, 151
100. Brandborg, L. L., Tankersley, C. B., Gottlieb, S., Barancik, M. and Sartor, V. E. (1967). Histological demonstration of mucosal invasion by *Giardia lamblia* in man. *Gastroenterology*, **52**, 143
101. Douglas, S. D., Goldberg, L. S. and Fudenberg, H. H. (1970). Clinical, serologic and leukocyte function studies on patients with idiopathic 'acquired' agammaglobulinemia and their families. *Am. J. Med.*, **48**, 48
102. Freundlich, E. (1957). Agammaglobulinemia. Report of a case. *J. Pediat.*, **50**, 475
103. Stites, D. P., Levin, A. S., Lauer, B. A., Costom, B. H. and Fudenberg, H. H. (1973). Selective 'dysgammaglobulinemia' with elevated serum IgA levels and chronic salmonellosis. *Am. J. Med.*, **54**, 260
104. Gitlin, D., Janeway, C. A., Apt, L. and Craig, J. M. (1959). Agammaglobulinemia. In *Cellular and humoral aspects of the hypersensitive states.* H. S. Lawrence (ed.) p. 375 (New York: Hoeber–Harper)
105. Cederbaum, S. D., Niwayama, G., Stiehm, E. R., Neerhout, R. C., Ammann, A. J. and Berman, W. (1974). Combined immunodeficiency presenting as the Letterer–Siwe syndrome. *J. Pediat.*, **85**, 466
106. Gitlin, D. and Craig, J. M. (1963). The thymus and other lymphoid tissues in congenital agammaglobulinemia. 1. Thymic alymphoplasia and lymphocytic hypoplasia and their relation to infection. *Pediatrics*, **32**, 517
107. Hitzig, W. H. (1968). The Swiss type of agammaglobulinemia. In *Immunologic deficiency diseases in man.* R. A. Good and D. Bergsma (eds.) *Birth Defects Original Article Series, NY*, **Vol. IV, No. 1**, 82
108. Hitzig, W. H., Barandun, S. and Cottier, H. (1968). Die schweizerische Form der Agammaglobulinämie. *Ergebn inn Med. Kinderheilk*, **27**, 79
109. Rosen, F. S. (1971). The thymus gland and the immune deficiency syndromes. In *Immunological diseases.* M. Samter, (ed.) **Vol. 1**, p. 497 (Boston: Little, Brown and Company)
110. Workshop report on combined immunodeficiency disease and ADA deficiency (1975). In New York State Department of Health. *Birth Defects*

Institute Symposium IV: Combined immunodeficiency disease and adenosin deaminase deficiency. A molecular defect. H. J. Meuwissen, R. J. Pickering, I. H. Porter and B. Pollara (eds.) (New York: Academic Press, Inc.)

111. DiGeorge, A. M. (1968). Congenital absence of the thymus and its immunologic consequences: concurrence with congenital hypoparathyroidism. In *Immunologic deficiency diseases in man.* R. A. Good and D. Bergsma (eds.) *Birth Defects Original Article Series, NY,* **Vol. IV, No. 1**, 116
112. Horowitz, S., Lorenzsonn, V. W., Olsen, W. A., Albrecht, R. and Hong, R. (1974). Small intestinal disease in T-cell deficiency. *J. Pediat.*, **85**, 457
113. Lux, S. E., Johnston, R. B. August, C. S., Say, B., Penchaszadeh, V. B., Rosen, F. S. and McKusick, V. A. (1970). Chronic neutropenia and abnormal cellular immunity in cartilage-hair hypoplasia. *New Engl. J. Med.*, **282**, 231
114. Nezelof, C. (1968). Thymic dysplasia with normal immunoglobulins and immunologic deficiency: Pure alymphocytosis, In *Immunologic deficiency diseases in man.* R. A. Good and D. Bergsma (eds.). *Birth Defects Original Article Series, NY,* **Vol. IV, No. 1**, 104
115. Rainier-Pope, C. R. and Watson, C. (1969). Thymic alymphoplasia: A case report. *S. Afr. Med. J.*, **43**, 1127
116. Aldrich, R. A., Steinberg, A. G. and Campbell, D. C. (1954). Pedigree demonstrating a sex-linked recessive condition characterized by draining ears, eczematoid dermatitis and bloody diarrhea. *Pediatrics*, **13**, 133
117. Kersey, J. H., Spector, B. D. and Good, R. A. (1973). Immunodeficiency and cancer. *Adv. Cancer Res.*, **18**, 211
118. Creagan, E. T. and Fraumeni, J. F. (1973). Familial gastric cancer and immunologic abnormalities. *Cancer*, **32**, 1325
119. Forssman, O. and Herner, B. (1964). Acquired agammaglobulinaemia and malabsorption. *Acta Med. Scand.*, **176**, 779
120. Hermans, P. E. and Huizenga, K. A. (1972). Association of gastric carcinoma with idiopathic late-onset immunoglobulin deficiency. *Ann. Int. Med.*, **76**, 605
121. Haerer, A. F., Jackson, J. F. and Evers, C. G. (1969). Ataxia-telangiectasia with gastric adenocarcinoma. *JAMA*, **210**, 1884
122. Ammann, A. J. and Hong, R. (1973). Selective IgA deficiency In *Immunologic disorders in infants and children*, E. R. Stiehm and V. A. Fulginiti (eds.) p. 199. (Philadelphia: W. B. Saunders Co.)
123. Fraser, K. J. and Rankin, J. G. (1970). Selective deficiency of IgA immunoglobulins associated with carcinoma of the stomach. *Aust. Ann. Med.*, **19**, 165
124. Miller, W. V., Holland, P. V., Sugarbaker, E., Strober, W. and Waldmann, T. A. (1970). Anaphylactic reactions to IgA: A difficult transfusion problem. *Am. J. Clin. Path.*, **54**, 618

125. Berendes, H., Bridges, R. A. and Good, R. A. (1957). A fatal granulomatosis of childhood. The clinical study of a new syndrome. *Minn. Med.*, **40**, 309
126. Carson, M. J., Chadwick, D. L., Brubaker, C. A., Cleland, R. S. and Landing, B. H. (1965). Thirteen boys with progressive septic granulomatosis. *Pediatrics*, **35**, 405
127. Landing, B. H. and Shirkey, H. S. (1957). A syndrome of recurrent infection and infiltration of viscera by pigmented lipid histiocytes. *Pediatrics*, **20**, 431
128. Holmes, B., Quie, P. G., Windhorst, D. B. and Good, R. A. (1966). Fatal granulomatous disease of childhood: an inborn abnormality of phagocytic function. *Lancet*, **i**, 1225
129. Johnston, R. B. and Baehner, R. L. (1971). Chronic granulomatous disease: Correlation between pathogenesis and clinical findings. *Pediatrics*, **48**, 730
130. Ament, M. E. and Ochs, H. D. (1973). Gastrointestinal manifestations of chronic granulomatous disease. *New Engl. J. Med.*, **288**, 382
131. Groll, A., Valberg, L. S., Simon, J. B., Eidinger, D., Wilson, B. and Forsdyke, D. R. (1972). Immunological defect in Whipple's disease. *Gastroenterology*, **63**, 943
132. Martin, F. F., Vilseck, J., Dobbins, W. O., Buckley, C. E. and Tyor, M. P. (1972). Immunological alterations in patients with treated Whipple's disease. *Gastroenterology*, **63**, 6

CHAPTER 4

Enteric infection and immunization

ROBERT L. CLANCY and JOHN BIENENSTOCK

Introduction

The principles of oral immunization were recognized more than 50 years ago, when Besredka[1] described a state of immunity following oral vaccines unrelated to circulating antibody, leading him to conclude that 'the plan in artificial vaccination, therefore, is to follow the route which the virus takes in its penetration into the body'. Detection of faecal antibody prior to its appearance in the circulation following human bacillary dysentery by Davies[2] in 1922, and the correlation of resistance to experimental cholera infection of guinea pigs with coproantibody by Burrows[3] in 1950, are representative of the early studies which supported Besredka's postulates. Identification of IgA as a more specific marker of a 'secretory immunoglobulin system' by Tomasi *et al.*[4] in 1965 stimulated a renewed interest in the local immune response and provided impetus to reopen the search for local vaccines to enhance mucosal resistance. The structure and function of secretory IgA has been extensively reviewed[5–12] independently, and in the context of local immunity.

Although the central theme in oral immunization is adaptive mechanisms of mucosal resistance, it must be recognized that many non-immunologic factors contribute to mucosal resistance and that these factors may modify the response to oral antigen. Thus many pathogens (e.g. *Salmonella typhi* and *Vibrio cholerae*) are sensitive to low pH. Gastric acidity and the rate of gastric emptying determine the dose of bacteria presented to the intestine. Within the intestinal lumen a number of soluble, cellular and microbial factors contribute to 'mucosal resistance'. In the first category would be included lactoferrin[13] an iron binding protein synthesized by neutrophils but also by glandular epithelial cells, and found particularly in secretions, and lysozyme. In the second category would be found phagocytes and lymphocytes potentially coming from the intestinal wall. The third category would include the interactions between the normal microbial flora. Finally, the mucous barrier and the glycocalyx must play important, albeit poorly understood, roles in resistance to infection, through mechanical interference with absorption to enterocytes.

Many of these non-specific factors may modify local immunity. These include the activation of mucosal immune mechanisms in germ free animals by colonizing bacteria[14], cross reactivity between potential pathogens and normal gut flora[15], auxillary role of soluble or cellular factors in specific reactions, e.g. the interaction of lysozyme with complement and IgA in mediating bacterial lysis[16] and enhanced phagocytosis through opsonisation by antibody, as well as perhaps a structural 'coat' of IgA antibody binding to mucus[17].

Functional anatomy of mucosal immune apparatus

Prior to a more specific discussion of models of oral immunization, it is relevant to make some general comments on the way ingested antigen is handled by the intestinal mucosa, and how an immune response is mounted in response to this antigen. Several of the concepts outlined here will be enlarged in subsequent discussion of models of oral immunization. Kraehenbuhl *et al.*[18] have shown that gammaglobulin enters the jejunal enterocyte by pinocytosis and is then transported through the cell to the intercellular space by a process of reverse pinocytosis. The protein then moves, presumably by diffusion, down to the base of the space where it may cross the basement membrane through gaps present in this structure. This route is also taken by smaller molecules such as horseradish peroxidase[19], and appears to be anatomically the reverse of that taken in the transport and secretion of IgA[20]. The demonstration that protein (including antibody) secretion shares a common transport process with protein absorption[21], has led to the suggestion that this may be an important control mechanism of antibody secretion by antigen[12]. Some evidence exists that antigen may be found in macrophages of the intestinal lamina propria after oral feeding of protein[22]. The fate of these macrophages, as well as the ingested antigen is not known. The Peyer's patches in the gut wall present an enigma since pinocytosis can be shown to occur in the specialized lymphoepithelial cells overlying these lymphoid aggregates[23] and yet evidence of antibody synthesis in these tissues has been hard to obtain. Thus, few of the follicular cells contain immunoglobulin in their cytoplasm, but the membranes of most stain with antisera to IgA or IgM[24]. The lack of direct demonstration of phagocytosis[25], the presence of extracellular bacteria especially in the dome[26], the difficulty in evoking a primary immune response *in vivo* in the Peyer's patch[27], and the restorative function of added 'adherent' cells *in vitro*[25], suggest a lack of normal antigen handling by macrophages. This postulate is consistent with the presence of a secondary response *in vivo*[28] and detection of an *in vitro* primary response only when 2-mercaptoethanol was added[25]. Studies of cell traffic suggest that T-lymphocytes migrate to the thymic-dependent areas as well as the dome epithelium[29], while small B-lymphocytes, as well as a few thymidine labelled, presumed B-blasts[30] from the thoracic duct, migrate to the dome of the patch. B-blasts from the thoracic duct lymph as well as the mesenteric lymph nodes migrate to the intestinal lamina propria where they become IgA producing cells[31,32]. The fate of Peyer's patch lymphocytes is less clear, but their known potential to differentiate into IgA-containing plasma cells when injected into irradiated rabbits[33] as well as the clustering of IgA-containing plasma cells in the mucosa beside Peyer's patches[34], strongly suggests that these lymphocytes are destined to become mucosal plasma cells. A second exit route for Peyer's patch lymphocytes may be into the gut lumen, as suggested by scanning electronmicroscopy[35] which demonstrates sheets of lymphocytes on the luminal surface of some patches. The function of lymphocyte transport into, or out of, the gut lumen is unclear, but such traffic could provide a mechanism of sensitization to ingested antigens restricted to the lumen, as well as an important effector system. The role of Peyer's patch T-lymphocytes is less clear as they appear to have restricted T-lymphocyte functions[36]. They can co-operate with B-lymphocytes[37], and as such may provide an important control mechanism in the differentiation of IgA cell precursors.

It is possible, therefore, that absorbed antigen interacts with antigen sensitive cells in Peyer's patches and the draining mesenteric nodes, that sensitized cells leave rapidly by the efferent lymphatics, that lymphocytes with surface IgG and IgM receptors seed systemic lymphoid tissue especially the spleen, that those cells with IgA receptors home to the gut mucosa, perhaps via the Peyer's patches which provide for differentiation and amplification. The 'loop' would provide a survival advantage as oral immunization would prime the animal for both a systemic and a local response. Cross reactivity between potential pathogenic bacteria and normal flora, e.g. *Escherichia coli*, and *H. influenza*[15], would enhance the protective effect of this sytem. A negative feedback would be provided by secretion of local specific antibody, which Walker *et al.*[38] have shown to significantly reduce absorption of soluble antigens in an everted intestinal loop system in rats.

It has been extensively shown that IgA cell precursors will home to the intestinal lamina propria in the apparent absence of antigen[39]. IgA cell precursors from the Peyer's patches also home in smaller numbers to the bronchial lamina propria and it is possible, as discussed later, that there exists a common mucosal system in which cells sensitized at one mucosal site may populate another mucosa[34]. Such a system would explain the presence of high titres of IgA anti-blood group substance antibody in the colostrum and there is also experimental support recently for this explanation[40]. About 10% of the cells in the small gut epithelium have the morphology of lymphocytes, and have been called thelio-lymphocytes, by Fichtelius[41]. This cell population develops in the absence of antigen, being present in both germ free animals and in fetal gut transplanted beneath the renal capsule of syngeneic recipients[42]. In the chicken it is reduced after either thymectomy or bursectomy[43], and kinetic studies show a different turnover time compared with lymphocytes in the lamina propria[44]. The origin and fate of these lymphocytes is not clear, though 'homing' experiments using thoracic duct T 'blasts' demonstrated homing to the gastrointestinal epithelium[31,45]. Many of the epithelial lymphocytes contain granules with staining characteristics similar to those of mast cells[46]. Such cells obtained from the rabbit can be degranulated with phytohaemagglutinin with the consequent release of histamine[47]. It is possible, therefore, that the epithelium provides both a population of cells capable of reacting with antigen, and a mechanism for increasing the permeability of the mucosa which could facilitate interaction of luminal antigen with specific antibody and sensitized cells. This may be relevant to the phenomenon described by Bellamy and Nielsen[48] who showed in the systemically hyperimmunized pig that antigen placed in the intestinal lumen produces a rapid accumulation of neutrophils and their emigration into the lumen without evidence of tissue damage.

The concept of a local humoral antibody immune response has been well established at the mucous surfaces. The extension of this concept to include a local cell-mediated immune response has been made particularly by Waldmann and his colleagues in their studies of the respiratory tract of both experimental animals and man[49], by using a variety of viral agents and soluble proteins. So far, this question of a local cell mediated immune mechanism in the gut has not been addressed but must remain a possibility.

Some evidence exists for the presence of memory in the respiratory tract local secretory immune system although this question remains controversial[50]. No evidence exists, surprisingly, to support the presence of memory in the secretory immune system of the gut. This has important implications since it suggests that the continued presence of antigen may be important to maintain local immunity. The problem is further compounded by the observations that depending on the antigen, dose, and timing, tolerance may be achieved by oral immunization, as discussed later. Thus the complex nature of the local immune response and its physiology and control are at best incompletely understood.

Models of oral immunization

The common denominator of oral immunization is the way in which antigen given by mouth is handled, which in turn determines the characteristics of the local and/or the systemic immune response. To provide logical regimens of oral immunization it is necessary, therefore, to understand the way in which the mucosa handles, and responds to, oral antigen. We shall attempt to discuss oral immunization in terms of a number of models of antigen handling, stressing what is known, and not known, about the physiology of the local immune response.

Non-microbial antigen

Advantages provided by review of this model include the considerable amount of knowledge gained on the physiology of local immunity from its study, the lack of complicating pathology often seen in infectious models, and the extension of the concept of oral immunization to include tolerance under certain specified conditions.

Pattern of antigen handling: Despite a host of physical barriers intact macromolecules and even particles such as starch and bacteria, pass through the intestinal mucosa and may be found in the peripheral circulation. From the intercellular space, antigen may enter either the portal or lymphatic systems. Some proteins appear to be preferentially transported via the lymphatics, and can then be detected in the peripheral blood[51]. The fate of protein entering the portal vein in immune animals is determined by the relative proportions of antigen and antibody. Thus in antibody excess, soluble complexes are removed by the liver, while in antigen excess this clearance mechanism is less efficient[52]. The nature of the antigen may largely determine its fate following absorption. Of particular interest is the handling of certain haptens such as DNCB. This antigen is mainly confined to the intestinal wall[53] and indirect evidence (see below) suggests that it is slowly released into the portal system. Localization after oral feeding of a soluble protein such as BSA, does not appear to occur in the Peyer's patches[27] at any time after ingestion. Flagellin, however, has been shown to localize to the mucosa in non-immune animals[54], but the role of cross reacting antibody here cannot be excluded.

In summary antigens of a wide size range can be absorbed from the intestine, especially in the early postnatal period. Depending on the amount, size and chemical nature of the antigen, it may be localized to the gut, or transported to the peripheral blood via the portal or lymphatic systems. The mode of handling of antigen probably determines the characteristics of the immune response. Processing of fed antigen by cells and its interaction with antigen sensitive lymphocytes is poorly understood.

Immune response: Farr, Rothberg and Kraft[55,56] have developed a rabbit model to study the immune response to ingested protein. Bovine serum albumin (BSA) is given in the drinking water at a concentration known to result in subimmunogenic circulating levels of antigen. Antibody to BSA was detected in peripheral blood after 10 days' feeding. A log rate of increase of antibody concentration occurred during the next 2 months, and levels then remained steady for as long as antigen was ingested. It could be shown that these animals were maximally immunized and that immunochemical characteristics of circulating antibody including immunoglobulin class and the kinetics of the response closely resembled those of parenterally immunized animals. Of particular interest was that the cellular basis of the systemic immune response to oral antigen included a migration of antigen reactive cells (lymphocytes capable of stimulation by antigen) to peripheral tissues[57]. An orderly progression of appearance of antibody producing cells in mesenteric lymph node and subsequently spleen has been shown[58]. Rothberg *et al.*[57] suggested that these cells originated in the lamina propria, and were seeded to systemic tissues. However, we have been unable to detect significant numbers of antigen binding or antigen reactive cells in the lamina propria after oral immunization with 0·1 % BSA[59].

Variations in antigen, animal and conditions of immunization, modify the systemic response. Thus ferritin fed to germ free C3H mice[60], and particulate killed toxoplasma fed to rabbits[61], were followed by circulating antibody of predominantly IgA class. However, feeding of most antigens to conventionally raised animals and man, results in a systemic immune response similar to that found after parenteral injection of antigen.

The observations in the above BSA model are all over a short period of time. In normal humans, absorption of protein antigen becomes less with increasing age[62], and many adults appear to be 'non-responsive' to antigen fed over long periods, even when challenged parenterally[63]. These observations relate to practical issues in oral immunization such as the optimal age for immunization and the timing of booster doses of antigen to avoid tolerance (discussed below).

Oral administration of DNCB to guinea pigs produces systemic and local tolerance. Animals fail to react to antigen injected into the mucosa whereas following systemic sensitization a delayed-type hypersensitivity occurs in both skin and gut[64]. Following ingestion of the hapten antigen appears to be mainly bound to the small intestine[53]. A similar state of tolerance can be induced by injection of minute amounts of hapten into the portal vein[65], but bypass of the liver by portal–systemic shunt results in systemic immunity[66]. A similar experiment with sheep red cells gave analogous results[67]. Further, André and co-workers[68] have shown that tolerance after oral feeding may be critically governed by the timing of the antigen administration. By appropriate experiments they showed that either tolerance or systemic immunization could be achieved.

In summary, study of non-microbial oral immunization models suggest that local immunization without systemic 'priming' may be unusual, that local immunization involves a systemic loop with an amplification mechanism, that local antibody operates a negative feed-back through inhibiting antigen absorption, and that this system provides an optimal mechanism for handling extrinsic antigen. Secondly, a major clinical potential for oral immunization is suggested by the induction of hyporesponsiveness to certain ingested antigens. Much further study on the cellular basis of the mucosal immune response, the mechanisms of orally induced non-responsiveness, and the influence of antigen and immunizing regimens on these phenomena, is urgently needed.

VIRAL ANTIGEN

Although a given organism may be primarily localized at a mucosal site, the actual dissemination of the relevant antigens or even small numbers of the organism cannot ever be excluded. However, the effect of a local antigenic load or disease resistance as prevention of functional changes in target tissues, may be hallmarks of the efficacy of a local immune response to an organism.

Patterns of antigen handling and its relationship to the pathogenesis of disease: Local immune mechanisms may be expected to interrupt pathogenic sequences in three general models of virus infection of the gut mucosa. Firstly, virus replication may be restricted to the gut mucosa. One example of such restricted infection is transmissible gastroenteritis of swine which has considerable economic importance due to its high infectivity and mortality in suckling pigs. The virus damages the intestinal epithelium, resulting in villous atrophy and malabsorption[69].

Secondly, following an initial phase of replication in the gut mucosa, the virus may disseminate to target organs, the distribution of which determines the clinical features of disease. Human enterovirus infections with this natural history include poliovirus, and Coxsackie virus. In both the above groups, local immune mechanisms effectively prevent the mucosal phase essential to both production of disease and establishment of the carrier state.

The third model relates to persistent faecal excretion of a virus which is not maintained by an essential mucosal phase. Although poorly understood, human hepatitis would appear to behave in this way. There is no evidence for an essential phase of mucosal replication, despite the fact that both hepatitis A and B virus may be transmitted via the oral route. Hepatitis B antigen is commonly detected in many secretions, and faecal excretion of antigen may continue for months after resolution of clinical disease.

Immune response

(i) *General*

Much indirect data[70] support the postulate that the viral neutralizing ability of secretory IgA at the mucosal surface prevents colonization and subsequent disease, but the relationship to recovery from virus infection is less clear. Thus IgA-rich colostrum prevents virus colonization (reviewed below), and in the enterovirus infections due to poliovirus, echovirus, and Coxsackie virus, coproantibody is restricted to the IgA class, and its presence bears little relationship to serum titres but correlates closely with cessation of virus excretion[70]. Much more is known about IgA antibody and its correlation with resistance to further challenge by particular viruses in the respiratory tract. By analogy many conclusions can be drawn in the gut, but it is important to recognize that there are many gaps in this body of information.

Clearly other specific (e.g. cell mediated immune mechanisms) as well as non-specific (e.g. interferon) mechanisms contribute to the outcome of the virus–host relationship, but the contribution of these factors is poorly understood. Thus regardless of the mechanisms involved in resistance following oral immunization against various enterovirus infections, IgA antibody has become a marker of immunity.

(ii) *Virus restricted to gut mucosa* (as determined by the distribution of pathology)

Study of this model raises two concepts relevant to oral immunization. Firstly, despite the apparent restriction of virus to the gut mucosa (spread of small numbers of virus cannot be excluded), a significant local immune response can be detected in the secretions of extraintestinal glandular tissues, which is reflected in higher titres of IgA antibody in colostrum than is found in serum. Similar observations were made with rabbit colostral antibody following ingestion of DNP-pneumococci[40]. These observations suggest either the selective concentration of IgA antibody, the selective localization of absorbed antigen, or the 'homing' of cells activated in the gut-associated lymphoid tissues. The studies of Crabbé *et al.*[60] support the last alternative, since they demonstrated exclusively IgA secreting cells in extraintestinal sites of germ-free mice following oral immunization with ferritin. Less conclusive support is found in experiments with conventional animals although a greater proportion of IgA response occurs after oral feeding[58]. This concept is an extension of our postulate for immunization to ingested protein, discussed above, and we have suggested above that a common mucosal system may exist based on the selective population of mucosal membranes by lymphocytes destined to differentiate into IgA secreting cells. Support comes from our demonstration that lymphocytes from the aggregated lymphoid tissues of the rabbit gut (Peyer's patches) and bronchus (BALT, or bronchus associated lymphoid tissue), both tend to populate, selectively with IgA containing cells, the mucosa of the gut and bronchus of irradiated recipients[34]. The failure to detect virus antibody in secretions distal to the site of local immunization may reflect the relatively low sensitivity of the techniques used, as judged by the low antibody titres[71]. The implications of a 'mucosal system' are far reaching as it could extend the indications for oral immunization to prophylaxis of infections at any mucosal site, e.g. gonorrhoea involving the urogenital tract.

Secondly, the efficacy of passive immunization is demonstrated. Thus a high degree of passive immunity in the suckling pig correlated with the presence of IgA antibody in mammary secretions[72,73]. Colostral IgG antibody following parenteral immunization proved less effective[51]. Passive antibody is equally effective in the prevention of colonization of enterovirus species that disseminate following mucosal replication[74].

Despite this effectivity it is hard to see passive immunization playing a major role in human subjects, although maternal oral immunization may ensure good protection to breast-fed infants[75] against a number of gastrointestinal or even respiratory tract infections. It is clear that milk and colostral secretions provide much more than antibody since they are a potent source of non-specific immune substances such as lactoferrin, as well as lymphocytes and macrophages[76].

(iii) *Virus that disseminates following mucosal replication*

The best studied model of immunity to enterovirus-induced systemic disease is resistance following the oral attenuated (Sabin) or the inactivated systemic (Salk) poliovaccines. Both oral and parenteral vaccines give similar serum levels of IgM, IgG, and IgA antibody[77] and provide excellent protection against systemic disease. However antibody can only be consistently detected in nasopharyngeal and alimentary tract secretions after oral vaccination[77,78]. Inactivated vaccine taken orally stimulates only a localized, low titre, transient antibody response (circulating antibody), and a second oral dose is not associated with an anamnestic response[78]. Ingestion of live vaccine, however, stimulates synthesis of IgA polioantibody which can be detected widely in secretions and is associated with circulating antibody. Antibody can be detected in secretions for 2–3 weeks and stable titres persist for the duration of the follow-up period which is now over 5 years[77]. Other than providing the most successful example of oral vaccination in clinical practice, the poliovaccine model has been used to provide data pertinent to oral vaccination. Firstly, the aggregated lymphoid tissue associated with the oropharynx contributes significantly to the local production of antibody. Thus removal of the tonsils and adenoids is associated with a 3–4 fold reduction in local antibody titres, and this reduction is more marked in young children[79]. Secondly IgA has been shown not to be essential to resistance to enterovirus. Thus effective titres of antibody in the IgM and IgG class replaced IgA antibody in secretions of IgA deficient subjects[80] explaining their normal response to enterovirus infections. Thirdly, in some instances regional differences in mucosal resistance follow local immunization, and this correlates with a variation in the regional production of secretory antibody. Thus attenuated virus placed in the distal limb of double barrelled colostomies stimulated a good antibody response in the secretions of the distal colon, minimal antibody in the proximal colon, and no detectable response in nasopharyngeal secretions[71]. The presence of antibody correlated with resistance to colonization by attenuated poliovirus. Fourthly, the presence of antibody in alimentary secretions of subjects given oral, but not parenteral, vaccine effectively prevented establishment of a carrier state in those enterovirus infections dependent upon an initial phase of mucosal replication[78].

Finally, the observation that local resistance stimulated by inactivated poliovaccine prevented subsequent colonization by live vaccine and the stimulation of circulating antibody[80], draws attention to the critical problem of the timing and combination of vaccines in an attempt to stimulate maximum resistance. The polio model clearly demonstrates the advantage of live replicating and therefore persistent, antigen over inactivated virus, in that it stimulates a more marked, more extensive, and more persistent local resistance, as well as stimulating effective systemic immunity. Repeated local immunization with non-replicating antigen may induce a state of tolerance[68] or be associated with typical primary responses[78] depending on the antigen, time course of immunization, etc. The apparent advantage in terms of host resistance of live versus dead virus vaccines is supported by the long term immunity which follows certain natural virus infections, and live vaccines such as smallpox and yellow fever. Inherent problems of any live vaccine include fragility of antigen, the ever-present dangers of passage of adventitious agents, and the risk of mutation back to virulence of the virus. Thus variation of immunization protocol either to improve effectivity of inactivated vaccines or reduce the dangers of live vaccines, needs exploration. An approach of particular interest is the combination of local and systemic immunization, as exemplified by a study with attenuated rubella vaccines[81]. While intranasal vaccination with live RA-27 virus stimulated IgA antibody in the local secretions of most recipients, challenge with wild virus was followed by detectable virus shedding in one-third of the vaccinated group. Parenteral immunization with the HPV-77 virus was followed by little antibody in nasal secretions, but when followed by intranasal RA-27 was associated with a significant booster effect in both secretions and serum. The potential priming of the mucosal system by inactivated parenteral vaccines, followed by local immunization with replicating antigen may prove a useful approach to stimulate a high degree of persistent resistance to infection, and minimize the dangers of attenuated vaccines.

(*iv*) *Shedding of virus-?unrelated to mucosal replication*

Hepatitis A and an unknown proportion of hepatitis B virus are transmitted through the faecal–oral route, and in disease due to hepatitis B virus, antigen can commonly be detected in faeces. The asymptomatic chronic carrier of hepatitis B antigen may also excrete infectious antigen. The local immune response is characterized by IgA coproantibody which however is only detected in those excreting large quantities of antigen, and only after a delay of several months[82]. No clear termination of either the systemic carrier state or of virus excretion appeared to correlate with appearance of coproantibody. The pathogenesis of disease, the mechanisms of virus persistence, and what constitutes an appropriate host response to terminate infection in hepatitis B infection, are poorly understood. It is not clear whether mucosal replication precedes systemic spread in those cases where virus is ingested. Thus stimulation of local immunity by oral vaccination may potentially play a role in prevention of mucosal colonization by hepatitis virus, although a role in termination of carrier status is less clear. If virus replication reponsible for both disease and secretion of virus is in extraintestinal tissue as would appear likely, parenteral immunization may be the logical approach once vaccines become available. It is further evident that no explanation is available currently for the observation of the co-existence of the hepatitis B antigen in faeces with IgA antibody[82]. This may suggest either that the antigenic load locally is too great, that the excretion of viral antigen is irrelevant to the site of replication, or that the crucial resistance mechanism locally is not mediated by the IgA system.

Bacterial antigen—non-invasive bacteria

Pattern of antigen handling: Natural infection due to *Vibrio cholerae* is limited to man. Experimental infection of the rabbit[83], and dog[84] reproduces the spectrum of human disease. Organisms multiply rapidly in the lumen of the small intestine in close association with epithelial cells. The flux of isotonic fluid into the gut lumen which characterizes choleraic disease, results entirely from an enterotoxin which stimulates membrane-bound adenylate cyclase of the rapidly dividing crypt epithelial cells.

Adherence of *Vibrio cholerae* to the gut epithelium is essential to the pathogenesis of clinical disease, but neither invasion of the mucosa nor ultrastructural evidence of damage to the epithelium[85] or the basement membrane has been observed.

Escherichia coli induces human disease with clinical characteristics resembling either cholera or shigella dysentery. The pattern of disease is determined by the way in which antigen is handled, which in each case closely resembles handling of *V. cholerae* or shigella organisms respectively[86]. In turn, the pattern of handling is determined by the age of the patient, and the serotype of the *E. coli*.

Immune response: Detection of both systemic and local antibody[87] following natural infection indicates that either the techniques used to demonstrate tissue cholera antigen were insensitive (since it is not found beyond the basement membrane), or that lymphocyte–bacteria interaction occurs at the epithelial cell surface. As the spectrum of immune response following cholera resembles that of invasive or absorbed antigen[88] it is possible that sensitization to exogenous antigen may occur in the lumen or at the epithelial level.

Natural and experimental[89] cholera stimulates circulating and coproantibody which acts on the organism and/or its exotoxin at the level of the gut mucosa to determine resistance. However the source of coproantibody, the relative contribution of antibacterial (mostly IgG) and antitoxin antibody (mostly IgA)[89], and the possible contribution of other factors are all unclear[90]. Thus Burrows *et al.*[3] in 1950 showed that resistance to experimental cholera in guinea pigs is better correlated with the presence of coproantibodies than with serum levels of anticholera antibody. Also the cholera stool is a rich source of IgA[91] containing up to 1·5 g in 24 hours. A role for systemic immunity is suggested by the inverse relationship between serum antibody titres and the likelihood of developing cholera[91], and by the protection of experimental animals from disease by passive administration of hyperimmune antisera[90]. Curlin *et al.*[92] used a cross-perfusion technique between dogs immunized by either the parenteral or the oral route, and non-immune animals, to demonstrate that circulating antibody could protect the gut of non-immunized dogs from the biological effects of cholera exotoxin, and that antitoxin activity did not reside in the gut mucosa. The biologic significance of this study is not clear as locally derived antibody could have been washed from the gut lumen, and antitoxin antibody may be a poor index of natural resistance. There is good evidence that antibacterial antibody plays a major role in determining resistance to cholera following ingestion of organisms. Thus antibacterial coproantibody is found following natural cholera[88], it can be regularly detected in the gut lumen after experimental infection[88], resistance to infection correlates with circulating vibriocidal antibody[91], and resistance has been largely shown to be type specific[93] suggesting that the cell wall antigens characteristic of the two major subtypes—Unaba and Ogawa—play a major role in the production of immunity. The mechanism by which antibacterial antibody prevents disease is not clear. Complement-dependent vibriocidal antibody can be detected *in vitro*[88], but there is little complement in the gut lumen[94]. Antibody, including IgA, prevents adsorption of vibrios to the intestinal mucosa, and thus prevents the proliferation essential to the pathogenesis of cholera[94]. This latter mechanism of prevention of epithelial colonization may be a crucial functional role of IgA in resistance to many bacteria.

Although antitoxin antibody has not been demonstrated regularly following cholera[88], systemic antibody following parenteral administration of toxoid rapidly and efficiently neutralizes a challenge of cholera exotoxin in animal loop preparations, whether it be circulating or added to the bowel lumen[92].

Study of the weanling piglet model has provided much information on the pathogenesis, genetics, and immunity in the cholera-like illness caused by *E. coli*, with very similar findings to those seen in *V. cholerae* infection[86]. Oral administration of streptomycin-dependent *E. coli* to patas monkeys gave good protection, which was associated with serotype-specific coproantibody[49]. Oral immunization of human infants with desoxycholate extracts of prevalent *E. coli* strains was attempted in a field trial following demonstration of protection with this antigen in mice. Although a seroconversion rate of 40% occurred in 11 000 infants, no epidemic has yet occurred to test resistance[86].

Bacterial antigen—local invasion

Antigen handling—(shigella): Ingestion of small numbers of bacteria (10^1–10^2) is followed by rapid proliferation in the small intestine, and penetration of the epithelial cells of the large intestine with subsequent mucosal ulceration. The mechanism of necrosis is not understood, but follows bacterial multiplication and an inflammatory response within the mucosa. Systemic spread of infection is uncommon.

Immune response: Clinical dysentery is followed by long-term type-specific resistance. The importance of local factors is emphasized by the failure of parenteral immunization with killed vaccines to prevent disease[86], and the detection of coproantibody before the appearance of serum antibody[2]. The importance of a restricted local immunity to shigella toxin following ingestion of killed organisms was first recognized by Shiga in the early 1900s[95]. Despite the historic interest of this model no advance in our knowledge of the mechanism of resistance has occurred in 50 years and advances have been restricted to quantitative studies of oral vaccination in humans.

Considerable effort has been made to develop avirulent live vaccines, which include strains that survive poorly in man, e.g. streptomycin-dependent mutants[96], and interspecies hybrids[97]; strains that have lost somatic antigen, e.g. smooth–to–rough mutations; and strains with impaired penetrance of epithelial cells[98]. It should be noted that Besredka during World War I immunized hundreds of thousands of military recruits by the oral route against dysentery with documented success[99]. The most recent extensive studies in man have been those of Mel *et al.* in Yugoslavia[100,101] where about 30 000 people have been orally immunized with streptomycin-dependent strains of *Shigella flexneri*. Side effects were minimal and no reversion to virulence was detected in over 3000 stools tested. Despite similar rates of intestinal colonization with wild shigella in both immunized and control subjects, and no increase in serum antibody titre, a protection rate of 85–100% was achieved[96,100,101]. Experimental infection of humans with moderately large numbers of organisms demonstrated significant immunity with both mutant-hybrids and streptomycin-dependent attenuated vaccine[100]. Oral immunization of monkeys with a polyvalent hybrid strain shigella vaccine, prevented dysentery after challenge with virulent strains, though serum antibody but not coproantibody was detected using the sensitive technique of haemagglutination[101]. The failure of parenteral vaccination to prevent dysentery in this system emphasizes a critical role for local factors.

In summary, bacterial dysentery offers one of the most hopeful areas for effective oral vaccination in the future despite the fact that the pathogenesis and the mechanisms of adaptive resistance are so poorly understood.

Bacterial antigen—systemic invasion

Antigen handling and its relationship to the pathogenesis of disease: Typhoid fever is representative of a group of systemic disorders termed the 'enteric fevers'. *Salmonella typhi* is naturally pathogenic only for man. Animals are susceptible to certain serotypes of *Salmonella*, and those with systemic disease resembling human typhoid fever such as *S. typhimurium* and *S. enteritidis* of rodents, have been extensively studied as models of human disease. Irrespective of the route of infection the prerequisites of disease are local multiplication, bacteraemia, hepatosplenic multiplication, followed by a secondary bacteraemia with subsequent localization and multiplication of bacteria in target tissues, especially within the gastrointestinal tract. Characteristics of infection include localization and multiplication within macrophages[102], associated with histiocytic proliferation, and depletion of lymphocytes from lymphoid tissue following an initial inflammatory response in these tissues[103]. Of relevance to oral immunization is the way *Salmonella* organisms are handled at the mucosal level. Carter *et al.*[104] have recently performed careful quantitative studies to follow the early distribution of an intragastric inoculum of virulent *S. enteritidis* in normal mouse intestine. Data on the primary site of *Salmonella* infection had been conflicting, with Schlewinski *et al.*[105] demonstrating a very early systemic infection of mice following ingestion of large doses of *S. typhimurium*, suggesting rapid absorption from high in the intestine, which in turn supported previous observations made in man[106]. Others, however, concluded that the primary site of *Salmonella* infection was the small and large intestine, prior to dissemination[107,108]. The study of Carter *et al.*[104] demonstrated by dye injection that lymphatic vessels drain areas of small intestine to regional Peyer's patches which in turn link with mesenteric lymph nodes, and that although more than 99% of organisms were eliminated from the gut within hours, lethal systemic infection still occurred. In this study, no 'early' bacteraemia could be detected. The primary site of bacterial penetration involved the distal ileum and bacteria rapidly passed to the local Peyer's patches where they divided and subsequently passed to draining lymph nodes, ultimately to reach the spleen and liver. Although bacterial proliferation and inflammatory changes occur in the mucosa in germ free animals[109] it is less clear that similar bacterial growth occurs in the ileum of conventional animals.

Immune response: Most studies of immunity to *Salmonella* have involved laboratory animals under a variety of non-physiological conditions. Protection of mice from an oral challenge with *Salmonella* organisms has been demonstrated for *S. enteritidis*, with a live vaccine using temperature sensitive mutants[110], and for *S. typhimurium*, using repeated high doses (10^{10} organisms) of a killed vaccine[111]. In the latter study similar systemic resistance was demonstrated following systemic vaccination, but a reduction of positive faecal cultures only occurred after oral vaccination. The immune status of man following either natural infection or immunization is less clear. Thus a constant proportion of an exposed population (second infections in World War II or experimental infection) tends to become ill regardless of whether they have had typhoid fever[112]. These figures can however be interpreted as reflecting some immunity. Killed vaccines do seem to reduce mortality by delaying the establishment of bacteria in target organs[112], and recent extensive field trials of attenuated oral vaccines do seem to indicate reduction of the incidence of disease in endemic areas[112]. Protection correlates only slightly with the levels of antibody (especially 'H'). though relapses are not uncommon in patients with high antibody titres[113] and no correlation was demonstrated in volunteers between resistance and antibody titre. Field trials with oral vaccination against typhoid fever are conflicting. Hornick *et al.*[112] presented an encouraging preliminary report of a field trial with multiple doses of orally administered live streptomycin-dependent *S. typhi* vaccine. The protective effect of this vaccine appeared superior to either an oral killed vaccine, or the commercial parenteral vaccine as judged by both incidence of disease and the number of positive stools. A second trial almost identical to the first failed to confirm these observations[86]. Vaccines have also been developed against 'core' antigens of several groups of enterobacteria[114] and have been shown to protect animals against cross reacting species, as well as against ribosomal extracts of salmonellae[115] which also have been effective in animal models.

It is clear that much is unknown about the immunity and pathogenesis of the enteric fevers. Activated macrophages and cell mediated immunity may play an important role. Local immune mechanisms could play an important part in interrupting the pathogenic sequence by limiting infection to the mucosa and in eradicating the carrier state. Preliminary field trials of live oral vaccination indirectly support this concept[112].

The 'normal bacterial flora'—its relevance to oral immunization

The juxtaposition of a normal gut flora and a local immune apparatus is an apparent paradox, the resolution of which is important both to the concept of oral immunization and its implementation. Several factors affect the host bacteria relationship at a mucosal surface. Firstly, the bactericidal mechanisms characteristic of systemic immunity require both ancillary factors (complement and phagocytes) and appropriate antibody, the former of which are limited in mucosal secretions[94]. Secondly, non-immunological factors promote a highly efficient removal of bacteria from mucous membranes. Of particular importance in the gut is the 'flush' mechanism provided by peristaltic contraction, and the continual desquamation of the cellular substrate for bacterial attachment. The available data suggest that local immunity promotes resistance to bacterial infection by augmenting this 'removal' mechanism. Freter's group has made several key observations[94,116,117]. Firstly it was observed that the number of live vibrios within the gut lumen was increased in immunized animals compared with non-immune controls, with the reverse pertaining to the mucosal lining. Subsequent studies confirm that antibody hinders the attachment of bacteria to epithelial cells, which is essential to colonization of the mucosa[118]. Secondly, it was shown that antibody in the presence of a viable mucosal surface inhibited the growth rate of attached bacteria[117]. Thirdly, the cholera model was used to demonstrate in germ-free mice that in this situation the vibrio grew rapidly to simulate 'normal' flora without a pathogenic effect[119], and that previous oral or systemic immunization had little effect on the caecal organism count. If however the germ-free host was given mixtures of facultative anaerobes or aerobes to simulate normal flora, a much slower growth rate was noted due to bacterial 'antagonism', but the effect of previous immunization in reducing the vibrio count was significantly greater. Another synergistic effect of a normal flora on local immune mechanisms is the protection of IgG and IgM from digestion by reducing enzyme concentration[88], but secretory IgA is clearly more resistant to proteolysis than these classes of antibody[5].

We have already referred to the possibility that the amount of antibody being secreted, by sharing a common metabolic pathway in the epithelial cell with antigen pinocytosis, may limit the antigen load taken up by the enterocyte[12]. Antibody also prevents proliferation, and may further interfere with uptake by enterocytes as well as prevent epithelial colonization. The amount, nature and persistence of antigen in the lumen of the gut may also control the amount of antibody provided through a feedback mechanism involved in the oral tolerance system, as yet very incompletely understood.

Normal intestinal flora provide systemic blood group isoagglutinins as was so elegantly shown by feeding experiments in man by Springer[120]. Robbins[121] has shown that oral feeding of bacteria cross-reacting with pneumococci will prevent morbidity and mortality of rabbits subsequently challenged with otherwise lethal doses of organisms. Coupled with the concept of a common mucosal circulation of cells, this could prove to be an immunization approach of the future.

Clearly a local immune response plays an important role in determining the normal bacterial flora, and can be thought of as providing a constant immunologic selection pressure. Thus secretions contain low levels of antibody against indigenous bacteria[122], bacteria obtained from secretions are coated with antibody[123], and the predominant 'normal' species may be analogous to the vibrio in monoassociated mice[124]. Miller *et al.*[125] used monoinfected germ-free mice with a specific *V. cholerae* serotype to demonstrate that in non-immune animals, mutants replace the initial serotype after 2 weeks, and that this switch was accelerated in immunized animals. Similarly, *E. coli* serotypes of gut flora change with time[126].

What determines bacterial virulence is poorly understood, but differential growth rates or nutritional requirements do not appear to account for pathogenicity. It is more reasonable to consider the pathogen as representing a novel serotype with a temporary selective advantage[118]. Here small numbers of bacteria would rapidly increase and would stimulate an exaggerated immune response which would cause selective elimination and immunity. Antibody to K88 or 'attachment antigen' of *E. coli* pathogenic to pigs, prevents infection[86] emphasizing the importance of the attachment to the mucosal substrate for colonization to occur. If for some reason colonization was a slower process, the reduced immune response may lead to a different balance characteristic of the 'carrier state' which may persist for weeks or months before elimination or seroconversion.

Brief consideration of the normal flora of the oral cavity illustrates physiology, pathology, and potential for manipulation by oral immunization. Thus regional colonization of the oral cavity is determined by the capacity of different bacterial species to adhere to various oral substrates[118], as organisms divide slowly and would otherwise be removed. The presence of antibody against resident bacteria in local secretions[122], the coating of these bacteria with antibody[123] and the low numbers of bacteria attached to epithelial cells scraped from the oral mucosa compared with the high numbers found using antibody-free bacteria and washed cells[123], reflect the operation of local antibody in controlling colonization of the oral cavity.

One normal inhabitant of the oral cavity, *Streptococcus mutans* is cariogenic[127]. This process requires attachment to teeth which is mediated by dextran polymers synthesized by bacterial enzyme from sucrose[128]. Bacterial accumulation leads to plaque formation which is associated with caries[127]. Maximal stimulation of local antibody against *S. mutans* in both conventional and germ-free rats has significantly reduced bacterial colonization, plaque formation, and caries[129]. This exciting observation indicates the potential of oral immunization for modifying the resident bacterial flora once the physiology is better understood.

Intestinal parasites

Introduction: Many parasites have an intestinal phase essential either to the pathogenesis in the host, or the spread of infestation. Thus stimulation of local resistance through oral immunization would appear a logical level to interrupt the intricate life cycle of these organisms. The capacity of many parasites to persist within the host for months or years indicates that a complex but delicate balance of factors related to reduced immunogenicity, suppression of the host response, or evasion of efferent immune mechanisms allows parasite persistence. The best studied model of parasitic disease is that of the rat nematode, *Nippostrongylus braziliensis*[130] which will be discussed here to illustrate adaptive mechanisms of expulsion and adaptation, the understanding of which is basic to development of successful immunization.

Pattern of antigen handling and its relationship to the pathogenesis of disease: The life cycle of *N. braziliensis* in its definitive host closely resembles that of most nematodes. The third larval stage enters the skin, migrates through the lungs, ascends the bronchial tree and passes into the intestine within 48 hours of entering the host, where it matures into an adult worm. Eggs are passed from day 6 for 6–10 days when 'self-cure' occurs in the form of rapid worm expulsion[131]. The antigenic determinants necessary for an effective immune response have not been settled, but seem to be largely secretion products of the terminal larval form and the adult worm, rather than structural antigens of the worm itself.

Immune response to antigen: The immune response to *N. braziliensis* antigen can best be examined in terms of its sequelae following a secondary infestation. Two patterns are recognized: The first follows a single inoculation and is characterized by (i) less larval forms reaching the gut, (ii) reduced fecunditity of mature worms, and (iii) an accelerated rejection of mature worms. The second pattern follows repeated administration with small doses of worms giving rise to a large stable 'adapted' intestinal worm population[130].

(i) Mechanisms related to worm elimination

The rapid and complete elimination of *N. Braziliensis* from the small intestine of the rat invokes two steps: (1) antibody action followed by (2) cellular action[130,131].

The immunological hallmark of parasitic infection is the production of IgE antibodies and an infiltrate of eosinophils and amine-containing cells (mast cells and basophils) at the site of infection[132]. Many helminths not only stimulate IgE antibodies against their own antigens, but non-specifically potentiate the IgE response to unrelated antigens[133]. IgE-secreting plasma cells are concentrated in mucous membranes[134] and are ideally placed to contribute to mucosal resistance. Granular lymphocytes (discussed above) may provide a pool of amine-containing cells essential for the expression of IgE at the mucosal surface. The IgE system is closely linked to T-lymphocytes as the latter appear to act as a control mechanism in the induction of an IgE antibody response[135], basophils share a membrane marker with T-lymphocytes[136], and are degranulated with mitogens specific for these cells[47]. Blood and tissue eosinophilia, markers of IgE-mediated reactions, may be linked to a similar control mechanism, as mobilization of the eosinophil from the bone marrow is also T-lymphocyte dependent[137]. One possible mechanism of mucosal resistance mediated by IgE is pathotopic potentiation. This phenomenon, originally described by Fazekas de. St

Groth[138], describes the influx of serum-borne immunity to a non-specifically stimulated site.

In nematode infections, the appearance of homocytotropic antibody postdates antibody-induced worm damage, but precedes worm expulsion[130]. The rapid accumulation of mast cells in the intestinal mucosa correlates closely with worm elimination[132]. Thus activation of the IgE-amine containing cell system correlates closely with the lymphocyte-dependent second phase of worm elimination. Thymectomy plus anti-lymphocyte serum prevents worm expulsion, which can be corrected by transfer of lymphocytes obtained from the mesenteric lymph node of immune animals[139]. T-lymphocytes could thus facilitate recruitment of one or other component of the IgE system, or the transfer of T-lymphocytes into the gut lumen could follow permeability changes induced by amines released from mast cells. Further study of the cellular component of the rejection mechanism in immature rats, showed that bone-marrow derived cells are also required[130]. The nature of this cell, and the mechanism of its action, remain to be demonstrated.

(*ii*) *Mechanism of worm adaptation*

Adaptation appears to involve both host and parasite. Thus the adapted worm is less immunogenic, less susceptible to the cellular component of the rejection process and has a reduced capacity to produce eggs[140]. Studies of mice with an adapted worm population indicate that the host has an impaired capacity to expel an unrelated nematode[130]. Finally certain parasites appear to 'block' rejection by incorporating host protein into their surface layers[141].

Worm adaptation provides a major difficulty in the development of oral vaccines in man. Other problems include antigen preparations. Most protective helmith antigens are secreted, and contained in low concentration in worm extracts. Effective vaccines, e.g. against dog hookworm, are prepared by irradiating the infective larvae to abort development to sexually mature forms. The strong heterologous immunity associated with this nematode has been exploited to obtain protective immunity in other systems. The problem in man, however, remains identification of protective immune mechanisms, clarification of the way by which helminths 'evade' immune destruction, and identification of stages of the life cycle in which immunity may be most effective.

ACKNOWLEDGEMENTS

Supported by the Ontario Department of Health and the Medical Research Council of Canada.

REFERENCES

1. Besredka, A. (1927). *Local immunization*, p. 181 (Baltimore: Williams and Wilkins)
2. Davies, A. (1922). Serological properties of dysentery stools. *Lancet*, **ii**, 1009
3. Burrows, W., Deupree, N. G. and Moore, D. E. (1950). The effect of X-irradiation on fecal and urinary antibody response. *J. Infect. Dis.*, **87**, 169
4. Tomasi, T. B., Tan, E. M., Solomon, A. and Prendergast, R. A. (1965). Characteristics of an immune system common to certain external secretions. *J. Exp. Med.*, **121**, 101
5. Tomasi, T. B. and Bienenstock, J. (1968), Secretory immunoglobulins. In *Advances in Immunology*, **9**, 1. Dixon and Kunkel (eds.) (New York: Academic Press Inc.)
6. Heremans, J. F. (1968). Immunoglobulin formation and function in different tissues. *Curr. Top. Microbiol. Immunol.*, **45**, 131
7. Tomasi, T. B. and Grey, H. M. (1972). Structure and function of Immunoglobulin A. *Progr. Allergy*, **16**, 81
8. The secretory and immunologic system (1970). D. Dayton, P. A. Small, R. M. Chanock, H. E. Kaufman and T. B. Tomasi (eds.) (US Dept. Health, Education, and Welfare)
9. Brandtzaeg, P. (1973). Structure synthesis and external transfer of mucosal immunoglobulins. *Ann. Immunol.* (*Inst. Pasteur*), **124C**, 417
10. Shearman, D. J. C., Parkin, D. M. and McClelland, D. B. L. (1972). The demonstration and function of antibodies in the gastrointestinal tract. *Gut*, **13**, 483
11. Heremans, J. F. and Vaerman, J-P. (1971). Biological significance of IgA antibodies in serum and secretions. In *Progress in Immunology*, B. Amos (ed.) p. 875 (New York: Academic Press)
12. Bienenstock, J. (1976). The physiology of the local immune response and the gastrointestinal tract. (England: Churchill, Livingstone) In press
13. Masson, P. L., Heremans, J. F. and Schonne, H. (1969). Lactoferrin, an iron-binding protein in neutrophilic leukocytes. *J. Exp. Med.*, **130**, 643
14. Crabbé, P. A., Bazin, H., Eyssen, H. and Heremans, J. F. (1968). The normal microbial flora as a major stimulus for proliferation of plasma cells synthesising IgA in the gut. *Int. Arch. Allergy*, **34**, 362
15. Robbins, J. B., Parke, J. C., Schneerson, R. and Whisnant, J. K. (1973). Quantitative measurement of 'natural' and immunization-induced

Haemophilus influenza type b capsular polysaccharide antibodies. *Pediatr. Res.*,**7**, 103
16. Adinolfi, M., Glynn, A. A., Lindsay, M. and Milne, C. M. (1966). Serological properties of IgA antibodies to *E. coli* present in human colostrum. *Immunology* (*Lond.*), **10**, 517
17. Heremans, J. F. (1975). In *The immune system and infectious diseases.* (Basel: Karger) In press
18. Kraehenbuhl, J. P. and Campiche, M. A. (1969). Early stages of intestinal absorption of specific antibodies in the newborn. *J. Cell. Biol.*, **42**, 345
19. Warshaw, A. L., Walker, A., Cornell, R. and Isselbacher, K. J. (1971). Small intestinal permeability to macromolecules. Transmission of horseradish peroxidase into mesenteric lymph and portal blood. *Lab. Invest.*, **25**, 675
20. Tourville, D. R., Adler, R. H., Bienenstock, J. and Tomasi, T. B. (1969). The human secretory immunoglobulin system. Immunohistological localization of A, secretory 'piece.' and lactoferrin in normal human tissues. *J. Exp. Med.*, **129**, 411
21. Kagnoff, M. F., Serfilippi, D. and Donaldson, R. M. (1973). *In vitro* kinetics of intestinal secretory IgA secretion. *J. Immunol.*, **110**, 297
22. Dolezel, J. and Bienenstock, J. (1971). Immune response of the hamster to oral and parenteral immunization. *Cell. Immunol.*, **2**, 326
23. Bockman, D. E. and Cooper, M. D. (1973). Pinocytosis by epithelium associated with lymphoid follicles in the bursa of Fabricius, appendix and Peyer's patches. An electron microscopic study. *Am. J. Anat.*, **136**, 455
24. Rudzik, O., Clancy, R. L., Perey, D. Y. E., Bienenstock, J. and Singal, D. P. (1975). The distribution of a rabbit thymic antigen and membrane immunoglobulins in lymphoid tissue, with special reference to mucosal lymphocytes. *J. Immunol.*, **114**, 1
25. Kagnoff, M. F. and Campbell, S. (1974). Functional characteristics of Peyer's patch lymphoid cells. 1. Induction of humoral antibody and cell mediated allograft reactions. *J. Exp. Med.*, **139**, 398
26. Masson, P. and Regaud, C. (1918). Sur l'existence de nombreux microbes vivant à l'état normal dans le tissu des follicules lymphoides de l'intestin, chez le lapin. *C. R. Soc. Biol.*, **81**, 1256
27. Bienenstock ,J. and Dolezel, J. (1971). Peyer's patches: Lack of specific antibody-containing cells after oral and parenteral immunization. *J. Immunol.*, **106**, 938
28. Veldkamp, J., Van der Gaag, R. and Willers, J. M. N. (1973). The role of Peyer's patch cells in antibody formation. *Immunology*, **25**, 761
29. Waksman, B. H. (1973). The homing pattern of thymus-derived lymphocytes in calf and neonatal mouse Peyer's patches. *J. Immunol.*, **111**, 878
30. Howard, J. C., Hunt, S. V. and Gowans, J. L. (1972). Identification of marrow-derived and thymus-derived small lymphocytes in the lymphoid tissue and thoracic duct lymph of normal rats. *J. Exp. Med.*, **135**, 200

31. Guy-Grand, D., Griscelli, C. and Vassalli, P. (1974). The gut-associated lymphoid system: nature and properties of the large dividing cells. *Eur. J. Immunol.*, **4**, 435
32. Moore, A. R. and Hall, J. G. (1972). Evidence for a primary association between immunoblasts and small gut. *Nature* (*Lond*,), **239**, 161
33. Craig, S. W. and Cebra, J. J. (1971). Peyer's patches an enriched source of precursors for IgA-producing immunocytes in the rabbit. *J. Exp. Med.*, **134**, 188
34. Rudzik, O., Clancy, R. L., Perey, D. Y. E., Day, R. and Bienenstock, J. (1975). Repopulation with IgA containing cells of bronchial and intestinal lamina propria after transfer of homologous Peyer's patches and bronchial lymphocytes. *J. Immunol.*, **114**, 1599
35. Johnston, N. and Bienenstock, J. (1976). In preparation
36. Perey, D. Y. E. and Guttman, R. D. (1972). Peyer's patch cells: Absence of graft-versus–host reactivity in mice and rats. *Lab. Invest.*, **27**, 427
37. Katz, D. H. and Perey, D. Y. E. (1973). Lymphocytes in Peyer's patches: Analysis of the constituent cells in terms of their capacities to mediate functions of mature T and B lymphocytes. *J. Immunol.*, **111**, 1507
38. Walker, W. A., Isselbacher, K. J. and Bloch, K. J. (1973). Intestinal uptake of macromolecules. II. Effect of parenteral immunization. *J. Immunol.*, **111**, 221
39. Halstead, T. E. and Hall, J. G. (1972). The homing of lymph-borne immunoblasts to the small gut of neonatal rats. *Transplantation*, **14**, 339
40. Montgomery, P. C., Rosner, B. R. and Cohn, J. (1974). The secretory antibody response. Anti-DNP antibodies induced by dinitrophenylated type III pneumococcus. *Immunol. Comm.*, **3**, 143
41. Fichtelius, K. E. (1968). The gut epithelium—a first level lymphoid organ? *Exp. Cell. Res.*, **49**, 87
42. Ferguson, A. and Parrott, D. M. V. (1972). The effect of antigen deprivation on thymus-dependent and thymus-independent lymphocytes in the small intestine of the mouse. *Clin. Exp. Immunol.*, **12**, 477
43. Bäck, O. (1970). Studies on the lymphocytes in the intestinal epithelium of the chicken. IV. Effect of bursectomy. *Int. Arch. Allergy Appl. Immunol.*, **39**, 342
44. Darlington, D. and Rogers, A. W. (1966). Epithelial lymphocytes in the small intestine of the mouse. *J. Anat.*, **100**, 813
45. Sprent, J. and Miller, J. F. A. P. (1972). Interaction of thymus lymphocytes with histoincompatible cells. II. Recirculating lymphocytes derived from antigen-activated thymus cells. *Cell. Immunol.*, **3**, 385
46. Collan, Y. (1972). Characteristics of non-epithelial cells in the epithelium of normal rat ileum. *Scand. J. Gastroenterol.*, **7** (**Suppl. 18**), 1
47. Day, R. P. and Bienenstock, J. (1976). In preparation
48. Bellamy, J. E. C. and Nielson, N. O. (1974). Immune mediated emigration of neutrophils into the lumen of the small intestine. *Infect. Immun.*, **9**, 615

49. Waldman, R. H. and Ganguly, R. (1974). Immunity to infections on secretory surfaces. *J. Infect. Dis.*, **130**, 419
50. Nash, D. R. and Holle, B. (1973). Local and systemic cellular immune responses in guinea pigs given antigen parenterally or directly into the lower respiratory tract. *Clin. Exp. Immunol.*, **13**, 573
51. Alexander, H. L., Shirley, K. and Allen, D. (1936). The route of ingested egg white to the systemic circulation. *J. Clin. Invest.*, **15**, 163
52. Thomas, H. C. and Vaez-Zadeh, F. (1974). A homeostatic mechanism for the removal of antigen from the portal circulation. *Immunology*, **26**, 375
53. Silverman, A. S. and Pomeranz, J. R. (1972). Studies on the localisation of hapten in guinea pigs fed picryl chloride. *Int. Arch. Allergy*, **42**, 1
54. Hunter, R. L. (1972). Antigen trapping in the lamina propria and production of IgA antibody. *J. Reticuloendo, Soc.*, **11**, 245
55. Farr, R. S., Dickinson, W. and Smith, K. (1960). Quantitative aspects of oral immunisation against bovine serum albumin. *Fed. Proc.*, **19**, 199
56. Rothberg, R. M., Kraft, S. C., Farr, R. S., Kriebel, G. W. and Goldberg, S. S. (1971). Local immunologic responses to ingested protein. In *The secretory immunologic system.* D. H. Dayton, P. A. Small, R. M. Chanock, H. E. Kaufman and T. B. Tomasi (eds.) p. 293 (Washington D.C.: U.S. Govt. Printing Office)
57. Rothberg, R. M., Kraft, S. C. and Michalek, S. M. (1973). Systemic immunity after local antigenic stimulation of the lymphoid tissue of the gastrointestinal tract. *J. Immunol.*, **111**, 1906
58. Dolezel, J. and Bienenstock, J. (1971). γ A and non γ A immune response after oral and parenteral immunization of the hamster. *Cell. Immunol.*, **2**, 458
59. Clancy, R. L. and Bienenstock, J. (1975). Unpublished observations
60. Crabbé, P. A., Nash, D. R., Bazin, H., Eyssen, H. and Heremans, J. F. (1969). Antibodies of the IgA type in intestinal plasma cells of germ-free mice after oral or parenteral immunization with ferritin. *J. Exp. Med.*, **130**, 723
61. Strannegard, O. (1967). The formation of toxoplasma antibodies in rabbits. *Acta Pathol. Microbiol. Scand.*, **71**, 439
62. Rothberg, R. M. and Farr, R. S. (1965). Anti-bovine serum albumin and anti-alpha lactalbumin in the serum of children and adults. *Pediatrics*, **35**, 571
63. Korenblat, P. E., Rothberg, R. M., Minden, P. and Farr, R. S. (1968). Immune responses of human adults after oral and parenteral exposure to bovine serum albumin. *J. Allergy*, **41**, 226
64. Strauss, H. and Bienenstock, J. (1975). Unpublished observations
65. Battisto, J. R. and Miller, J. (1962). Immunological unresponsiveness produced in adult guinea pigs by parenteral introduction of minute quantities of hapten or protein antigen. *Proc. Soc. Exp. Biol. Med.*, **111**, 111
66. Cantor, H. M. and Dumont, A. E. (1967). Hepatic suppression of

sensitization to antigen absorbed into the portal system. *Nature* (*Lond.*), **215**, 744

67. Triger, D. R., Cynamon, M. H. and Wright, R. (1973). Studies on heptic uptake of antigen. I. Comparison of inferior vena cava and portal vein routes of immunization. *Immunology*, **25**, 941
68. André, C., Bazin, H. and Heremans, J. F. (1973). Influence of repeated administration of antigen by the oral route on specific antibody-producing cells in the mouse spleen. *Digestion*, **9**, 166
69. Haelterman, E. O. and Hooper, B. E. (1967). Transmissible gastroenteritis of swine as a model for the study of enteric disease. *Gastroenterology*, **53**, 109
70. Ogra, P. L. (1971). The secretory immunoglobulin system of the gastrointestinal tract. In *The Secretory Immunologic System*. P. A. Small, D. H. Dayton, R. M. Channock, H. E. Kaufman and T. B. Tomasi (eds.) p. 259 (US Dept. of Health, Education, and Welfare)
71. Ogra, P. L. and Karzon, D. T. (1969). Distribution of poliovirus antibody in serum, nasopharynx, and alimentary tract following segmental immunisation of lower alimentary tract with poliovaccine. *J. Immunol.*, **102**, 1423
72. Saif, L. J., Bohl, E. H. and Gupta, R. K. (1972). Isolation of porcine immunoglobulins and determination of the immunoglobulin classes of transmissible gastroenteritis viral antibodies. *Infect. Immunity*, **6**, 600
73. Bohl, E. H., Gupta, R. K., Olquin, M. V. and Saif, L. J. (1972). Antibody responses in serum, colostrum, and milk of swine after infection or vaccination with transmissible gastroenteritis virus. *Infect. Immunity*, **6**, 289
74. Katz, M. and Plotkin, S. A. (1968). Oral polio immunisation of the newborn infant; a possible method for overcoming the interference by ingested antibodies. *J. Pediat.*, **73**, 267
75. Brown, E. H. and Bailey, E. H. (1957). Infantile gastroenteritis; Changing needs in treatment. *Lancet*, **ii**, 1218
76. Beer, A. E., Billingham, R. E. and Head, J. (1974). The immunologic significance of the mammary gland. *J. Invest. Derm.*, **63**, 65
77. Ogra, P. L., Karzon, D. T., Righthand, F. and MacGillivray, M. (1968). Immunoglobulin response in serum and secretions after immunisation with live and inactivated poliovaccine and natural infection. *New Eng. J. Med.*, **279**, 893
78. Ogra, P. L. and Karzon, D. T. (1969). Polio virus antibody response in serum and nasal secretions following intranasal inoculation with inactivated poliovaccine. *J. Immunol.*, **102**, 15
79. Ogra, P. L. (1971). Effect of tonsillectomy and adenoidectomy on nasopharyngeal antibody response to poliovirus. *New Eng. J. Med.*, **284**, 59
80. Ogra, P. L. and MacGillivray, M. H. (1972). Serum and secretory antibody response to viral infections in immunoglobulin deficiency syndromes. *Ped. Res.*, **6**, 379

81. Ogra, P. L., Wallace, R. B., Umana, G., Ogra, S. S., Kerr Grant, D. and Morag, A. (1974). Implications of secretory immune system in viral infections. In *The immunoglobulin A system. Adv. Exp. Med. Biol.*, **45**, 271
82. Ogra, P. L. (1973). Immunologic aspects of hepatitis-associated antigen and antibody in human body fluids. *J. Immunol.*, **110**, 1197
83. De, S. N. and Chatterje, D. N. (1953). An experimental study of the mechanism of action of *Vibrio cholerae* on the intestinal mucous membrane. *J. Path. Bact.*, **66**, 559
84. Sack, R. B. and Carpenter, C. C. J. (1969). Experimental canine cholera. II. Production by cell-free culture filtrates of *Vibrio cholerae*. *J. Infect. Dis.*, **119**, 150.
85. Elliott, H. L., Carpenter, C. C. J., Sack, R. B. and Yardley, J. H. (1970). Small bowel morphology in experimental canine cholera. A light and electron microscopic study. *J. Lab. Invest.*, **22**, 112
86. Oral Enteric Bacterial Vaccines. (1972). *Wld. Hlth. Org. techn. Rep. Ser.*, **No. 500**, 19
87. Freter, R., De, S. P., Mondal, A., Shrivastava, D. L. and Sunderman, F. W. (1965). Coproantibody and serum antibody in cholera patients. *J. Infect. Dis.*, **115**, 83
88. Fubara, E. S. and Freter, R. (1972). Availability of locally synthesized and systemic antibodies in the intestine. *Infect. Immunity*, **6**, 965
89. Kaur, J., McGhee, J. R. and Burrows, W. (1972). Immunity to cholera: the occurrence and nature of antibody-activity immunoglobulins in the lower ileum of the rabbit. *J. Immunol.*, **108**, 387
90. Carpenter, C. C. and Pierce, N. F. (1969). Possible role of secretory antibodies in cholera; in Kaufman secretory immunologic system. In *Vero Beach Proc.* p. 281 (Washington: US Govern. Print. Office) 1971
91. Mosley, W. H. (1969). The role of immunity in cholera. A review of epidemiological and serological studies. *Texas Rep. Biol. Med.*, **27**, 227
92. Curlin, G. T. and Carpenter, C. C. J. (1970). Antitoxic immunity to cholera in isolated perfused canine ileal segments. *J. Infect. Dis.*, **1215**, 132
93. Neoh, S. H. and Rowley, D. (1972). Quoted in: *Oral Enteric Bacterial Vaccines. Wld. Hlth. Org. techn. Rep. Ser.*, **No. 500**, 19
94. Freter, R. (1969). Studies of the mechanism of action of intestinal antibody in experimental cholera. *Texas Rep. Biol. Med.*, **27**, 299
95. Tomasi, T. B. (1969). Quoted in: *The concept of local immunity and the secretory system.* In *The secretory immunologic system.* (US Dept. of Health, Education and Welfare)
96. Mel, D. M., Papo, R. G., Terzin, A. L. and Vuksic, L. (1965). Studies on vaccination against bacillary dysentery. 2. Safety tests and reactogenicity studies on a live dysentery vaccine intended for use in field trials. *Bull. Wld. Hlth. Org.*, **32**, 637
97. Formal, S. B., LaBrec, E. H., Kent, T. H. and Falkow, S. (1965). Abortive intestinal infection with an *Escherichia coli–Shigella flexneri* hybrid strain. *J. Bact.*, **89**, 1374

98. Schneider, H. and Formal, S. B. (1963). Spontaneous loss of guinea pig virulence in a strain of *Shigella flexneri* 2a. *Bact. Proc.*, **63**, 66
99. Besredka, A. (1927). *Local immunization.* (Baltimore: Williams and Wilkins)
100. Mel, D. M., Arsic, B. L., Nikolic, B. D. and Radovanic, M. L. (1968). Studies on vaccination against baccillary dysentery. 4. Oral immunization with live monotypic and combined vaccines. *Bull. Wld. Hlth. Org.*, **39**, 375
101. Mel, D. M., Gangarosa, E. J., Arsic, B. L., Radovanic, M. L. and Litvinjenko, S. (1971). Effectiveness of oral live attenuated *Shigella* vaccines. In *Proc. of the Symposium on Bacterial Vaccines* (Zagreb)
102. Blanden, R. V., Mackaness, G. B. and Collins, F. M. (1966). Mechanisms of acquired resistance in mouse typhoid. *J. Exp. Med.*, **124**, 585
103. Stuart, A. E. and Collee, J. G. (1967). Selective lymphoid deletion and generalised lymphoid depletion in mouse typhoid. *J. Path. Bact.*, **94**, 429
104. Carter, P. B. and Collins, F. M. (1974). The route of enteric infection in normal mice. *J. Exp. Med.*, **139**, 1189
105. Schlewinski, E. W. Graben, N., Funk, J. *et al.* (1971). Orale Immunisierung mit Nichtvermehrungsfahigen Mikroorganismen oder ihren Antigenen. 13. Persorption und Sekretion von Microorganismen im Tierversuch. *Zentralbl. Bakteriol.*, **218**, 93
106. Sprinz, H. E., Gangarosa, E., Williams, M., Hornick, R. B. and Woodward, T. E. (1966). Histopathology of the upper small intestines in typhoid fever. *Am. J. Dig. Dis.*, **11**, 615
107. Ozawa, A., Goto, J., Ito, T. and Shibata, H. (1973). Histopathological and biochemical responses of germ free and conventional mice with *Salmonella* infection. In *Germ free research, Biological Effect of Gnotobiotic Environments.* J. B. Heneghan (ed.), (New York: Academic Press Inc.)
108. Collins, F. M. (1970). Immunity to enteric infection in mice. *Infect. Immunol.*, **1**, 243
109. Ruitenberg, E. J., Guinee, P. A. M., Kruyt, B. C. and Berkvens, J. M. (1971). *Salmonella* pathogenesis in germ free mice. *Br. J. Exp. Pathol.*, **52**, 192
110. Fahey, K. J. and Cooper, G. N. (1970). Oral immunisation in experimental salmonellosis. *Infect. Immunity*, **2**, 183
111. Waldman, R. H., Grunspan, R. and Ganguly, R. (1972). Oral immunisation of mice with killed *S. typhimurium* vaccine. *Infect. Immunity*, **6**, 58
112. Hornick, R. B., Greisman, S. E., Woodward, T. E., Dupont, T. E., Dawkins, A. T. and Snyder, M. J. (1970). Typhoid fever: pathogenesis and immunological control. *New Eng. J. Med.*, **283**, 686 and 739
113. Watson, K. C. (1957). The relapse state in typhoid fever treated with chloramphenicol. *Amer. J. Trop. Med.*, **6**, 72
114. Luderitz, O. (1972). Quoted in: *Oral Enteric Bacterial Vaccines. Wld. Hlth. Org. techn. Rep. Ser.*, **No. 500**, 24

115. Venneman, M. R. and Bigley, N. J. (1969). Isolation and partial characterization of an immunogenic moiety obtained from *Salmonella typhimurium*. *J. Bact.*, **100**, 140
116. Freter, R. (1972). Parameters affecting the association of vibrios with the intestinal surface in experimental cholera. *Infect. Immunol.*, **6**, 134
117. Freter, R. (1970). Mechanisms of action of intestinal antibody in experimental cholera. II. Antibody-mediated antibacterial reaction at the mucosal surface. *Infect. Immunol.*, **2**, 556
118. Gibbons, R. J. (1974). Bacterial adherance to mucosal surfaces and its inhibition by secretory antibodies. In *The immunoglobulin A system. Adv. Exp. Med. Biol.*, **45**, 315
119. Freter, R. (1974). In *The immunoglobulin A system. Adv. Exp. Med. Biol.*, **45**, 349
120. Springer, G. F. and Horton, R. E. (1969). Blood group isoantibody stimulation in man by feeding blood group-active bacteria. *J. Clin. Invest.*, **48**, 1280
121. Robbins, J. (1975). In *The immune system and infectious diseases.* (Basel: Karger) In press
122. Williams, R. C. and Gibbons, R. J. (1972). Inhibition of bacterial adherence by secretory immunoglobulin A: a mechanism of antigen disposal. *Science*, **177**, 697
123. Brandtzaeg, P., Fjellanger, J. and Gjeruldsen, S. T. (1968). Adsorption of immunoglobulin A onto oral bacteria *in vivo*. *J. Bacteriol.*, **96**, 242
124. Sack, R. B. and Miller, C. E. (1969). Progressive changes of vibrio serotypes in germfree mice infected with *Vibrio cholerae*. *J. Bacteriol.*, **99**, 688
125. Miller, C. E., Wong, K. H., Feeley, J. L. and Forlines, M. E. (1972). Immunological conversion of *Vibrio cholerae* in gnotobiotic mice. *Infect. Immunol.*, **6**, 739
126. Cooke, E. M., Ewins, S. and Shooter, R. A. (1969). Changing faecal population of *Escherichia coli* in hospital medical patients. *Br. Med. J.*, **4**, 593
127. Scherp, H. W. (1971). Dental caries: prospects for prevention, combined utilization of available and imminent measures should largely prevent this ubiquitous disease. *Science*, **173**, 1199
128. McCabe, M. M. and Smith, E. E. (1973). Origin of the cell-associated dextransucrase of *Streptococcus mutans*. *Infect. Immunol.*, **7**, 829
129. Genco, R. J., Evans, R. T. and Taubman, M. A. (1974). Specificity of antibodies to *S. mutans*; significance in inhibition of adherence. The immunoglobulin A system: In *Adv. Exp. Med. and Biol.*, **15**, 327
130. Ogilvie, B. M. and Love, R. J. (1974). Co-operation between antibodies and cells in immunity to a nematode parasite. *Transpl. Rev.*, **19**, 147
131. Dineen, J. K., Ogilvie, B. M. and Kelly, J. D. (1973). Expulsion of *Nippostrongylus braziliensis* from the intestine of rats: Collaboration between humoral and cellular components of the immune response. *Immunology*, **24**, 467

132. Ogilvie, B. M. (1967). Reagin-like antibodies in rats infected with the nematode parasite *Nippostrongylus braziliensis*. *Immunology*, **12**, 113
133. Orr, T. S. C. and Blair, A. M. J. N. (1969). Potentiated reagin response to egg albumin and conalbumin in *Nippostrongylus braziliensis* infected rats. *Life Sci.*, **8**, 1073

CHAPTER 5

Celiac disease and gastrointestinal food allergy

ANNE FERGUSON

Introduction

Food intolerance has many manifestations and as many causes—psychological aversion to the sight, smell or taste of food, maldigestion and malabsorption syndromes, toxic effects of food additives or contaminants, and true allergy, when the clinical disease is the result of an immunologically mediated hypersensitivity reaction to a dietary antigen. In the case of gastrointestinal food allergy, an immunological basis has been inferred from positive family history of allergy, the presence of serum, secretion or reaginic antibodies to food allergens, tests of lymphocyte function and immunological effects of food challenge. Although the same type and range of evidence in favour of gluten hypersensitivity is present for celiac disease, there is still debate as to whether this permanent gluten intolerance has a biochemical or an immunological basis. However, the clinical, pathological and immunological features of these two diseases are so similar that the conclusion that both are due to hypersensitivity or allergy to foods seems inescapable.

The first part of this chapter deals with the range of types of immune responses to foods, factors which can influence these, and the experimental evidence that a local immune reaction can influence small intestinal structure and function. This forms the theoretical background to a discussion of the clinical immunology of celiac disease and food allergy, and of a working model of local intestinal hypersensitivity mechanisms.

The concept of hypersensitivity reactions

The term allergy when first introduced meant[1] altered host reactivity to an antigen[1] and thus was synonymous with the word immunity as used today. The term which best covers immunologically mediated disease is hypersensitivity, in which in a previously immunized host, tissue damage results from the immune reaction to a further dose of antigen. Hypersensitivity reactions may be mediated by antibodies or by lymphocytes, and are classified in four broad groups[1].

Type I, immediate hypersensitivity: This results when an antigen reacts with reaginic antibody (usually IgE) on the surface of mast cells, with the release of vasoactive substances such as histamine. The reaction takes place within minutes of exposure to antigen.

Type II, cytotoxic hypersensitivity: This is due to the reaction of an antibody with a cell surface antigen, or with an antigen or hapten which has become attached to the cell surface. For cell lysis to occur, other factors such as complement, or K (killer) cells, may be required. The time scales of these cytotoxic reactions are variable.

Type III, late hypersensitivity, Arthus reaction: In this reaction, tissue damage is mediated by antigen–antibody complexes, particularly the soluble complexes formed in slight antigen excess which fix and activate the C3 component of complement, and attract neutrophil polymorphs to the site. This type of reaction is at maximum a few hours after exposure to antigen.

Type IV, delayed hypersensitivity, cell mediated immunity: This is the result of interaction between antigen and primed thymus-dependent lymphocytes. Most of the manifestations are produced via lymphokines-soluble factors secreted by these lymphocytes on contact with antigen, and which cause local inflammation, attract other lymphocytes and macrophages to the site, enhance phagocytosis and increase macrophage metabolism. This type of reaction takes place 1–2 days after antigen exposure.

Celiac disease and food allergy defined

Celiac disease in childhood has been defined by a working party of the European Society for Paediatric Gastroenterology[2]. This is a permanent condition in which the mucosa of the upper small intestine is flat and there is usually biochemical evidence of malabsorption. When the child takes a diet free of wheat, rye, barley and oat gluten, mucosal architecture and absorption return to normal and subsequent reintroduction of gluten to the diet will be followed by recurrence of mucosal abnormalities. Celiac disease in adults is also a permanent condition in which there is a flat mucosa in the upper small intestine, usually malabsorption, and a clinical response to gluten withdrawal. However, adult celiacs differ from children in that it is rare to find complete restoration of the jejunal mucosa to normal on a gluten-free diet. Furthermore, the morphological effects of gluten challenge are seen within hours in adult celiac patients, whereas in children, morphological relapse may be delayed for up to 2 years after the reintroduction of gluten to the diet[3]. Yet despite these minor differences, it is now generally accepted that celiac disease is a single entity, no matter what the age of the patient at diagnosis.

Food allergy: This term encompasses all the effects of hypersensitivity to food antigens. The route of immunization may be by ingestion, but also by inhalation (e.g. of avian antigens, milk droplets) or by injection (e.g. intradermal skin tests, injection of egg antigens with viral vaccines). Subsequent antigen challenge may also be via any of these routes, and the harmful immune reaction can be localized at the site of challenge, at a single remote site (e.g. the lungs) or systemically.

In *gastrointestinal food allergy*, the subject of this chapter, the usual site of both sensitization and of challenge is the small intestine. In contrast to celiac disease, this is a transient condition and many foodstuffs have been implicated, including cows' milk, eggs, soya protein, rice and wheat. The typical clinical picture is of a child aged less than 6 months who presents with diarrhea and failure to thrive or malabsorption[4]. Histology of the proximal small intestine usually shows partial or subtotal villous atrophy[4–6] and there is an immediate clinical and histological response to withdrawal of the appropriate dietary antigen. Challenge with the offending foodstuff shortly after the initial illness will cause the return of symptoms and of the jejunal abnormality. However, after a period of time the child usually outgrows the allergy and subsequent challenge has no effect. Food allergy in older children and adults is usually associated with reactions outwith the gastrointestinal tract (e.g. asthma, angioneurotic edema). However, in some adults food allergy causes a protein losing enteropathy or malabsorption which responds to withdrawal of the food allergen concerned[7].

Induction and recall of immune reactions to food antigens

Spectrum of immune responses

The primary immune response to an antigen is influenced by the dose, physical properties and route of administration of the antigen, and by the immune status of the host—this latter factor being a combination of age, heredity, and adjuvant or immunosuppressive agents in the environment. Several different results can be produced by antigen exposure.

Immunity: Heightened response to the antigen, due to one or more immunoglobulin classes of antibody and/or to specific cell-mediated immunity, with or without associated immunological memory, and often conferring protection to the invasive or pathogenic effects of the antigen.

Hypersensitivity: This has been discussed above; it is present when in a previously immunized person, tissue damage results from subsequent exposure to the antigen.

Tolerance: A specific non-reactivity of lymphoid cells to the given antigen. This is the usual response to contact with antigens in early fetal life, but has also been produced in adult animals by feeding of proteins or hapten (or, more accurately, feeding of antigens produced non-reactivity to the same substance when subsequently administered parenterally)[8,9].

No immune response: This differs from tolerance in that the host, unless immunodeficient, retains the capacity to mount a normal immune response to the antigen. Obviously, this would be the response to an antigen which has been completely destroyed (e.g. by digestion) before it can meet immunocompetent cells.

Usual response to feeding of antigen: All the present evidence suggests that the usual responses to feeding of an antigen are the secretion of IgA class antibody and a systemic state of tolerance (see Chapter 2). Neither of these is associated with harmful immune reactions and, indeed, systemic tolerance is incompatible with a hypersensitivity state. Clearly, the development of hypersensitivity—type I, II, III or IV—implies a breakdown of or alteration in the usual immune response to an orally administered antigen.

Foods as antigens

In Britain, recent changes in infant feeding habits have produced a situation where not only are most babies fed cows' milk from birth, but in addition mixed feeding with cereals, egg and fruits is often started in the first month of life[10]. This early introduction of cereal feeding has advanced the age of presentation of celiac disease[11] so that it must be considered in the differential diagnosis of diarrhea in an infant. It also complicates the management of some children with gastrointestinal food allergy who may be allergic to many foods. However, cows' milk allergy remains by far the most common type of food allergy in infants, and is the only type which has been extensively studied.

Cows' milk contains five main proteins—bovine serum albumin (BSA), bovine gamma globulin (BGG), α lactalbumin (αLA), β lactoglobulin (βLG) and casein[12]. BSA and BGG are highly immunogenic proteins and have been extensively used in immunological research; experiments in thymus-deprived mice have shown that all the milk proteins are thymus-dependent antigens[13], i.e. co-operation between T- and B-cells is required for subsequent antibody production by B-cells. Purified milk proteins can be purchased commercially, and although the separation process may alter some of their properties, these proteins have proved very useful in laboratory tests for detection of antibodies or cell mediated immunity to cows' milk.

Wheat proteins comprise four main classes—globulins, albumins, gliadin and glutenin. Glutenin is a macromolecule which confers the visco-elastic properties to dough. The gliadins are a complex group of proteins, rich in glutamic acid and in proline. Some immunized animals and celiac patients have serum antibodies to a dozen or more separate antigenic determinants of crude gliadin[14], and pure α, β and γ gliadin can be prepared in gramme quantities[15]. Although the toxicity of α gliadin for celiac patients is established[16], possible harmful effects of the other fractions have yet to be defined. This subject is discussed further in the section on celiac disease.

Other food allergens: Most foods studied have been shown to contain one or more allergens, e.g. eggs, bananas, nuts, tomatoes, fish[17,18]. The effects of cooking or digestion may be to destroy these allergens, but may also reveal new antigenic sites, allergy to which may be missed if skin tests are done using only the intact food substances.

ANTIBODIES TO FOODS IN SERUM

The presence, in serum, of IgG antibodies to a food implies that immunogenic molecules have been absorbed from the lumen of the gastrointestinal tract, have passed via the lamina propria, lymph or the portal circulation, to be phagocytosed and processed by macrophages in the spleen and lymph nodes, and that plasma cells are secreting specific antibody into the extracellular fluid compartment. Serum antibodies of IgA class may have a similar origin (e.g. from plasma cells in the mesenteric lymph nodes) but an alternative source is the secretion by IgA immunoblasts during their traffic in the lymph and blood, before they finally home to the lamina propria of the gut.

Small amounts of antibody to many food antigens (mainly IgG class) have been detected in the serum of normal human children and adults, by using sensitive techniques such as passive haemagglutination, immunofluorescence and radioimmunoelectrophoresis. Antibodies to cows' milk are present in the serum of most bottle-fed human infants, up to the age of 3 years[19,20] (Figure 5.1) and the relative titres of antibody to the five main proteins also vary with age and disease. Very young children (aged 2 months) have antibody to casein but not to the other milk proteins[20]; patients with IgA deficiency and with celiac disease tend to have high titres of antibody to bovine immunoglobulin (BGG)[20,21].

Abnormally high titres of serum anti-food antibodies are present in the serum in many gastrointestinal diseases, and can be demonstrated by relatively insensitive techniques such as precipitation in gel. Antibodies to many animal, avian and cereal antigens can be detected but the need for a soluble preparation of antigen is a limitation, especially in tests for anti-cereal antibodies. In most groups of patients who have anti-food precipitins in the serum, the incidence of anti-ruminant antibodies is highest, followed by anti-avian antibodies, with a low incidence of anti-cereal antibodies. Table 5.1 summarizes the results of these tests in patients with celiac disease, inflammatory bowel disease and oral ulceration. Two important points emerge from these results. The presence of serum precipitins to a food does not indicate clinical intolerance or allergy to that food—many patients with celiac disease have high titres of anti-milk or anti-egg antibodies, but are not intolerant of these foods. Also, although an occasional blood donor or patient with inflammatory large bowel disease has serum antibodies to milk or egg,

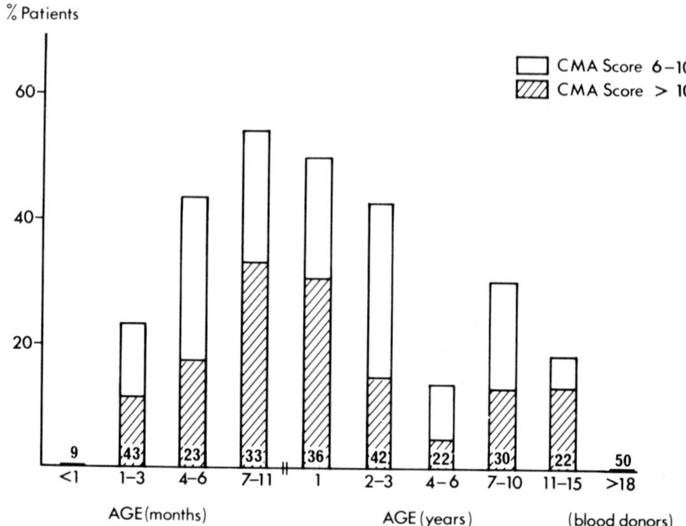

FIGURE 5.1 The influence of age on serum antibodies to cows' milk, in children investigated for possible gastro-intestinal or allergic disease (celiac patients excluded). The cows' milk antibody (CMA) score is derived from the sum of scored titres of antibody to the five cows' milk proteins—titre 1 in 16 scores 1, 1 in 32 scores 2, etc. Per cent of patients with scores of 6–10 and >10 are shown for each age group and the number of patients is indicated at the foot of each column

precipitins to cereals have only been found in patients with celiac disease, cystic fibrosis and IgA deficiency. Detection of anti-gluten or anti-wheat precipitins should lead to further investigation of the patient by sweat test and jejunal biopsy.

Thus, the presence of serum food antibodies in low titre is merely evidence that the patient is still eating the food and that sufficient immunogenic material is crossing the gut epithelium to stimulate immunocytes. High titres of antibody and precipitins to food antigens are evidence of very high antigen dosage (e.g. undigested proteins in cystic fibrosis) or of undue permeability of the gastrointestinal tract epithelium (e.g. celiac disease) but do not indicate allergy to the food.

Antibodies to foods in intestinal secretions

There are a number of technical problems associated with the measurement of secretory immunoglobulins and antibodies. For example, IgG is slowly degraded in intestinal secretions stored at −20 °C[22] and so

Table 5.1 INCIDENCE OF PRECIPITINS TO FOOD ANTIGENS IN THE SERUM OF PATIENTS WITH GASTROINTESTINAL DISEASE

Diagnosis	*Number of patients studied*	*Precipitin test positive with*		
		cereal antigens (e.g. wheat extract)	*ruminant antigens (e.g. cows' milk)*	*avian antigens (e.g. egg)*
Normal adult	20	—	—	—
Blood donors	50	—	1	—
Ulcerative colitis	50	—	1	—
Crohn's disease	13	—	2	—
Irritable bowel syndrome	18	—	—	—
Aphthous ulcers	25	—	2	4
Adult celiac disease (untreated)	6	2	4	2
Adult celiac disease (gluten-free diet)	30	3	7	7
Childhood celiac disease (untreated)	33	21	25	6
Age matched non-celiac children	38	2*	4	—

* Two infants with cystic fibrosis

the most reliable investigations are those which have been done using freshly obtained material. The first reports of anti-food coproantibodies (in stools or intestinal secretions) suggested that they had a major role in the pathogenesis as well as in the diagnosis of celiac disease and gastrointestinal food allergy. Katz and his colleagues reported the presence of coproantibodies to gluten in all of 12 celiac patients studied but in none of 51 controls[23] and Self *et al.* reported coproantibodies to milk, egg and other antigens in children with allergy to these proteins[24]. However, other groups have failed to confirm the specificity of such coproantibodies. Milk antibodies are present in the stools of three-quarters of normal children[25], and in children with non-specific diarrheas[26]. With a precipitin technique, we detected anti-cereal antibodies in secretions of 80% of celiac children, but also in 43% of children with other conditions[27], and Mawhinney who studied adults with an immunofluorescent technique, detected antibody to gluten fraction III in the intestinal secretions of 64% of celiac patients, but also in 31% of normal adults[28]. Clearly, in normal children and in adults there is a local humoral immune response to foods as well as to commensal gut bacteria, orally administered vaccines and various enteric infections. However, just as has been found in serum antibody tests, the incidence of coproantibodies (to various foods), the titres of these antibodies, and the range of foods to which antibodies are present, have all been higher in patients with celiac disease compared with controls[27,28].

The immunoglobulin classes of coproantibodies to milk proteins and to gluten have been studied by radioimmunoelectrophoresis[25], radioimmunodiffusion[19] and by immunofluorescence[28]. All these techniques have shown that most secreted anti-food antibody is of the IgA class, whereas most of the serum antibody to the same antigens is IgG[19,28]. Table 5.2 summarizes some of our unpublished results on antibodies to the milk proteins BSA and BGG.

Where are the plasma cells which are secreting anti-food antibodies? It might be thought that fairly large numbers of such cells would be found in the gut mucosa, especially in conditions such as celiac disease and food allergy where the lamina propria is packed with plasma cells. In fact, the most painstaking of searches have demonstrated some plasma cells containing antibody to ovalbumin[29] and a very few plasma cells with antibody to gliadin antigens[30]. This merely serves to show that the cells in question have been diluted by enormous numbers of plasma cells making antibody to other gut-associated antigens—there are around 430 000 plasma cells/mm^3 in the lamina propria of normal human small intestine[31].

IgA antibodies block absorption of antigen from the gut lumen, and most patients with IgA deficiency have high titres of serum antibody to milk[21,32]. However, in celiac disease and food allergy there are often high titres of anti-food antibodies both in serum and secretions. A qualitative defect of IgA in celiac disease has been postulated[33], but on flimsy evidence. More likely, the IgA blocking antibodies are unable to compensate entirely for the considerable destruction of the mechanical barrier to absorption which is normally formed by the sheet of enterocytes.

Reaginic antibodies to foods

These can be detected by using the *in vivo* technique of skin testing for

Table 5.2 IMMUNOGLOBULIN CLASS OF ANTIBODIES TO BSA AND BGG DETECTED BY RADIOIMMUNODIFFUSION (USING [^{125}I]-BSA AND [^{125}I]-BGG)

Diagnosis	*No. of specimens examined*	*Nature of specimen*	*Antibody to BSA detected by RID*	*Ig class of antibody to BSA*			*Antibody to BGG detected by RID*	*Ig class of antibody to BGG*		
				IgG	*IgA*	*IgM*		*IgG*	*IgA*	*IgM*
Normal adult	3	Serum	0	—	—	—	0	—	—	—
Adult celiac disease (gluten-free diet)	18	Serum	0	—	—	—	1	1	1	1
Childhood celiac disease (untreated)	13	Serum	5	3	4	1	12	12	10	8
Age matched non-celiac children	18	Serum	3	2	2	—	14	7	8	11
IgA deficiency	3	Serum	0	—	—	—	3	3	—	1
Childhood celiac disease (untreated)	15	Upper intestinal secretions	4	0	3	1	9	0	9	3
Age matched non-celiac children	9	Upper intestinal secretions	2	1	2	1	3	1	3	3

immediate hypersensitivity, by the *in vitro* radioallergosorbent technique[34], or by rat mast cell degranulation[35]. Immediate hypersensitivity to foods is relatively uncommon even in atopic people. When it is present the hypersensitivity reaction may take place locally in the gut, but more often the antigen is absorbed and reacts with antibody on the surface of mast cells in other parts of the body. Atopy in the patient or his family, and positive skin tests to foods are present in a majority of patients with gastrointestinal protein allergy[36] but these are not features of celiac disease[37].

Cell-mediated immunity to foods

Specific cell-mediated immunity (CMI) can be detected by skin tests for delayed hypersensitivity and by *in vitro* techniques such as blast transformation in, and lymphokine secretion by, lymphocytes when cultured in the presence of antigen. Peripheral blood leucocytes are often used in these tests, and we have recently shown, by using an organ culture technique, that the properties of intestinal lymphocytes can also be studied[38].

There is no evidence of CMI to foods in normal human beings or in animals. Intradermal injection of gluten causes local lymphocyte infiltration in the skin of normal subjects and of celiac patients, but by the usual criteria of CMI—macroscopic inflammation at 1–2 days—the results are negative[39]. At least two groups have failed to produce gluten-related blast transformation in the peripheral blood lymphocytes of celiac patients[40,41], but Holmes *et al.* demonstrated blast transformation in 16% of their celiac patients on a normal diet and in 32% of celiac patients on a gluten-free diet[42]. However, the lymphocytes of some celiac children also transform to blast cells when cultured with cows' milk antigens[43], so, if indeed this is a test of CMI, it indicates delayed hypersensitivity to foods other than gluten in celiac disease. Studies in children with cows' milk allergy have been more fruitful, for in many such children, peripheral blood lymphocytes are stimulated by cows' milk antigens[44,45] and it has even been suggested that this test can be used as a diagnostic criterion[46].

The small intestinal mucosa contains many lymphocytes and their numbers are increased in celiac disease[47,48] and in cows' milk allergy[49]. One way to prove or disprove the existence of sensitized lymphocytes in the mucosa is to culture fragments of intestine in the presence and absence of antigen, and to demonstrate antigen induced lymphokine secretion[48]. We carried out this experiment in patients with celiac disease and with other conditions, and found secretion of a leukocyte migration inhibition factor when intestine from 5 of 6 untreated celiac patients was cultured with α-gliadin[38] (Figure 5.2). This preliminary work indicates that it is possible to detect local intestinal CMI, and the technique should be appropriate to studies of local immunity to antigens other than gluten.

Factors which influence induction of immunity to foods

In considering the theoretical aspects of the immunology of food hypersensitivity, the induction of an abnormal immune response must be accepted as the main aetiological factor. This is now recognized to be an important and fruitful area of research, but there is still a dearth of published work on the subject.

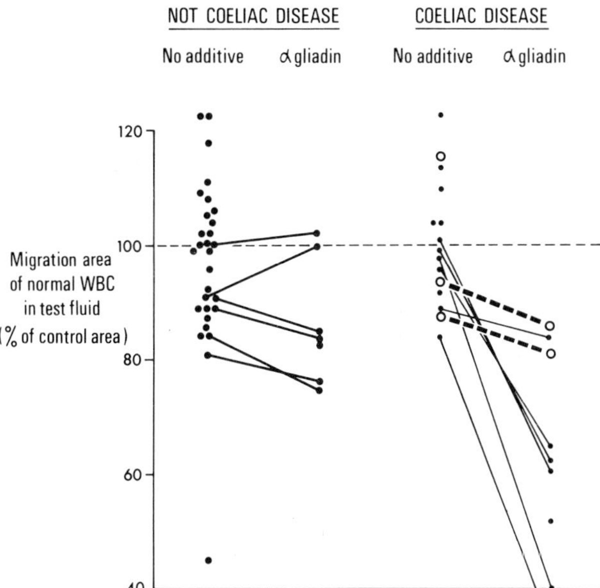

FIGURE 5.2 Migration of normal human white bloodcells in test culture medium, expressed as percentage of area of migration in previously unused culture medium. Test culture media had previously been used for 5-hour culture of fragments of jejunal biopsy specimens with and without added α-gliadin (0.5 mg/ml). Three celiac patients on a gluten-free diet are shown as open circles

Immune capacity can influence the responses to systemically administered antigens, and is likely also to be important in gastrointestinal immunity. Immune status can be assessed by using a battery of investigations of non-specific, humoral and cell-mediated immunity[50]. This background capacity to respond to antigens is impaired in old age, after some viral infections (e.g. measles), by cytotoxic drugs, steroids, and some antibiotics, by radiotherapy, and, of course, in patients with congenital and acquired immune deficiency diseases.

IgA deficiency, per se, probably does not cause gastrointestinal disease. However, there is an association between the presence of IgA deficiency and the development of certain diseases such as autoimmune disease and celiac disease[51]. Even in the absence of these associated diseases, IgA-deficient persons usually have high titres of serum antibodies to milk antigens[21,32] (investigations of antibodies to other foods have not been published). An important role for IgA in early infancy has been proposed by Taylor *et al.*[52], who investigated the inheritance of atopy. In a prospective study of newborn children of atopic mothers, they found that a group of babies who became atopic in the first year of life had abnormally low serum levels of IgA at the age of three months. These workers postulated that an inherited and transient IgA deficiency was the factor which allowed induction of reaginic antibodies to allergens in the babies' environment.

Amount of food in proximal small intestine: The final concentration of immunogenic food in the intestine depends on many factors—the amount eaten, the effects of gastric acid, pepsin, bile and pancreatic enzymes, and the rate of removal of food either by absorption or by peristalsis. The lack of pancreatic enzymes and thus the presence of large amounts of food antigen in the proximal intestine, is probably the reason for the presence of precipitins to foods in the serum of children with cystic fibrosis[27,53].

Permeability of the gut epithelium: This is clearly a critical factor in controlling the amount of food absorbed as intact molecules. In health, there are probably several routes of penetration of antigen, at extrusion zones, at the tips of the villi, through the enterocytes via pinocytotic vesicles, and by persorption—the passage of large particles between enterocytes. Increased permeability may occur in the neonatal period[54] and in gastrointestinal diseases. Ulceration of the buccal mucous membrane will allow direct absorption of small amounts of food proteins, especially those which are in solution when ingested (the proteins of milk). Multiple small ulcers elsewhere in the gastrointestinal tract may be important, although there is no evidence of increased permeability to foods or other antigens in peptic ulceration. Finally, widespread damage to the sheet of enterocytes, with extensive extrusion zones and breaks in the adhesion of the cells to one another, may allow ingress of very large amounts of food antigen, and also will produce protein-losing enteropathy.

Route of removal of antigens from the mucosa: After antigens have crossed the epithelial barrier, they may be handled in several ways. There are many reticuloendothelial cells in the lamina propria, cells which have a role in phagocytosis of food and microbial antigens. These materials may leave the mucosa in the blood capillaries, to go via the portal vein to the liver where they are taken up and destroyed by Kupffer cells with little or no subsequent immune response. However, if antigens leave the gut in the lymph they will make close contact with lymphocytes, can be phagocytosed and processed by reticuloendothelial cells in the mesenteric lymph nodes, and this will result in the induction of specific humoral and/or cellular immune responses. Whether and to what extent antigen is also absorbed into the Peyer's patches is still disputed.

Pre-existing immunity: If a person or animal is already 'primed' for example for IgG or IgE antibody production, then even if there is no circulating antibody, the immune response to a further dose of antigen will be enhanced—a manifestation of immunological memory. In addition, passively acquired immunity to foods may be present when the mother has a disease such as celiac disease or ulcerative colitis in which serum antibodies to foods are present and which, if of the IgG class, will cross the placenta. It is not known whether immune complexes would be formed in the gut mucosa of the infant who had passively acquired antibodies to cows' milk, and who was then fed cows' milk.

Adjuvants are substances which non-specifically enhance or modify the immune response to an antigen. In experimental immunology, antigens are usually administered mixed with the adjuvant, e.g. in a water in oil emulsion. However, many microbial products have adjuvant activity—mycobacterial cell walls, endotoxin, pertussis. Lymphokines produced by activated T-cells have been shown to enhance the induction of CMI to other antigens[55], and the products of several helminth parasites will potentiate IgE synthesis[56].

Timing of exposure to a new food antigen: Since the presence of bacteria or parasites in the gut may have an adjuvant effect, the temporal relationships between changes in diet and the state of microbial colonization of the gut may be very relevant in the development of the local and systemic immune responses to foods. With the optimal diet of breast milk, secretory IgA coats the intestine with 'antiseptic paint' and also allows for a slowly progressive microbial contamination of the child's intestine long before exposure to food antigens. However, most children in our society are fed cows' milk which is a complex mixture of several proteins whose immunogenicity may be altered by freeze-drying or by heating. The daily dose of milk proteins ingested by an infant may be 15–20 g. Perhaps more important than the dose of protein is that in babies bottle-fed from birth, the timing of first exposure to milk antigens coincides with the onset of microbial colonization of the gut after birth. Furthermore, in prospective studies now in progress on the long-term effects of acute gastroenteritis in infants, evidence is accumulating that such an infection may be the trigger which produces immunization of a child to cows' milk, so that subsequent feeding with cows' milk after recovery from the acute infectious illness will cause malabsorption due to gastrointestinal milk allergy[57].

Local hypersensitivity in the small intestine in animal models

Hypersensitivity reactions of types I, III and IV can be produced artificially in the mucosa of the small intestine. This now gives a tool for the investigation of the ways in which a local immune response can affect the macrosopic, microscopic and fine structure of the intestine; functional aspects such as cell production, cell loss, and absorption; and intestinal permeability and antigen handling. The published literature on this subject is still scanty; however, there is sufficient information to define the morphological features of these hypersensitivity reactions, and to compare the findings in these animal models with the results of antigen challenge in human food hypersensitivity states.

Local immediate hypersensitivity: This has been produced in rats by immunization with antigen (ovalbumin) together with pertussis as an adjuvant, so that reaginic antibodies are formed; and then producing anaphylaxis by intravenous injection of the antigen[58]. In laboratory rats, perhaps because of the presence of sufficient mast cells in the normal small intestinal mucosa, anaphylaxis causes changes in the small intestine as well as in other parts of the body. These are separation of the individual epithelial cells from the basement membrane by sub-enterocyte blebs, the formation of fluid filled spaces underneath the basement membrane, especially at the tips of the villi, and the out-pouring of extracellular fluid into the lumen of the gut[58]. In some unpublished experiments we produced similar lesions in mice and rats (Ferguson and Macdonald), and it is important to emphasize that the effects are on the extracellular fluid compartment, and that no changes in the cellular constituents of the lamina propria or in the epithelium were seen in our experiments or in the earlier work by Barth *et al*[58].

Arthus reaction: This has been produced experimentally in several ways, either by actively immunizing animals so that they produce high titres of serum antibody, or by passive immunization with rabbit antiserum. After feeding of antigen, or instillation of high concentrations into Thiry–Vella loops of intestine, three effects have been seen (Ferguson and Macdonald, unpublished). When the challenging dose is fairly low, this procedure has produced no morphological changes in the small intestine. However, in around half of the experiments so far carried out, at about 4 hours after antigen challenge large numbers of polymorphonuclear leukocytes accumulate in the small blood vessels of the gut, in the lamina propria, between the epithelial cells, and even within the gut lumen. Similar penetration of the gut by polymorphs was reported by Bellaway[59]. He found no evidence of functional derangement in association with the cellular infiltrate and made the interesting suggestion that this might be a mechanism for the attraction of polymorphs to a site of inflammation, as part of a non-specific protective immune response. In a few of our experiments in which animals, actively or passively immunized, were subsequently challenged with high doses of antigen in a Thiry–Vella loop, the local Arthus reaction resulted in necrosis of the epithelium with ulceration, complete denudation of the villi and subsequently, a return to normal morphology. So far no studies on the effects of a local Arthus reaction on intestinal function or permeability have been reported.

Delayed hypersensitivity reactions: The effects of local CMI on the intestine has been studied by using models in which the intestine itself is the antigen—rejection of allografts of small intestine—and also in graft–versus–host reaction where, by using appropriate genetic combinations of donor and host, injected lymphoid cells mount an immune response against the host. The morphology of rejection of mouse small intestine has been studied in grafted fetal intestine implanted under the kidney capsule and therefore never exposed to microbial antigens or to foods[61,62]. In this model the first sign of rejection is infiltration of the lamina propria with lymphocytes, and shortly thereafter there is a significant increase in the length of the crypts of Lieberkhün, followed by a lymphocyte infiltration of the epithelium and atrophy of the villi with exfoliation of sheets of epithelial cells into the lumen of the transplanted tissue (Figure 5.3). At the late stage of rejection the mucosa ulcerates and the graft comprises only a sheet of smooth muscle heavily infiltrated with lymphocytes and plasma cells. This mouse allograft model is known to be a thymus-dependent reaction[61],

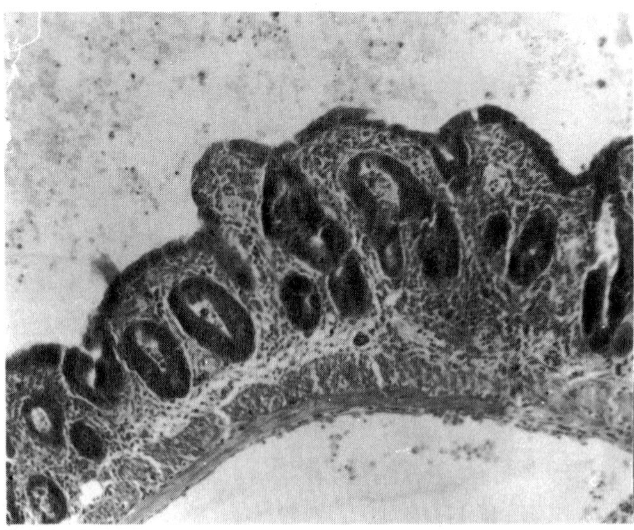

FIGURE 5.3 A cell-mediated immune reaction in the intestinal mucosa—rejection of an allograft of mouse small intestine

and rejection and the associated morphological damage occur several days before the appearance of antigraft antibodies in the serum, thus confirming that the reaction is cell mediated[63]. Finally, since the tissues transplanted are fetal and have never been exposed to foods or microbial antigens, all of the morphological changes observed can be attributed to the rejection process.

Studies in graft–versus–host disease[64] and also in allografts of intestine in larger animals[65] have shown similar morphological changes to those described above. However, at a late stage of rejection of unsterile grafts, there is polymorph infiltration of the mucosa with evidence of superadded bacterial infection[65].

The functional effects of this type of immune reaction have been demonstrated both in allografts of small intestine in large animals and in graft–versus–host disease. They result in malabsorption[66] disaccharidase deficiency[66], protein losing enteropathy[67] and changes in bile salt metabolism[68].

There is some evidence that the presence of a local CMI reaction directed against antigens other than those of the intestine will also cause villous atrophy and crypt hyperplasia. In the case of the local enteropathy associated with parasite infection (*Nippostrongylus braziliensis* in rats) the villous atrophy and crypt hyperplasia associated with this infection have been shown to be thymus dependent[69]. Thus the morphological changes are produced by the immune response to the parasite and not by the toxic products of the organisms themselves. Nevertheless, both humoral and cell mediated immune responses to this parasite are thymus-dependent, so that the absolute proof that the changes in intestinal structure are the result of the CMI reaction is still awaited.

Immunology of celiac disease

Several lines of investigation point to the possibility that an immunological dysfunction may be the primary cause of celiac disease. However, whether further work shows the basic defect to be immunological or biochemical, there can be no doubt that as a result of the intense local inflammation and increased permeability, secondary changes in immune status take place in many patients; these changes may involve cellular and humoral mechanisms and may result either in immune deficiency or in enhanced immunity to intestinal and other antigens.

Immunology and heredity in celiac disease

Celiac disease is familial with an incidence of around 10% in asymptomatic first degree relatives of celiac patients[70]. Autoimmune disease and IgA deficiency are also found in relatives of celiacs[71]. A few years ago the association between celiac disease and a genetic marker (the histocompatibility antigen HL-A8) was established independently by two groups[72,73] and has been confirmed in many other series. Although HL-A8 individuals are 10 times more likely to have celiac disease than those without the antigen, and the frequency of HL-A8 in any racial group is a good marker of predisposition to celiac disease[74], the association is by no means complete, and even in Britain, one in five celiac patients does not have the HL-A8 antigen. In addition, in a few families celiac disease has been found to segregate with an HL-A antigen other than 8[75]; in some large family studies, sibs of celiacs who share the same haptotype do not have the disease[75]; and discordance for celiac disease in identical twins has been reported[76]. All of this indicates that there is a gene near to the HL-A locus, inheritance of which predisposes to the development of celiac disease, but that other factors (genetic and environmental) are involved in development of the disease in genetically predisposed individuals. The likely candidate for the 'celiac disease' gene is one of the immune response (Ir) genes, which are linked to histocompatibility loci in man and animals. It has now been established that there is an association between HL-A haplotype and humoral immune responses to viruses[77], foods[78] and ragweed antigens[79].

Environment is probably as important as genetics where the cause of celiac disease in an individual patient is considered for although the incidence of the disease in the county of Galway is 1 in 300 births[80], the number of celiac children born each year varies, and none of the children born in the county in 1964 have subsequently been found to have the disease[81]. Although celiac disease is very common in Scotland and in Ireland, it is rare in the north-eastern states of the USA, even though many of these Americans are of Scottish or Irish descent.

Despite the considerable amount of recent work on HL-A and celiac disease, the genetics of the immune response to gluten (and to other foods) are as yet scarcely explored. This point can be illustrated by consideration of the spectrum of genes involved in the production of the IgG class antibody response to a suitable dose of antigen:

(i) Genes coding for the light and heavy polypeptide chains, their incorporation into an IgG molecule, and the rates of synthesis and secretion of IgG by individual plasma cells.

(ii) One or more genes which code for the capacity to recognize an antigen as foreign and immunogenic.

(iii) Control of several stages in the maturation of marrow stem cells to B-cells, and of the switch from IgM to IgG production during the immune response.

(iv) Factors (some genetic) which determine the intensity of the immune response to a defined antigen dose—as reflected by peak titres of antibody in the serum.

(v) The genetic predisposition which directs the immune response along the standard (IgM, IgG or IgA) pathway, rather than, as in atopic persons, towards IgE production and in other individuals, towards a cell mediated immune response.

Immune status in celiac disease

A complete assessment of immune status should include morphological examination of lymphoid tissues, tests of non-specific immunity (i.e. polymorphs and reticuloendothelial system function), measurements of immunoglobulins and specific antibodies in serum and in secretions, tests of lymphocyte function and of specific CMI to defined antigens and serial observation of the development of an immune response to a new antigen. As yet, there is no published work in which even half of this assessment has been done in a series of celiac patients. However, many single aspects of immune status have been examined and reported.

The reticuloendothelial (*RE*) *system and functional asplenia:* Idiopathic atrophy of the spleen in adult celiac disease was first recognized in 1923[82], and has been confirmed in many centres since then. This is a true 'functional asplenia' in that the spleen, although still present as a small organ weighing 5–30 g, is thickly encapsulated with fibrous tissue and the red pulp (where the phagocytic cells are normally to be found) is replaced by bands of fibrous tissue. By using clearance of radiolabelled, heat-damaged red cells from the circulation as a test of splenic function, we found that around 40% of adult celiac patients were asplenic[83]; all of these patients had typical hyposplenic features on routine examination of blood films in the haematology department. That this asplenia is probably unique to celiac disease (at least in the West of Scotland) was shown by a further study in which all patients found to have hyposplenic blood films (on routine in- and out-patient haematological studies) were investigated. In a 6-month period 18 previously unrecognized asplenic patients were detected. Further investigation showed that in 16 cases the spleen had been removed in the course of upper abdominal surgery. The remaining two patients (both presenting with gynaecological problems) were further investigated and found to have celiac disease[84].

The asplenia of celiac disease is often dismissed as but one feature of a generalized immunological deficiency in this disease. However, the presence of asplenia has not been found to correlate with any other clinical, haematological, pathological or immunological features, or with associated diseases or complications[83] (Table 5.3) with the possible exception of chronic ulcerative jejuno-ileitis.

The reason for destruction of the spleen in a third of patients with

Table 5.3 CLINICAL AND LABORATORY DETAILS OF PATIENTS WITH ADULT CELIAC DISEASE, RELATED TO SPLEEN FUNCTION

	Normal spleen function	*Asplenia (splenic atrophy)*
Number of patients	18 (4 male)	13 (4 male)
Age at diagnosis of celiac disease (mean)	47·3 yr.	49·9 yr.
History of celiac disease in childhood	8	5
Presented as adult with full-blown malabsorption syndrome	5	3
At diagnosis, faecal fat > 10g/day	6	4
Folate deficiency	13	8
Metabolic bone disease	8	5
Previous treatment with steroids	5	5
Serum IgG (mean)	1709 mg/100 ml	1445 mg/100 ml
Serum IgA (mean)	335 mg/100 ml	325 mg/100 ml
Serum IgM (mean)	68 mg/100 ml	89 mg/100 ml
Autoimmune disease	1	3
Skin disease	4	2
History of tuberculosis	3	4
Lymphoma	1	1
Benign ileal ulceration	—	1

celiac disease is still undefined. In other circumstances the spleen may atrophy because of intra-arterial thrombosis (thrombocythaemia), multiple small infarcts (sickle cell disease) and local irradiation (after Thorotrast exposure). Whatever the cause, absence of this important component of the RE system should be recognized, for asplenic patients have an increased risk of developing a variety of blood-borne infections including meningococcal and pneumoccal septicaemia, Babesosis and malaria.

Humoral immunity: Immunoglobulin levels in serum and intestinal secretions vary with the age, clinical state and treatment of celiac patients. Low serum levels of IgG and increased secretion of IgG may simply reflect a degree of protein-losing enteropathy[85]. The very high levels of serum IgA, which fall to normal after gluten withdrawal[86,87] are probably produced in part by increased traffic of IgA immunoblasts through the vascular compartment, and by the increased number of IgA plasma cells in affected areas of the small intestine. The reason for the low level of serum IgM in celiac disease[88,89] is more difficult to explain. Abnormally low numbers of IgM plasma cells were found in the bone marrow of some patients[90] which suggests that there may, indeed, be a deficiency in this, the most primitive compartment of humoral immunity.

Isolated IgA deficiency is present in around 1 in 50 patients with celiac disease[87,89], but there is no association with other immune deficiency states (although giardiasis, with partial villous atrophy in a hypogammaglobulinaemic child or adult may produce malabsorption, there is no response to gluten withdrawal).

In the intestinal secretions, it is usual to find increased amounts of IgG, IgA and IgM[90,91]. This is paralleled by increased numbers of these three classes of immunocytes in the mucosa[30,90,91,92] by increased synthesis of IgA and IgM by cultured fragments of jejunal biopsies from celiac patients[93], and by high titres of antibody (both in serum and secretions) to foods and other antigens normally present in the gut lumen[27].

Cell-mediated immunity: The peripheral blood lymphocyte count is low in untreated celiac disease[94]; there are reduced numbers of circulating T-cells as assessed by rosetting technique[95] and peripheral blood lymphocyte responsiveness to phytohaemagglutinin may be impaired[96].

These tests all show a moderate reduction in the peripheral blood T-lymphocyte function, which could result either from loss of T-cells into the gut lumen, or redistribution of these cells, for example by accumulation of T-lymphocytes in the small intestinal mucosa and mesenteric lymph nodes. Nevertheless patients with celiac disease do not have clinical evidence of T-cell deficiency—for example they are not unduly susceptible to viral and fungal infections.

Immune responses after immunization: The functions of afferent and efferent limbs of the immune response can be studied by measuring titres of antibody, or specific cell-mediated immunity, after immunization with a new antigen. However, unless such studies are performed in patients who have been treated with a gluten-free diet and who have normal intestinal morphology (as can be attained in most children) then any abnormalities detected may be secondary to the continuing inflammation and increased permeability of the small intestine. From the four reports so far in the literature it is clear that although most of the celiac patients studied in this way have been treated by gluten withdrawal, morphological appearances of the jejunum at the time of immunization experiments are not reported. The studies carried out fall into three groups.

(i) Tetanus toxoid was given intramuscularly to 14 patients with celiac disease by Pettingale[97]. He found that two of the five patients who received primary immunizations failed to produce detectable serum antitoxin, as measured by the *in vivo* mouse protection test, and that the nine patients who were re-immunized produced significantly lower serum antitoxin levels than controls. IgA responses in celiac patients were not impaired, but occurred earlier in celiacs than controls; however, in the celiac patients, IgM responses were significantly low. Beale *et al.*[33] used three injections of tetanus toxoid at monthly intervals to immunize their patients, and they reported normal titres of antitoxin in five treated and five untreated celiac patients.

(ii) Oral polio vaccine (containing types I, II and III viruses) was given to five treated and five untreated celiac patients by Beale *et al.*[33], as three monthly doses. One month later they measured serum antibodies by virus neutralization, a technique which does not differentiate IgG, IgA and IgM antibody activities. The antibody response to Type I virus was definitely subnormal in three of the 10 patients, a subnormal response to Type II was found in one patient and subnormal response to Type III in six patients. However, from their figures, all 10 patients had a normal response to at least one of the viruses in the vaccine. It was unfortunate that these authors drew unwarranted conclusions (which have been widely quoted) from this very small study in which no measurements of IgA responses were, in fact, made. Mawhinney and Love[98] have now reported the results of a well designed study of the serum antibody responses to a single dose of oral type II polio vaccine in 38 celiac patients and 39 age- and sex-matched controls. They used an indirect immunofluorescence technique to measure the antibody responses within the three main immunoglobulin classes, and found celiac patients have a much higher incidence of antibody response than controls, the response being mainly IgA class in both groups of patients.

(iii) Intravenous immunization with the bacteriophage $\phi \times 174$ has been used by Baker *et al.*[99] to study the serial responses of eight celiac patients after primary and secondary immunization with this completely new antigen. The technique used allowed differentiation of IgM antibody from other classes (by fractionation on sucrose density gradients). They found that both the primary and secondary antibody responses were abnormally low in celiac patients. The impairment correlated with the clinical state and also with the size of the spleen as measured on the abdominal scan after intravenous injection of technetium[99] (although none of their patients was asplenic). They also found that celiac patients had an impaired ability to switch from IgM to IgG antibody production in the secondary response.

The findings outlined above speak for themselves. There is definite evidence of abnormal IgG and IgM responses in celiac disease; IgA antibody responses to oral polio virus are probably enhanced, and there have, as yet, been no studies on the development of specific cell-mediated immunity (for example to dinitrochlorobenzene) in celiac patients.

Associated immunological diseases: The incidence of autoantibodies (for example to gastric and thyroid antigens) is high in adults with celiac disease and dermatitis herpetiformis[100,101], but these autoantibodies have not been found in the serum of celiac children[89].

Clinical autoimmune disease may also occur in some of these patients[102,103] and the patients with autoantibodies often also have abnormal serum immunoglobulins[101]. An antibody which reacts with connective tissue (antireticulin antibody) has been found in the serum of 70% of untreated celiac patients (children and adults)[89,99,104,105], in 30% of treated celiacs[105] and also in 25% of patients with Crohn's disease [104,105]. Since reticulin is present in foods, it is quite conceivable that the antireticulin antibody is merely another food antibody and although it is easy to measure and may have limited value as part of a screening programme, it is unlikely to be of any fundamental importance in the pathogenesis of celiac disease or as the cause of autoimmune disease in general.

The high incidence of malignancy in celiac disease, and in particular lymphoma[106,107], may be associated with the established immunological aberrations—some patients with lymphoma have been found to have exceptionally high levels of serum IgA although treated with a gluten-free diet[87]. Oncogenic viruses, or other carcinogens, may penetrate the abnormal gut mucosa more readily than normal intestine. Alternatively, since the proliferation and traffic of gut associated lymphoid cells in celiac disease must be many times higher than in a normal person, it is conceivable that the incidence of malignant transformation in this population of cells is increased in parallel.

Lymphoid cells of the intestinal mucosa in untreated celiac disease

The movement of lymphoid cells into, from and within the mucosa takes place against a background of rapid enterocyte turnover. Although in a normal human being the mature enterocyte is probably present at the epithelial surface for about 3 days this is certainly not so in celiac disease, where the length of time an enterocyte remains at the mucosal surface may only be a few hours. This means that since most jejunal biopsies are taken in the fasting patient, the cells which cover the surface at the time of biopsy have been formed in the crypts and have covered the surface during a period when the patient has been fasting. In several artificial 'gluten challenge' experiments, serial biopsies have been taken within a few hours of a dose of gluten (see below) and some of the findings which are observed, such as polymorph infiltration, might well be seen in sporadically taken jejunal biopsies from ordinary celiac patients. However, since the defined parameters of abnormality in the mucosa have been based on biopsies taken after an overnight fast, these will be considered first.

Intraepithelial lymphocytes: Lymphocytes in the intestinal mucosa are present both in the lamina propria and within the epithelium. The intraepithelial (IE) lymphocytes can readily be counted and normal values defined both in children and adults (in our hands between six and 40 lymphocytes per 100 epithelial cells)[47,108]. Virtually all patients with celiac disease so far reported have been found to have abnormally high counts of IE lymphocytes, and IE lymphocytes counts fall when the patient follows a gluten-free diet[47,48,108–111] (Table 5.4). High IE

Table 5.4 COUNTS OF INTRAEPITHELIAL LYMPHOCYTES IN CELIAC DISEASE [47,108]

Diagnosis	*Number of patients*	*IE lymphocyte count**	
		mean	*range*
Normal adult, ND	40	21	10–39
Celiac adult, ND	20	78	32–165
Celiac adult, GFD	20	42	23–108
Normal child, ND	7	20	14–25
Celiac child, ND	13	59	37–92
Celiac child, GFD	3	28	19–41

ND–normal diet.
GFD–gluten-free diet
*lymphoctyes per 100 epithelial cells

lymphocyte counts do not always parallel abnormalities in villi and crypts for in some treated patients, the mucosa is still flat although the number of IE lymphocytes is in the normal range and in other treated celiacs, the mucosa may appear fairly normal apart from a high IE lymphocyte count[47]. In addition, in other conditions which produce partial villous atrophy (such as acute gastroenteritis) the number of IE lymphocytes may be normal or even low[108]. Thus, it must be accepted that IE lymphocyte infiltration is a feature of celiac disease which is related to the presence of gluten in the diet but is not directly the cause of the mucosal lesion. In this context, it is interesting that there is accumulating evidence that IE lymphocytes are T-cells (see Chapter 1). No measurements, or even estimates, have been made of the total number of IE lymphocytes in the whole small intestine. However, since in celiac disease the IE lymphocyte counts are usually two or three times higher than normal, and the area of surface epithelium in celiac disease is reduced by a factor of five or more, the size of the population of IE lymphocytes in celiac disease is unlikely to be increased and, indeed, may be decreased.

Lamina propria lymphoid cells: In the lamina propria (LP) there are several lymphoid cell types, including lymphocytes, plasma cells, macrophages, eosinophils and mast cells. Just as for the epithelium, the cellular population of the LP is continually changing and in addition, the proportion of total mucosal volume which is occupied by LP increases considerably when there is partial or subtotal villous atrophy. Lamina propria differential counts are difficult and time consuming to perform, and, of course, are somewhat subjective.

The results are usually expressed as a number of cells/mm^2 of section and so depend on factors such as the thickness of the section and the amount of shrinkage due to fixation. Another important factor is that the density and relative proportions of lymphoid cells vary at different levels of the mucosa, with highest total density and the maximum proportion of plasma cells being found at the base of the mucosa among the crypts[112]. Despite these sources of variation, essentially similar trends have been reported in several studies of differential cell counts in the LP of biopsies from normal people and patients with celiac disease[109,112–115] (Table 5.5). They all agree that the most striking change in untreated celiac disease is an increase in the number of plasma cells, both in absolute numbers and as the proportion of LP cells. The number of LP lymphocytes per unit area is lower than normal in untreated celiac disease, and no striking changes in other cell types have been identified. In view of the above-mentioned lack of uniformity in plasma cell distribution, it is worth noting that plasma cell counts (on H & E stained sections) of jejunum from normal subjects have been of the same order as that reported by Paul Crabbé in 1965[31], based on 3-dimensional analyses of intestinal cell content.

Table 5.5 COUNTS OF TOTAL CELLS, LYMPHOCYTES AND PLASMA CELLS IN THE LAMINA PROPRIA OF JEJUNAL BIOPSIES (MEAN VALUES)

		Total cells per mm²			*Lymphocytes per mm²*			*Plasma cells per mm²*		
			Celiac disease			*Celiac disease*			*Celiac disease*	
Reference	*Technical aspects*	*Controls*	*ND*	*GFD*	*Controls*	*ND*	*GFD*	*Controls*	*ND*	*GFD*
Holmes *et al.*[109]	5 μm sections counts done within 150 μ of epithelium	5702	13 412	9584	1948	1172	2004	1974	10 498	6148
Ferguson *et al.*[114]	5 μm sections	6650	13 400	9562	2248	1168	2004	1962	9020	5948
Ferguson *et al.*[115]	5 μm sections '3 areas' counted	7413	—	—	2971	—	—	1050	—	—
Lancaster-Smith *et al.*[113]	5 μm sections counts between muscularis mucosa and epithelium	—	—	—	1714	1499	1556	2028	5908	3187
Montgomery & Shearer[112]	5 μm sections counts in deep part of mucosa	11 021	15 996	—	3482	2235	—	1117	7425	—
Crabbé *et al.*[31]	Fluorescent antibody technique with photography and planimetry	—	—	—	—	—	—	2250 (assuming 5μ sections)		

ND—normal diet
GFD—gluten-free diet

Several groups have used immunofluorescence to identify the Ig class of plasma cells in celiac disease. A number of technical factors may influence the results of this type of study—for example the specificity and avidity of the antisera, the dilution of conjugate which is used in the study and the subjective decision of the observer as to whether a cell is positive or negative. Clearly, the thickness of a section will almost directly correlate with the number of positive cells per unit area. In addition, such technical factors as the proper orientation of specimens and the way in which the area of lamina propria is assessed are important. Either double labelling techniques or photography are necessary for the valid comparison of numbers of cells of different Ig classes per unit area of LP. Most studies have shown that the numbers of plasma cells of all three classes (IgG, IgA and IgM) are increased in celiac disease, and that the increase in IgM cells tends to be greater than the increase in IgA cells[30,90–92,116,117].

Can any inference be drawn as to the total population changes in the gut LP in celiac disease? The reduced LP lymphocyte counts have been taken to indicate a possible partial immunodeficiency, or to result from loss of lymphocytes from the LP via the epithelium into the gut lumen[109]. The technique of Baklien *et al.*[118] can be used to study immunocyte distribution in the intestine as a whole—they use a double labelling technique and count the numbers of each cell type in a block of mucosa 6 μm thick and 500 μm long, the third dimension being variable—the depth from epithelium to muscularis mucosa. With this method the increase in immunocyte counts per block of mucosa in celiac disease is by a factor of 2 for IgA, 3 for IgM and 9 for IgG[30]. Thus, the total number of plasma cells per block of mucosa increases to between 2·5 and 3 times the normal value. In celiac disease, the average increase in the density of plasma cells/mm^2 is by a factor of $\times$ 5 (from Table 5.4, approximate increases are $\times$ 5, $\times$ 3, $\times$ 7, and $\times$ 4·5 in the four series). Thus, although the proportion of mucosa taken up by LP is increased in celiac disease, and the LP cells are more tightly packed, unit area counts tend to overestimate the real increase in the numbers of plasma cells in the gut as a whole. They will thus tend to overestimate the total numbers of other LP cell types. In celiac disease, LP lymphocyte counts/mm^2 are 65% of normal (60%, 85%, 70% and 50% from Table 5.4). Thus by comparing their numbers with plasma cells it can be deduced that the reduction in total mucosal LP lymphocytes is even more profound than is suggested by the raw figures—they are probably only 30–40% of the normal number of LP lymphocytes in a block of mucosa from a patient with celiac disease.

Extracellular immunoglobulins and secretory piece: It is appropriate here to mention the studies on the location of extracellular immunoglobulins and secretory component in the mucosa. This has been studied by immunofluorescence[119] and by the more accurate techniques of peroxidase labelling and electron microscopy[120]. The peroxidase work has shown that there is an increase in the amount of IgA in the mucosa in patients with celiac disease but this is found in relatively similar distribution to the IgA of normal mucosa—inside plasma cells, in the extracellular fluid spaces and in small vacuoles within the enterocytes[120], and has not confirmed the earlier suggestion that deposition of IgA in the basement membrane is an important and unique feature of celiac disease[119]. Secretory piece is present in the apical part of the enterocytes and is not among the proteins detected in the lamina propria.

Immunity to foods in celiac disease

Much of the background work on immunity to foods in celiac disease has been discussed in the first part of this chapter, and the 'stop–go' pattern of the investigation of this subject should deter any research worker from making extravagant claims that one or other type of immune response to gluten is the cause of the disease. More than 10 years ago it was reported that patients with celiac disease have serum antibodies to gluten[121] but they also have antibodies to many other foods[27]. In the late 1960s, the claim was made that patients with celiac disease were unique in having antibodies to gliadin in the intestinal secretion[23]. Once again, further studies showed that they also had secretion antibodies to foods to which they were not intolerant[27,28] and many normal children and adults also had secretion antibodies to gliadin as assessed by precipitin tests[27] and immunofluorescence[28]. Recently we have produced evidence of local cell-mediated immunity to gliadin in celiac disease[38] but we have not yet followed this up by experiments to demonstrate local CMI to other foods[48], and, indeed, Jos[43] has referred to his unpublished work which indicates that celiac children may also have CMI to cows' milk proteins.

If there is some type of abnormal immunity to gliadin in celiac disease, can it be in terms of immunoglobulin class of antibody? Falchuk, Gebhard and Strober[122] suggest that the abnormality in celiac disease is a predisposition to form IgA antibodies to gluten, that an IgA-gluten complex has the capacity to adhere to normal enterocytes, especially if they express the HL-A8 antigen on the enterocyte surface, and that this immune complex–surface antigen association then produces damage to the enterocyte. This theory is based on several pieces of evidence. The cell surface antigen HL-A8 is common in celiac disease[73,74] (but, of course, is present in only four out of five Caucasian celiacs); cultured jejunal biopsies from celiac patients synthesize and secrete abnormally large amounts of IgA and IgM into the culture medium[93] and among the materials secreted is a substantial amount of protein with anti-gliadin activity (i.e. material which binds to a gliadin–sepharose column)[123]; and that when a biopsy from a celiac patient has been cultured with gliadin, the culture medium contains a humoral factor which is enteropathic to biopsies from patients with celiac disease in remission (so far this enteropathic effect has been assessed only by changes in the alkaline phosphatase content of the tissue)[124]. This series of experiments has certainly provided evidence that a soluble mediator is secreted by (untreated) celiac mucosa in response to gluten exposure, and that this mediator can produce tissue injury. Falchuk and his colleagues consider that the humoral factor is an IgA-gluten complex (even though, as reviewed by Bazin in Chapter 2, IgA antibodies have never been shown to cause tissue injury). We consider that their findings equally support our theory that much of the tissue injury may be due to secretion of an enteropathic lymphokine by T-cells in celiac intestine[38,48].

A further abnormal antibody which could be implicated in celiac disease is lymphocyte-dependent antibody (LDA). This is antibody of the IgG class, which although present in extremely low titres, can, if attached to a cell surface, render a cell liable to be destroyed by the non-specific K or killer cell (the lymphocytic or monocytic nature of which is still disputed)[125]. LDAs can be produced readily in rabbits by standard immunization procedures; many LDA autoantibodies and anti-tumour antibodies have now been found; thus it would not be surprising if LDA's to gliadin and other foods were present in patients who had high titres of other types of antibody, as in celiac disease. It has been suggested that patients with celiac disease are unique in having LDA to gliadin assessed by three different techniques[126]. However, in this work the only controls examined were eight normal adults and eight patients with 'other gastro-intestinal diseases'. If LDA to gliadin has an important role to play in the pathogenesis of celiac disease, these preliminary findings should have, by now, been confirmed by 'blind' studies in larger series and by the findings of negative results in studies of children and adults with other food allergies, gastro-intestinal infections and inflammatory bowel diseases. Such supporting evidence has not yet been reported or published.

Changes in the immunology of celiac disease after gluten withdrawal

The immune status of celiac patients, as assessed in many ways, usually returns to normal after gluten withdrawal. Serum levels of IgA fall[86,87], and although sequential studies of peripheral blood lymphocyte function have not been reported, blood lymphocyte counts do tend to rise[94]. Studies of immune response to tetanus toxoid, polio vaccine and coliphages, discussed in an earlier section, were mainly carried out in treated celiac patients and provided evidence that immune responses to these antigens are not completely normal even after gluten withdrawal. Splenic atrophy, which is present in one-third of adult celiacs[83], persists despite dietary treatment. The numbers of lymphoid cells in the intestinal mucosal also return towards normal (but rarely completely) and the values for IE lymphocyte counts, LP plasma cells and LP lymphocytes are intermediate between those in normal subjects and in untreated celiac patients[47,48,109–111,113,114] (Table 5.5). Antibodies to foods are reduced in titre or disappear after a patient follows a gluten-free diet for a few months[27,127]. This is so for antibodies to foods such as milk which the patient continues to take, as well as to gluten, an antigen to which he or she is no longer exposed[127,128].

Fragments of jejunal biopsies can be maintained in organ culture for 2 or 3 days, and this *in vitro* system mimics, in some ways, gluten withdrawal *in vivo*. The general morphology of celiac biopsies tends to return towards normal during organ culture, with the reappearance of a healthy columnar epithelium of enterocytes[129]. We have studied the changes in lymphoid cells in such biopsies and have found that even after 24 hours of culture there are striking changes in the numbers and distribution of these cells[48,130]. Both in normal biopsies and in biopsies from celiac patients, counts of IE lymphocytes and LP plasma cells fall, but there is a rise in the number of LP lymphocytes. We have interpreted these findings as indicating that although there is a high density of lymphoid cells in celiac jejunum, for most of these cells the difference from normal (at least in terms of cell numbers) is quantitative but not qualitative; the plasma cells present on the day of jejunal biopsy may well be derived from immunoblasts which have entered the mucosa only one or two days previously; and the ultimate fate of IE lymphocytes would appear to be not to fall off into the lumen of the gut, but to penetrate the basement membrane and re-enter the lamina propria.

Immunology of gluten challenge

The clinical, morphological and immunological effects of gluten challenge vary considerably from patient to patient and the differences seem to be related to age of the patient, the strictness of the gluten-free diet in the period prior to challenge, and the degree of morphological abnormality of the jejunum at the time of challenge. Several types of experiments have been used, either controlled reintroduction of a small amount of gluten daily (e.g. a slice of bread)[131], instillation of a single large dose of gluten into the intestinal lumen[132] and daily feeding of large doses of wheat or gluten[113,133]. The harmful effects of the challenge substances have been demonstrated clinically (by the production of symptoms or biochemical malabsorption) and morphologically (by serial jejunal biopsy) for whole wheat[133], whole gluten[134], α gliadin[16,135] peptic tryptic digests of gluten (Frazer's fraction III[136]) and for the polypeptide component of fraction III with a molecular weight of 8000[137]. The low molecular weight components of fraction III (electrolytes, ammino acids and oligopeptides) are not toxic[137].

The immunological effects of challenge with a single dose of gluten: Challenge with 20 or 30 g of gluten may have no clinical effect, may cause malaise and abdominal pain a few hours later, but does not produce anaphylaxis. Induction of a clinical relapse does not normally occur. The changes in mucosal lymphoid cells after a gluten challenge have been documented in several studies, and the results are outlined in Table 5.6. In biopsies taken at 4 and 12 hours after challenge, there is polymorph infiltration of the lamina propria[132,138], thereafter the numbers of LP lymphocytes and plasma cells increase[113,132,138,139] and from 12 hours, IE lymphocyte counts are also high[48,113]. Immunofluorescent

Table 5.6 SEQUENCE OF CHANGES IN LYMPHOID CELLS OF JEJUNAL BIOPSIES FROM CELIAC PATIENTS, AT DIFFERENT TIMES AFTER A SINGLE DOSE GLUTEN CHALLENGE

Reference	*Technique used for assessment*	*Time after challenge* 2 hours	4–6 hours	12 hours	24 hours +
Shiner & Ballard[138]	Subjective grading of LP cell types	No change	↑ LP eosinophils	↑ LP eosinophils, polymorphs, mast cells	↑ LP lymphocytes, plasma cells
Shiner[139]	Subjective grading of LP cell types	No change	—	—	↑ LP lymphocytes, plasma cells
Doe *et al.*[132]	Subjective grading of LP cell types	—	↑ LP polymorphs	↑ LP polymorphs	—
Lancaster-Smith *et al.*[140]	Direct immuno-fluorescence with counts of plasma cells of IgG, IgM and IgA classes	—	—	—	↑ IgM and IgA cells
Lancaster-Smith *et al.*[113]	Counts of IE lymphocytes and LP lymphoid cells	—	—	—	↑ IE lymphocytes ↑ LP lymphocytes plasma cells
Ferguson[48]	Counts of IE lymphocytes	—	Normal IE lymphocytes	↑ IE lymphocytes	↑ IE lymphocytes

studies have shown that granular extracellular deposition of the complement component C3 and of IgA, IgM and IgG are most marked at 4 hours after challenge[132], and the region of the basement membrane is also stained to a variable extent with anti-IgA and anti-C3 conjugates[132,138]. These findings, together with the marked polymorph infiltrate at 4 hours, suggest that a local Arthus-type reaction has taken place in the intestinal mucosa. Further evidence for this is that the serum levels of several complement components fall within a few hours of gluten challenge (indicating complement consumption[132,141]); that C3 breakdown products have been found in the serum at 8 and 24 hours[141]; and that some patients have circulating immune complexes after gluten challenge[132]. It should be noted that in none of these studies has the nature of the antigen within the immune complexes been defined.

Immunological effects of controlled gluten challenge over several days: Daily feeding of gluten can induce clinical relapse, and whereas the effects of single dose gluten challenge on intestinal architecture are transient and inconstant, daily feeding of 20 to 30 g of gluten often results in partial or subtotal villous atrophy (in adult celiacs). Biopsies taken after 7 days of gluten feeding have shown increases in the numbers of IE lymphocytes and LP plasma cells[113,134] but no significant changes in LP lymphocytes were detected[113].

In vitro *gluten challenge:* Culture with gluten or its fractions has no effect on jejunal biopsies from normal subjects, but when biopsies from untreated celiac patients were cultured with gliadin digests, cytotoxicity, necrosis and ultrastructural damage to the enterocytes were observed[142] and the trend towards morphological improvement, which has been previously reported after culture of celiac biopsies[129,130] did not occur. Gliadin did not have a toxic effect on morphologically normal biopsies from celiac children in diet-induced remission, but the toxic effect was restored if the children had been challenged with gluten *in vivo* a few days prior to biopsy[142]. Furthermore, in some untreated celiac children, addition of partially digested casein *in vitro* also produced damage. This may or may not be related to the fact that children have evidence of CMI to milk proteins as assessed by blast transformation of peripheral blood lymphocytes[142]. These results are in keeping with the findings of Falchuk *et al.*[124] and with our own report[38] that only untreated or post-challenge jejunal biopsies secrete an enteropathic factor when cultured with gliadin. It remains to be shown whether this factor is an immunoglobulin, a lymphokine or is unrelated to immunological and hypersensitivity mechanisms.

Immunology of gastrointestinal food allergy

There is a paucity of immunological investigations in patients with gastrointestinal (GI) food allergy, due partly to the rarity of the disease, and also to the fact that most affected patients are seriously ill infants, in whom diagnosis may not be easy and treatment may be started empirically[5]. Only for cows' milk allergy have large series of patients been studied. Most of the research described below relates to the malabsorption syndrome in infancy with cows' milk intolerance. This is one end of the spectrum of GI food allergy, the other end being the chronic protein-losing enteropathy in an adult which is often associated with eosinophil infiltration of the gut[7].

Immunology and heredity in food allergy

Hereditary factors are present both in celiac disease and gastrointestinal food allergy, but through different mechanisms. In contrast to celiac disease, there is no association between HL-A8 and cows' milk allergy (CMA). In a Finnish series this antigen was found in 18% of the normal population, 87% of patients with celiac disease and 22% of children with CMA[143]. However, 70% of CMA patients have a family history of allergy or atopic disease (asthma, hayfever, eczema[144]). The onset of CMA after recovery from infectious gastroenteritis[57] indicates that environmental factors may also be relevant.

Immune status and immunity to foods

If protein-losing enteropathy is a predominant feature of the clinical illness in food allergy, then the patient will lose albumin, IgG and lymphocytes and sometimes also blood into the gut and he is likely to have evidence of immediate hypersenstivity to foods by skin testing. When the clinical picture is of a malabsorption syndrome[5,86,145], serum and secretion[5] levels of IgA and IgM may be raised. An association between IgA deficiency and food allergy has not been fully documented but I have seen one family of three IgA deficient brothers, two of whom had clinical evidence of cows' milk allergy when aged 2–4 months.

Most normal bottle-fed infants have low titres of antibody to cows' milk in the serum[19,20] and the titres of these antibodies are high, with positive precipitin tests, in cows' milk allergy[4,146] but also in patients with celiac disease[27], and several other conditions[145]. The significance of positive lymphocyte transformation tests with milk antigens[44] has been discussed above. A state of hypersensitivity to foods is not necessarily confined to those foods which harm the affected infant. Cows' milk allergic infants may also have serum precipitins to soya, cereal and egg antigens (Rossipal, personal communication).

Lymphoid cells of the intestinal mucosa in food allergy

The morphology of jejunal biopsies from untreated patients with CMA is more variable than in celiac disease—the usual finding is of partial villous atrophy, but some patients have only minor changes in villi and crypts and others have subtotal villous atrophy indistinguishable from celiac disease[4,5,6,146,147]. Formal quantitation of lymphoid cells has not been done but in all the reports mentioned above subjective assessment has shown increased numbers of lamina propria cells and IE lymphocytes. The increase in plasma cell infiltrate involves cells of the IgA, IgM and IgE classes[5,57,147].

The effect of elimination diets on the immunology of food allergy

After withdrawal of the offending foodstuff (e.g. by a return to human milk feeds) the patient's immune status and jejunal histology usually return to normal[4,5]. However, if cows' milk is replaced by another immunogenic food (e.g. soya) the child may then become allergic to this, and yet other foods[148]. Fortunately, this is not a common problem in food allergy, but when it does occur, prolonged intravenous feeding or use of an elemental diet may be lifesaving[4]. The recent report of long-term follow-up of 54 Finnish children with CMA[4] gives figures for the incidence of intolerance to other foods. Four of 35 children challenged with soya were clinically intolerant of this food, as were seven of 19 challenged with wheat and three of 17 challenged with Nutramigen. Furthermore, although cows' milk allergy is normally a transient condition, five of the 54 children had a flat jejunal mucosa and malabsorption at follow-up 2 years later; appropriate investigations showed that they had developed celiac disease subsequent to the recovery from cows' milk allergy.

Dietary challenge in food allergy

In gastrointestinal food allergy, by definition, dietary reintroduction of the appropriate food will reproduce malabsorption and jejunal biopsy changes only if performed shortly after the initial illness. The clinical and morphological effects of challenge in cows' milk allergy[5,49,147] and in soya allergy[149] have been reported. Even low doses (1–2 ml milk) may produce symptoms, and sequential biopsies show the early development of edema and haemorrhage followed within 24 hours by the appearance of a flat mucosa with increased numbers of plasma cells and with increased IE lymphocyte counts. These abnormalities persist during prolonged challenge and are accompanied by rises in the amounts of IgA and IgM in intestinal secretions and in the faeces and by a rise in serum IgA[5]. Just as in celiac disease sequential studies of serum complement levels have been shown that there is complement consumption and activation[141,150] after milk challenge. Thus, as well as immediate and delayed hypersensitivity reactions to challenge, there is probably also immune complex formation and deposition in the intestinal mucosa.

Conclusions: What is the primary immunological lesion in celiac disease?

There is clinical and experimental evidence that, although an animal or a man may be immune to antigens within the gut lumen, local hypersensitivity reactions do not usually occur. Defence against hypersensitivity lies partly in the sheet of columnar enterocytes which lines the healthy small intestine and partly in IgA which has excellent 'blocking' functions. Absorption of fluid from the gut lumen will dilute antigens and enhance their removal from the mucosa to the liver and lymph nodes with the result that, unless an antigen is complexed or bound in some way to tissue components, it will not remain in the gut mucosa for sufficient time to allow development of a delayed hypersensitivity reaction.

What is the evidence that celiac disease is merely one form of foop allergy? This is what is implied if a hypersensitivity mechanism is thought to be the cause. Several factors contribute to the development of food allergy of infants—a genetic predisposition to make IgE antibodies, feeding of large doses (in an immunological sense) of foreign proteins, and probably a trigger factor such as infection. Absorption of very small quantities (nanograms) of allergens, amounts which can cross an intact mucosa, will produce immediate hypersensitivity reactions; subsequently increased permeability of the mucosa will permit penetration of other antigens and also a protein-losing enteropathy. It may be the sudden ingress of large amounts of antigen which cause the development of IgM, IgG antibodies and cell-mediated immunity to foods in this condition. Alternatively, the spectrum of hypersensitivity reactions which develop in the initial immunization phase may vary from child to child.

In the case of celiac disease, it seems that when gluten in introduced into the diet, the person involved becomes systemically immunized and develops humoral (IgG, IgM) and cell-mediated immunity to the antigens of gluten, as well as the usual secretory IgA response. If one or more genetic factors associated with immune response are implicated, they can only be those which control the afferent limb of immunity to gluten or similar antigens, and thus influence the development of the immune response to orally administered antigen. Once a patient has been immunized, local hypersensitivity reactions due to both antibodies and to cells can explain most of the morphological and functional derangement in the jejunum in celiac disease. However, the exact mechanism whereby damage to individual enterocytes can occur has not been mimicked immunologically[62] and may, indeed, have a direct cytotoxic basis.

Nevertheless not all of the local immune reactions are directed against gluten. Only a few of the many plasma cells in the mucosa make antigluten antibody, and a period of intravenous feeding or starvation does not restore the mucosa to normal. The local immunity and/or hypersensitivity to many antigens, may simply reflect a hereditary tendency to develop humoral and cell-mediated immune reactions to any orally administered antigen; it may be the result of penetration of large amounts of immunogenic material through the very abnormal epithelium; or local immune complexes and lymphokines (which are likely to be present in high concentration as a result of the local immune response to gluten) may have an adjuvant effect, thereby enhancing yet other immune reactions in the intestinal mucosa.

ACKNOWLEDGEMENTS

Some of this work has been supported by a grant from The National Fund for Research into Crippling Diseases, The William Gibson Research Scholarship of the Royal Society of Medicine, and research facilities supplied by E. Merck Ltd.

REFERENCES

1. Gell, P. G. H. and Coombs, R. A. (1969). *Clinical aspects of immunology*. p. 575 (Oxford: Blackwell)
2. Meeuwisse, G. W. (1970). Diagnostic criteria in coeliac disease. *Acta Paediatr. Scand.*, **59**, 461
3. Schmerling, D. H. (1969). An analysis of controlled relapses in gluten-induced coeliac disease. *Acta Paediatr. Scand.*, **58**, 311
4. Kuitunen, P., Visakorpi, J. K., Savilahti, E. and Pelkonen, P. (1975). Malabsorption syndrome with cows' milk intolerance. Clinical findings and course in 54 cases. *Arch. Dis. Child.*, **50**, 351
5. Savilahti, E. (1973). Immunochemical study of the malabsorption syndrome with cows' milk intolerance. *Gut*, **14**, 491
6. Fontaine, J. L. and Navarro, J. (1975). Small intestinal biopsy in cow's milk protein allergy in infancy. *Arch. Dis. Child.*, **50**, 357.
7. Greenberger, N. and Gryboski, J. D. (1973). Allergic disorders of the intestine and eosinophilic gastroenteritis. In *Gastrointestinal disease*. M. H. Sleisenger and J. S. Fordtran (eds.) p. 1066 (Philadelphia: Saunders)
8. Pomeranz, J. R. (1970). Immunologic unresponsiveness following a feeding of picryl chloride. *J. Immunol.*, **104**, 1486
9. Thomas, H. C. and Parrott, D. M. V. (1974). The induction of tolerance to a soluble protein antigen by oral administration. *Immunology*, **277**, 631
10. Taitz, L. S. (1971). Infantile overnutrition among artificially fed infants in the Sheffield region. *Br. Med. J.*, **1**, 315
11. McNeish, A. S. and Anderson, C. M. (1974). Coeliac disease. The disorder in childhood. *Clinics in Gastroenterology*, **3**, 127
12. Rose, C., Brunner, J. R., Kalan, E. B., Larson, B. L., Melnychyn, P., Swaisgood, H. E. and Waugh, D. F. (1970). Nomenclature of the proteins of cows' milk: third revision. *J. Dairy Sci.*, **53**, 1
13. Shearer, B. (1974). B.Sc. thesis, University of Glasgow
14. Beckwith, A. C. and Heiner, D. C. (1966). An immunological study of wheat gluten proteins and derivatives. *Arch. Biochem. Biophys.*, **117**, 239
15. Patey, A. L. and Evans, D. J. (1973). Large scale preparation of gliadin proteins. *J. Sci. Food Agric.*, **24**, 1229
16. Hekkens, W. Th. J. M., Haek, A. J. and Willinghagen, R. G. (1970).

Some aspects of gliadin fractionation and testing by a histochemical method. In *Coeliac Disease.* C. C. Booth and R. H. Dowling (eds.) p. 11 (London: Churchill-Livingstone)

17. Lietze, A. (1969). Laboratory research in food allergy. 1. Food allergies. *J. Asthma Res.*, **7**, 25
18. Bleumink, E. (1974). Allergies and toxic proteins in food. In *Coeliac Disease.* W. Th. J. M. Hekkens and A. S. Pena (eds.) p. 46 (Leiden: Stenfert-Kroese)
19. Kletter, B., Gery, I., Freier, S. and Davies, A. M. (1971). Immune responses of normal infants to cows' milk. 1. Antibody type and kinetics of production. *Int. Arch. Allergy. Appl. Immunol.*, **40**, 556
20. Ferguson, A. (1976). Immunogenicity of cows' milk in man. The influence of age and disease on the distribution of antibodies to five cows' milk proteins. In press
21. Huntley, C. C., Robins, J. B., Lyerly, B. S. and Buckley, R. H. (1971). Characterisation of precipitating antibodies to ruminant serum and milk proteins in humans with selective IgA deficiency. *New Eng. J. Med.*, **284**, 7
22. Samson, R. R., McClelland, D. B. L. and Shearman, D. J. C. (1973). Studies on the quantitation of immunoglobulin in human intestinal secretions. *Gut*, **14**, 616
23. Katz, J., Kantor, F. S. and Herskovic, T. (1969). Intestinal antibodies to wheat fractions in coeliac disease. *Ann. Int. Med.*, **69**, 1149
24. Self, T. W., Herskovic, T., Czapek, E., Caplan, D., Schonberger, T. and Gryboski, J. D. (1969). Gastrointestinal protein allergy: immunologic considerations *JAMA*, **207**, 2393
25. Kletter, B., Freier, S., Davies, A. M. and Gery, I. (1971). The significance of coproantibodies to cows' milk proteins. *Acta Paediatr. Scand.*, **60**, 173
26. Davis, S. D., Bierman, C. W., Pierson, W. E., Maas, C. W. and Iannetta, A. (1970). Clinical nonspecificity of milk coproantibodies in diarrheal stools. *New Eng. J. Med.*, **282**, 612
27. Ferguson, A. and Carswell, F. (1972) Precipitins to dietary proteins in serum and upper intestinal secretions of coeliac children. *Br. Med. J.*, **1**, 75
28. Mawhinney, H. (1973). MD thesis, Belfast University
29. Crabbé, P. A. (1964). Ph.D. thesis, University of Leiden
30. Brandtzaeg, P. and Baklien, K. (1974). Bowel diseases involving local immunoglobulin systems. *Acta Pathol. Microbiol. Scand.* (*Suppl.*), **248**, 43
31. Crabbé, P. A., Carbonara, A. O. and Heremans, J. F. (1965). The normal human intestinal mucosa as a major source of plasma cells containing γA immunoglobulin. *Lab. Invest.*, **14**, 235
32. Buckley, R. H. and Dees, S. C. (1969). Correlation of milk precipitins with IgA deficiency. *New Eng. J. Med.*, **281**, 465
33. Beale, A. J., Parish, W. E., Douglas, A. P. and Hobbs, J. R. (1971). Impaired IgA responses in coeliac disease. *Lancet*, **i**, 1198

34. Turner, K. J., Baldo, B. A. and Hilton, J. M. N. (1975). IgE antibodies to *Dermatophagoides pteronyssinus, Aspergillus fumigatus* and β-lactoglobulin in sudden infant death syndrome. *Brit. Med. J.*, **1**, 357
35. Haddad, Z. H. and Korotzer, J. L. (1972). Immediate hypersensitivity reactions to food antigens. *J. Allergy Clin. Immunol.*, **49**, 210
36. Goldman, A. S., Anderson, D. W., Sellers, W. A., Saperstein, S., Kniker, W. T. and Halpern, S. R. (1963). Milk allergy. *Pediatrics*, **32**, 425
37. Hobbs, J. R., Hepner, G. W., Douglas, A. P., Crabbé, P. A. and Johannsson, S. G. O. (1969). Immunological mystery of coeliac disease. *Lancet*, **ii**, 649
38. Ferguson, A., MacDonald, T. T., McClure, J. P. and Holden, R. J. (1975). Cell-mediated immunity to gliadin within the small intestinal mucosa in coeliac disease. *Lancet*, **i**, 895
39. Asquith, P. (1974). Cell-mediated immunity in coeliac disease. In *Coeliac Disease*. W. Th. J. M. Hekkens and A. S. Pena (eds.) p. 242 (Leiden: Stenfert-Kroese)
40. Ansaldi, N., de Sanctis, C., Fabris, C. and Ponzone, A. (1970). Blastizzazione linfocitaria *in vitro* con fitoemogglutinina e con glutine in bambini affeti da morbo celiaco. *Minerva Pediatr.*, **22**, 1907
41. Morganroth, J., Watson, D. W. and French, A. B. (1972). Cellular and humoral sensitivity to gluten fractions in patients with treated nontropical sprue. *Am. J. Dig. Dis.* **17**, 205
42. Holmes, G. K. T., Asquith, P. and Cooke, W. T. (1972). Cell mediated mechanisms in adult coeliac disease. *Gut*, **13**, 324
43. Jos, J. (1974). In discussion. In *Coeliac Disease*. W. Th. J. M. Hekkens and A. S. Pena (eds.) p. 106 (Leiden: Stenfert-Kroese)
44. Borrone, C., Dagna-Bricarelli, F., Massimo, L., Fossati-Guglielmoni, A. and Durand, P. (1970). Lymphocyte transformation in milk allergy. *Acta Paediatr. Scand.*, **59**, 449
45. May, C. D. and Alberto, R. (1972). *In vivo* stimulation of peripheral lymphocytes to proliferation after oral challenge of children allergic to foods. *Int. Arch. Allergy Appl. Immunology*, **43**, 525
46. Fontaine, J. L., Navarro. J. and Polonovski, C. (1974). The intestinal biopsy in 20 cases of intolerance to cows' milk proteins in infancy. *Acta Paediatr. Scand.*, **63**, 652
47. Ferguson, A. and Murray, D. (1971). Quantitation of intraepithelial lymphocytes in human jejunum. *Gut*, **12**, 988
48. Ferguson, A. (1974). Lymphocytes in coeliac disease. In *Coeliac Disease*. W. Th. J. M. Hekkens and A. S. Pena (eds.) p. 265 (Leiden: Stenfert-Kroese)
49. Kuitunen, P., Rapola, J., Savilahti, E. and Visakorpi, J. K. (1973). Response of the jejunal mucosa to cows' milk in the malabsorption syndrome with cows' milk intolerance. *Acta Paediatr. Scand.*, **62**, 585
50. Graham-Pole, J., Willoughby, M. L. N., Aitken, S. and Ferguson, A. (1975). Immune status of children with and without severe infection during remission of malignant disease. *Br. Med. J.*, **2**, 467

51. Hong, R. and Ammann, A. J. (1972). Selective absence of IgA, autoimmune phenomena and autoimmune disease. *Am. J. Pathol.*, **69**, 491
52. Taylor, B., Norman, A. P., Orgel, H. A., Stokes, C. R., Turner, M. W. and Soothill, J. F. (1973). Transient IgA deficiency and pathogenesis of infantile atopy. *Lancet*, **ii**, 111
53. McFarlane, H., Holzel, A., Brenchley, P., Allan, J. D., Wallwork, J. C., Singer, B. E. and Worsley, B. (1975). Immune complexes in cystic fibrosis. *Br. Med. J.*, **1**, 423
54. Rothberg, R. M. (1969). Immunoglobulin and specific antibody synthesis during the first weeks of life of premature infants. *J. Pediatr.*, **75**, 391
55. Krejči, J., Pekarek, J. Svejcar, J. and Johanovsky, J. (1973). The effect of lymphokines on the development of delayed hypersensitivity to an unrelated antigen. *Immunology*, **25**, 875
56. Jarrett, E. E. E. (1972). Potentiation of reaginic (IgE) antibody to ovalbumin in the rat following sequential trematode and nematode infections. *Immunology*, **22**, 1099
57. Kilby, A., Walker-Smith, J. A. and Wood, C. B. S. (1975). Small intestinal mucosa in cows' milk allergy. *Lancet*, **i**, 531
58. Barth, E. E. E., Jarrett, W. F. H. and Urquhart, G. M. (1966). Studies on the mechanism of the self-cure reaction in rats infected with *Nippostrongylus braziliensis*. *Immunology*, **10**, 459
59. Bellaway, J. E. C. and Nielsen, N. O. (1974). Immune-mediated emigration of neutrophils into the lumen of the small intestine. *Infect. Immunol.*, **9**, 615
60. Ferguson, A. and Parrott, D. M. V. (1972). Growth and development of 'antigen-free' grafts of foetal mouse intestine. *J. Pathol.*, **106**, 95
61. Ferguson, A. and Parrott, D. M. V. (1973). Histopathology and time course of rejection of allografts of mouse small intestine. *Transplantation*, **15**, 546
62. MacDonald, T. T. and Ferguson, A. (1976). Hypersensitivity reactions in the small intestine. 2. The effects of allograft rejection on mucosal architecture and lymphoid cell infiltrate. *Gut*. In press
63. Elves, M. W. and Ferguson, A. (1975). The humoral immune response to allografts of small intestine in mice. *Brit. J. exp. Path.*, **56**, 454
64. Reilly, R. W. and Kirsner, J. B. (1965). Runt intestinal disease. *Lab. Invest.*, **14**, 102
65. Holmes, J. T., Klein, M. S., Winawer, S. J. and Fortner, J. G. (1971). Morphological studies of rejection in canine jejunal allografts. *Gastroenterology*, **61**, 693
66. Hedberg, C. A., Reiser, S. and Reilly, R. W. (1968). Intestinal phase of the runting syndrome in mice. II. Observations on nutrient absorption. *Transplantation*, **6**, 104
67. Cornelius, E. A. (1970). Protein-losing enteropathy in the graft–versus–host reaction. *Transplantation*, **9**, 247

68. Palmer, R. H. and Reilly, R. W. (1971). Bile salt depletion in the runting syndrome. *Transplantation*, **12**, 479
69. Ferguson, A. and Jarrett, E. E. E. (1975). Hypersensitivity reactions in the small intestine. 1. Thymus dependence of experimental 'partial villous atrophy'. *Gut*, **16**, 114
70. Asquith, P. (1974). Family studies in coeliac disease. In *Coeliac Disease*. W. Th. J. M. Hekkens and A. S. Pena (eds.) p. 322 (Leiden: Stenfert-Kroese)
71. Mawhinney, H. and Tomkin, G. H. (1971). Gluten enteropathy associated with selective IgA deficiency. *Lancet*, **ii**, 121
72. Falchuk, Z. M., Rogentine, G. N. and Strober, W. (1972). Predominance of histocompatibility antigen HL-A8 in patients with gluten-sensitive enteropathy. *J. Clin. Invest.*, **51**, 1602
73. Stokes, P. L., Asquith, P., Holmes, G. K. T., Mackintosh, P. and Cooke, W. T. (1972). Histocompatibility antigens associated with adult coeliac disease. *Lancet*, **ii**, 162
74. McNeish, A. S., Rolles, C. J., Nelson, R., Kyaw-Myint, T. O., Mackintosh, P. and Williams, A. F. (1974). Factors affecting the differing racial incidence of coeliac disease. In *Coeliac Disease*. W. Th. J. M. Hekkens and A. S. Pena (eds.) p. 330 (Leiden: Stenfert-Kroese)
75. Harms, K., Granditsch, Rossipal, E., Ludwig, H., Polymenidis, Z., Scholz, S., Wank, R. and Albert, E. D. (1974). HL-A in patients with coeliac disease and their families. In *Coeliac Disease*. W. Th. J. M. Hekkens and A. S. Pena (eds.) p. 215 (Leiden: Stenfert-Kroese)
76. Walker-Smith, J. (1970). Transient gluten intolerance. *Arch. Dis. Child.*, **45**, 523
77. Thomas, H. C., Holden, R., Ironside, J. and Sommerville, R. G. (1974). Viral and bacterial antibodies in primary biliary cirrhosis and other chronic liver diseases. *Gut*, **15**, 826
78. Scott, B. B., Swinburne, M. L., Rajah, S. M. and Losowsky, M. S. (1974). HL-A8 and the immune response to gluten, *Lancet*, **ii**, 374
79. Levine, B. B., Stember, R. H. and Fotino, M. (1972). Ragweed hay fever: genetic control and linkage to HL-A haplotypes. *Science*, **178**, 1201
80. Mylotte, M., Egan-Mitchell, B., McCarthy, C. F. and McNicholl, B. (1973). Incidence of coeliac disease in the West of Ireland. *Br. Med. J.*, **1**, 703
81. McCarthy, C. F. (1974). In discussion. In *Coeliac Disease*. W. Th. J. M. Hekkens and A. S. Pena (eds.) p. 326 (Leiden: Stenfert-Kroese)
82. Blumgart, H. L. (1923). Three fatal adult cases of malabsorption of fat with emaciation and anaemia and in two acidosis and tetany. *Arch. Int. Med.*, **32**, 113
83. Ferguson, A., Maxwell, J. D. and Hutton, M. M. (1969). Splenic function in adult coeliac disease. *Scot. Med. J.*, **14**, 261
84. Ferguson, A., Hutton, M. M., Maxwell, J. D. and Murray, D. (1970). Adult coeliac disease in hyposplenic patients. *Lancet*, **i**, 163

85. Jarnum, S., Kensen, K. B., Soltoft, J. and Westergaard, H. (1970). Protein loss and turnover of albumin, IgA and IgM in adult coeliac disease. In *Coeliac Disease*. C. C. Booth and R. H. Dowling (eds.) p. 163 (Edinburgh: Churchill-Livingstone)
86. Immonen, P. (1967). Levels of the serum immunoglobulins IgA, IgG and IgM in the malabsorption syndrome in children. *Ann. Paediatr. Fenniae*, **13**, 115
87. Asquith, P., Thompson, R. A., Cooke, W. T. (1969). Serum immunoglobulins in adult coeliac disease. *Lancet*, **ii**, 129
88. Hobbs, J. R. and Hepner, G. W. (1968). Deficiency of γM globulin in coeliac disease. *Lancet*, **i**, 217
89. Brown, I. L., Ferguson, A., Carswell, F., Horne, C. H. W. and MacSween, R. N. M. (1973). Autoantibodies in children with coeliac disease. *Clin. Exp. Immunol.*, **13**, 373
90. Douglas, A. P., Crabbé, P. A. and Hobbs, J. R. (1970). Immunochemical studies of the serum, intestinal secretions and intestinal mucosa in patients with adult coeliac disease and other forms of the coeliac syndrome. *Gastroenterology*, **59**, 414
91. Lancaster-Smith, M., Kumar, P., Marks, R., Clark, M. L. and Dawson, A. M. (1974). Jejunal mucosal immunoglobulin-containing cells and jejunal fluid immunoglobulins in adult coeliac disease and dermatitis herpetiformis. *Gut*, **15**, 371
92. Savilahti, E. (1972). Intestinal immunoglobulins in children with coeliac disease. *Gut*, **13**, 958
93. Falchuk, Z. M. and Strober, W. (1972). Increased jejunal immunoglobulin synthesis in patients with non-tropical sprue as measured by a solid phase immunoabsorption technique. *J. Lab. Clin. Med.*, **79**, 1004
94. Brandt, L. and Stenstam, M. (1975). Subnormal lymphocyte counts in adult coeliac disease. *Lancet*, **i**, 978
95. O'Donoghue, D. P., Lancaster-Smith, M. and Kumar, P. J. (1975). Depletion of thymus-dependent lymphocytes in adult coeliac disease. *Gut*, **16**, 392
96. Blecher, T. E., Brzechwa-Ajdukiewicz, A., McCarthy, C. F. and Read, A. E. (1969). Serum immunoglobulins and lymphocyte transformation studies in coeliac disease. *Gut*, **10**, 57
97. Pettingale, K. W. (1970). Immunoglobulin and specific antibody responses to antigenic stimulation in adult coeliac disease. *Clin. Sci.*, **38**, 16
98. Mawhinney, H. and Love, A. H. G. (1975). The immunoglobulin class responses to oral poliovaccine in coeliac disease. *Clin. Exp. Immunol.*, **22**, 47
99. Baker, P. G., Verrier-Jones, J., Peacock, D. B. and Read, A. E. (1975). The immune response to $\phi \times 174$ in man. III. Evidence for an association between hyposplenism and immunodeficiency in patients with coeliac disease. *Gut*, **16**, 538

100. Seah, P. P., Fry, L., Hoffbrand, A. V. and Holborow, E. J. (1971). Tissue antibodies in dermatitis herpetiformis and adult coeliac disease. *Lancet*, **i**, 834
101. Lancaster-Smith, M. J. and Strickland, I. D. (1971). Autoantibodies in adult coeliac disease. *Lancet*, **i**, 1244
102. Ferguson, A. and McNeish, A. S. (1970). Coeliac disease. *Scot. Med. J.*, **15**, 118
103. Goudie, R. B., Stuart-Smith, D. A., Boyle, I. T. and Ferguson, A. (1969). Serological diagnosis of idiopathic Addison's disease in patients on prolonged prednisolone therapy for steatorrhoea. *Lancet*, **i**, 186
104. Alp, M. H. and Wright, R. (1971). Autoantibodies to reticulin in patients with idiopathic steatorrhoea, coeliac disease and Crohn's disease and their relation to immunoglobulins and dietary antibodies. *Lancet*, **ii**, 682
105. Seah, P. P., Fry, L., Holborow, E. J., Rossiter, M. A., Doe, W. F., Magalhaes, A. F. and Hoffbrand, A. V. (1973). Antireticulin antibody: incidence and diagnostic significance. *Gut*, **14**, 311
106. Gough, K. R., Read, A. E. and Naish, J. M. (1962). Intestinal reticulosis as a complication of idiopathic steatorrhoea. *Gut*, **3**, 232
107. Harris, O. D., Cooke, W. T., Thompson, H. and Waterhouse, J. A. H. (1967). Malignancy in adult coeliac disease and idiopathic steatorrhoea. *Am. J. Med.*, **42**, 899
108. Ferguson, A., McClure, J. P. and Townley, R. R. W. (1976). Intra-epithelial lymphocyte counts in children with diarrhoea. *Acta Paed. Scand.* In press
109. Holmes, G. K. T., Asquith, P., Stokes, P. L. and Cooke, W. T. (1974). Cellular infiltrate of jejunal biopsies in adult coeliac disease in relation to gluten withdrawal. *Gut*, **15**, 278
110. Fry, L., Seah, P. P., McMinn, R. M. H. and Hoffbrand, A. V. (1972). Lymphocytic infiltration of epithelium in diagnosis of gluten sensitive enteropathy. *Br. Med. J.*, **3**, 371
111. Kumar, P. J., Silk, D. B. A., Marks, R., Clark, M. L. and Dawson, A. M. (1973). Treatment of dermatitis herpetiformis with corticosteroids and a gluten-free diet: a study of jejunal morphology and function. *Gut*, **14**, 280
112. Montgomery, R. D. and Shearer, A. C. I. (1974). The cell population of the upper jejunal mucosa in tropical sprue and post-infective malabsorption. *Gut*, **15**, 387
113. Lancaster-Smith, M., Kumar, P. J. and Dawson, A. M. (1975). The cellular infiltrate of the jejunum in adult coeliac disease and dermatitis herpetiformis following reintroduction of dietary gluten. *Gut*, **16**, 683
114. Ferguson, R., Asquith, P. and Cooke, W. T. (1974). The jejunal cellular infiltrate in coeliac disease complicated by lymphoma. *Gut*, **15**, 458
115. Ferguson, R., Allan, R. N. and Cooke, W. T. (1975). A study of the cellular infiltrate of the proximal jejunal mucosa in ulcerative colitis and Crohn's disease. *Gut*, **16**, 205

116. Pettingale, K. W. (1971). Immunoglobulin-containing cells in the coeliac syndrome. *Gut*, **12**, 291
117. Soltoft, J. (1970). Immunoglobulin-containing cells in non-tropical sprue. *Clin. Exp. Immunol.*, **6**, 413
118. Baklien, K., Brandtzaeg, P., Fausa, O. and Gjone, E. (1972). Mapping of immunocyte distribution in human intestinal mucosa. *Scand. J. Gastroenterol.* (*Suppl*), **16**, 13
119. Shiner, R. J. and Ballard, J. (1973). Mucosal secretory IgA and secretory piece in adult coeliac disease. *Gut*, **14**, 778
120. Jos, J. and Labbe, F. (1975). Ultrastructural localization of immunoglobulins in normal and coeliac intestinal mucosa using peroxidase-labelled antibodies. *Communication to the European Society for Paediatric Gastroenterology.*
122. Taylor, K. B., Thomson, D. L., Truelove, S. C. and Wright, R. (1961). An immunological study of coeliac disease and idiopathic steatorrhoea. *Br. Med. J.*, **2**, 1727
122. Falchuk, Z. M., Gebhard, R. L. and Strober, W. (1974). The pathogenesis of gluten sensitive enteropathy (coeliac sprue): organ culture studies. In *Coeliac Disease.* W. Th. J. M. Hekkens and A. S. Pena (eds.) p. 107 (Leiden: Stenfer-Kroese)
123. Falchuk, Z. M. and Strober, W. (1974). Gluten sensitive enteropathy: synthesis of anti-gliadin antibody *in vitro. Gut*, **15**, 947
124. Falchuk, Z. M., Gebhard, R. L., Sessoms, C. and Strober, W. (1974). An *in vitro* model of gluten sensitive enteropathy: the effects of gliadin on intestinal epithelial cells of patients with gluten-sensitive enteropathy in organ culture. *J. Clin. Invest.*, **53**, 487
125. Perlmann, P., Perlman, H. and Wigzell, H. (1972). Lymphocyte mediated cytotoxicity *in vitro.* Induction and inhibition by humoral antibody and nature of effector cells. *Transpl. Rev.*, **13**, 91
126. Ezeoke, A., Ferguson, N., Fakhri, O., Hekkens, W. Th. J. M. and Hobbs, J. R. (1974). Antibodies in the sera of coeliac patients which can co-opt K cells to attack gluten-labelled targets. In *Coeliac Disease.* W. Th. J. M. Hekkens and A. S. Pena (eds.) p. 176 (Leiden: Stenfert-Kroese)
127. Kenrick, K. G. and Walker-Smith, J. A. (1970). Immunoglobulins and dietary protein antibodies in childhood coeliac disease. *Gut*, **11**, 635
128. Carswell, F. and Ferguson, A. (1973). Plasma food antibodies during withdrawal and reintroduction of dietary gluten in coeliac disease. *Arch. Dis. Child.*, **48**, 583
129. Trier, J. S. and Browning, T. H. (1970). Epithelial cell renewal in cultured duodenal biopsies in coeliac sprue. *New Eng. J. Med.*, **283**, 1245
130. Ferguson, A., McClure, J. P. and Holden, R. J. (1976). The effects of *in vitro* culture on the lymphoid cells of human jejunum. In press
131. Hamilton, J. R. and McNeill, L. K. (1972). Childhood celiac disease: response of untreated patients to a small uniform daily dose of wheat gluten. *J. Pediatr.*, **81**, 885

132. Doe, W. F., Henry, K. and Booth, C. C. (1974). Complement in coeliac disease. In *Coeliac Disease*. W. Th. J. M. Hekkens and A. S. Pena (eds.) p. 189 (Leiden: Stenfert-Kroese)
133. Rubin, C. E., Brandborg, L. L., Flick, A. L., Phelps, P., Parmentier, C. and van Niel, S. (1962). Studies of celiac sprue: III. The effect of repeated wheat instillation into the proximal ileum of patients on a gluten-free diet. *Gastroenterology*, **43**, 621
134. Bayless, T. M., Rubin, S. E., Topping, T. M., Yardley, J. H. and Hendrix, T. R. (1970). Morphological and functional effects of gluten feeding on jejunal mucosa in coeliac disease. In *Coeliac Disease*, C. C. Booth and R. H. Dowling (eds.) p. 76 (Edinburgh: Churchill-Livingstone)
135. Kendall, M. J., Cox, P. S., Schneider, R. and Hawkins, C. F. (1972). Gluten subfractions in coeliac disease. *Lancet*, **ii**, 1065
136. Frazer, A. C., Fletcher, R. F., Ross, C. A. C., Shaw, B., Sammons, H. C. and Schneider, R. (1959). Gluten-induced enteropathy. The effect of partially digested gluten. *Lancet*, **ii**, 252
137. Dissanayake, A. S., Jerrome, D. W., Offord, R. D., Truelove, S. C. and Whitehead, R. (1974). Identifying toxic fractions of wheat gluten and their effect on the jejunal mucosa in coeliac disease. *Gut*, **15**, 931
138. Shiner, M. and Ballard, J. (1972). Antigen-antibody reactions in jejunal mucosa in childhood coeliac disease after gluten challenge. *Lancet*, **i**, 1202
139. Shiner, M. (1973). Ultrastructural changes suggestive of immune reactions in the jejunal mucosa of coeliac children following gluten challenge. *Gut*, **14**, 1
140. Lancaster-Smith, M., Kumar, P. J. and Clark, M. L. (1974). Immunological phenomena following gluten challenge in the jejunum of patients with adult coeliac disease and dermatitis herpetiformis. In *Coeliac Disease*, W. Th. J. M. Hekkens and A. S. Pena (eds.) p. 173 (Leiden: Stenfert-Kroese)
141. McNeish, A. S., Rolles, C. J. and Thompson, R. A. (1974). Complement and its degradation products after challenge with gluten in children with coeliac disease. In *Coeliac Disease*, W. Th. J. M. Hekkens and A. S. Pena (eds.) p. 197 (Leiden: Stenfert-Kroese)
142. Jos, J., Lenoir, G., de Ritis, G. and Rey, J. (1974). *In vitro* culturing of biopsies from children. In *Coeliac Disease*, W. Th. J. M. Hekkens and A. S. Pena (eds.) p. 91 (Leiden: Stenfert-Kroese)
143. Kuitunen, P., Tiilikainen, A. and Visakorpi, J. K. (1975). Histocompatibility antigens (HL-A) in cows' milk intolerance and malabsorption syndrome in children. *Communication to the European Society for Paediatric Gastroenterology*
144. Freier, S. (1974). Allergic mechanisms in intestinal cows' milk intolerance. *Acta Paediatr. Scand.*, **63**, 651
145. Freier, S. (1974). Paediatric gastrointestinal allergy. In *Clinical Immunology—Allergy in Paediatric Medicine*. J. Brostoff (ed.) p. 107 (Oxford: Blackwell)

146. Freier, S., Kletter, B., Gery, I. and Lebenthal, M. D. (1969). Intolerance to milk protein. *J. Pediatr.*, **75**, 623
147. Shiner, M., Ballard, J. and Smith, M. E. (1975). The small intestinal mucosa in cows' milk allergy. *Lancet*, **i**, 136
148. Cadranel, S., Rodesch, P., Mozin, M. J. and Loeb, H. (1974). Pitfalls in treatment of cows' milk intolerance: soy milk intolerance. *Arch. Paediatr. Scand.*, **63**, 563
149. Ament, M. E. and Rubin, C. E. (1972). Soy protein—another cause of flat intestinal lesion. *Gastroenterology*, **62**, 227
150. Matthews, T. S. and Soothill, J. F. (1970). Complement activation after milk feeding in children with cows' milk allergy. *Lancet*, **ii**, 893

CHAPTER 6

Autoimmune and inflammatory diseases of the gastrointestinal tract

D. P. Jewell and H. J. F. Hodgson

Introduction

This chapter concerns three diseases of the gut of unknown aetiology—pernicious anaemia, ulcerative colitis and Crohn's disease. In each there is mucosal inflammation which, by creating greater permeability to antigen present in the lumen, will stimulate local and systemic immune responses. It is therefore not surprising that many immunological phenomena have been described. Much interest has centred around the possibility that these diseases are caused by responses directed towards 'self-antigens', and around the mechanisms by which these responses might arise. These include mucosal inflammation itself which may alter mucosal antigens or reveal those previously sequestered, and the possession of common antigens by mucosa and intestinal micro-organisms. It also seems likely that the ability to mount these responses is partly genetically controlled.

Pernicious anaemia

The gastric mucosa is a complex structure containing many cell types—parietal cells producing acid and intrinsic factor, pepsinogen-producing chief cells, epithelial cells and mucus neck cells, which may be the stem cells[1]. In addition, the mucosa contains the endocrine APUD cells, which secrete a variety of polypeptide hormones.

All of these cells have been shown to contain specific antigens. Leaving aside the APUD cells, a specific antigen has been demonstrated in gastric epithelial cells[2] and antibodies raised in rabbits to purified pepsinogens will stain chief cells using immunofluorescent techniques[3]. Using isolated guinea pig parietal cells four antigens within the parietal cell have been defined, namely intrinsic factor, an antigen associated with the cell membrane, the canalicular antigen and a cytosol antigen[4]. These antigens appear to be entirely cell-specific but not species-specific. Although antibodies can be raised experimentally to all of these antigens, only antibodies to intrinsic factor and to the parietal call canalicular antigen have been found in human sera, even though the epithelial and chief cells are involved as much as the parietal cells in chronic inflammatory diseases of the gastric mucosa.

Although antibody to intrinsic factor and to the canalicular antigen are characteristic of pernicious anaemia, their pathogenicity as auto-antibodies is by no means established. Other factors may be important and evidence is now accumulating that lymphocytes from these patients may be sensitized to gastric antigens, implying that cell-mediated immune responses may also be involved in the pathogenesis of the disease. The strong association between pernicious anaemia and other diseases thought to be immunologically-mediated, such as thyroid disease, serves to emphasize the probable role of an underlying immunological mechanism in the pathogenesis of the gastric mucosal lesion.

As will become apparent in the following discussion, an atrophic gastritis may be caused by a number of mechanisms, not all of which are immunological, and the problem is to define whether a given immunological response is secondary to tissue damage or whether that response has a pathogenetic role.

Genetic influences

Studies of the relatives of patients with pernicious anaemia have shown that it is a familial disease[5-7]. The frequency of pernicious anaemia or the latent form of the disease has been estimated as about 20% amongst the families of patients although this is almost certainly an underestimate in view of the difficulties in diagnosing latent pernicious anaemia[5,7]. The disease affects first-degree relatives more commonly than the more remote relatives[6,8].

The relatives of patients with pernicious anaemia also show a higher frequency of antibodies both to the parietal cell canalicular antigen and to intrinsic factor, when compared with control subjects[6,7,9,10]. Female relatives show a higher incidence of antibodies than male relatives and, again, first-degree relatives show a higher frequency than second-degree relatives. Antibodies to thyroid were found more frequently in the relatives of patients than controls by Doniach and Roitt[9]. The Oxford study showed a similar trend although the differences did not reach statistical significance[7].

At the present time there are no published studies reporting the frequency of HL-A types in patients with pernicious anaemia and their relatives. Such information would be of great interest in view of the fact that HL-A1 and 8 are said to occur more commonly in thyroid disorders and diabetes; diseases which are associated with pernicious anaemia.

Associated diseases

Patients with pernicious anaemia have a higher incidence of other diseases which are associated with organ-specific antibodies. These other diseases include thyroid disorders (thyrotoxicosis, myxedema, Hashimoto's thyroiditis), Addison's disease, hypoparathyroidism, diabetes mellitus and vitiligo. Patients with pernicious anaemia also have an increased frequency of circulating autoantibodies associated with these diseases. The most striking example is that of the thyroid where

Table 6.1 THE FREQUENCY OF GASTRIC AUTOANTIBODIES

	No. tested	*Parietal canalicular antibody % positive*	*Intrinsic factor antibody % positive*	*Reference*
Healthy subjects	87	NT	0	6
	3492	4·8	NT	217
Pernicious anaemia	143	86	44	21
	137	83	70	23
	132	79·5	53	7
Atrophic gastritis	29	34	10	218
	48	44	0	219
Thyroid disease	300	22	5	220
	394	32	NT	40
Diabetes mellitus	671	20		224
(Insulin dependent)	380 (females)		3·4	224
	200	28	4	222
Addison's disease	35	40	20	225
	63	12	NT	226
Hypoparathyroidism	61	16	NT	227
Iron deficiency	47	17	NT	221
	64	20	NT	223

NT = not tested

up to 50% of patients with pernicious anaemia may have antibodies to thyroid[11]. Table 6.1 shows the frequency of the parietal canalicular antibody in the other organ-specific autoimmune disorders. It can be seen that the antibody occurs commonly in each of the disease categories, and that it is found in about 20–30% of patients regardless of the diagnosis. The factors which determine the appearance of the canalicular antibody in such a constant proportion of patients with these organ-specific autoimmune disorders are unknown, but it would be interesting to relate the presence of this antibody to HL-A status.

Antibodies to intrinsic factor

Patients with pernicious anaemia fail to absorb vitamin B_{12} because of very low levels of intrinsic factor in the gastric juice. Intrinsic factor is a glycoprotein having a molecular weight of approximately 60 000[12]. In man, it is secreted by the parietal cell[13,14] and, using immunofluorescent techniques, it appears to be situated peripherally within the cell[14]. Secretion may be stimulated by histamine or pentagastrin in healthy subjects, but in patients with chronic gastritis there is a reduction in the output of intrinsic factor[15]. The degree to which secretion is impaired, with a corresponding fall in the absorption of vitamin B_{12}, correlates with the severity of the gastric mucosal lesion[16].

In 1959, Taylor[17] described a factor in the sera of patients with pernicious anaemia which blocked the action of hog intrinsic factor in promoting B_{12} absorption. A similar factor was described by Schwartz[18]. This inhibitory factor was thought to be an antibody to intrinsic factor and this was confirmed by immunological and electrophoretic studies[19]. Subsequent work has shown that two antibodies to intrinsic factor occur. Type I or blocking antibody is directed towards the site on the intrinsic factor molecule which combines with vitamin B_{12} and it therefore prevents the free vitamin combining with intrinsic factor[6,20]. Type II or binding antibody reacts with a site on the intrinsic factor molecule which is distant from the vitamin B_{12} combining site[20–22]. This antibody can, therefore, combine with either free intrinsic factor or the intrinsic factor–B_{12} complex.

The Type I antibody occurs in the serum of about 70% of patients with pernicious anaemia[23,24], although, in one series from India, no intrinsic factor antibody was found in a group of patients with pernicious anaemia, even though the parietal cell canalicular antibody was present with the expected frequency[25]. Type II antibody occurs less commonly, being found in the serum of 35–40% of patients with pernicious anaemia[23,26].

Both the frequency and the height of the titre of Type II antibody are directly proportional to the concentration of Type I antibody, so that Type II antibody rarely occurs in the absence of Type I antibody[23]. These authors also found Type II antibody to be present more commonly in patients with blood group O than in patients with blood group A. On the basis of experimental work, Samloff and Turner[20] have suggested that the immunogenicity of the antigenic site for Type I antibody is greater than that for Type II and that the immunogenicity of both sites is potentiated by complexing with B_{12}. The immunoglobulin class of the serum antibodies is mainly IgG[27] and there is light-chain heterogeneity[28] indicating that they are not produced from a single clone of antibody-forming cells. IgA antibody of either type appears to be uncommon in serum.

Both types of antibody have been found in gastric juice and may occur with greater frequency than in serum[27,29,30]. Type I antibody may be entirely complexed to intrinsic factor in the gastric juice and, in these circumstances, may only be detected following acid dissociation of the complexes[31,32]. The immunoglobulin class of both types of antibody may be either IgG or IgA[27,32]. In addition, they may also be present as secretory IgA antibody[32,33]. However, there appears to be no correlation between the immunoglobulin class of the Type II antibody in serum and in the gastric juice, suggesting that the serum and juice antibodies may be formed at different sites. Similar data for Type I antibody is not available.

There is very little known about the sites of formation of these antibodies. However, using a double-labelling technique, it has been shown that Type II antibody of IgG class can be detected in the plasma cells of the gastric mucosa[27,34]. No IgA type II antibody was found within plasma cells which is an intriguing finding since IgA Type II antibody is frequently present in gastric juice and IgA-producing plasma cells predominate in the lamina propria.

Antibody to the parietal cell canaliculus

Following the discovery of circulating antibody to intrinsic factor in the sera of some patients with pernicious anaemia, evidence was obtained for another antibody which was commonly present in these sera and which was directed towards a parietal cell antigen distinct from intrinsic factor. This second antibody was detected by either complement fixation or immunofluoresence[21,35], although immunofluoresence provided the more sensitive test. The antigen to which the antibody is directed is specific to the parietal cell and does not cross-react with other tissues including the thyroid. However, it is not species-specific and is present in the parietal cells of a wide variety of species[36]. The antigen is found in the microsomal fraction of the cell[37] and Ward and Nairn[38] have shown that the greatest antigen activity is associated with smooth cytoplasmic membrane vesicles. The antigen has been localized to the microvillus membranes of the secretory canaliculus by electron microscopic examination of gastric mucosal sections to which canalicular antibody labelled with horse-radish peroxidase has been applied[39].

Protein and lipid are essential components of the antigen since it is destroyed by proteolytic enzymes (papain, trypsin), organic solvents (ethanol, butanol) and surface-active agents[37,38]. Attempts to isolate the pure antigen have been unsuccessful and it has, therefore, been presumed to be an insoluble lipoprotein associated with the cell membranes[37,38].

Antibody to the canalicular antigen is found in about 90% of sera from patients with pernicious anaemia[21,23,24,40] although it occurs less often in patients over the age of sixty[21,40]. Female patients have been reported to have a higher incidence of canalicular antibody than male patients[7]. They are usually of IgG immunoglobulin class, IgA antibody occurring less frequently[27].

Canalicular antibody is also present in gastric juice in patients with pernicious anaemia, although less frequently than in the serum. The immunoglobulin class of the antibody may be IgG or IgA and both classes of antibody may occur together[27]. As with intrinsic factor antibody, no correlation exists between the immunoglobulin class of the serum antibody and the antibody in gastric juice, but IgG antibody tends to be more common in serum and IgA antibody more common in the juice. Whether the IgA antibody in gastric juice is secretory IgA is not known. Plasma cells in gastric mucosa from patients with pernicious anaemia have been shown to produce canalicular antibody[41], but the immunoglobulin class of this locally produced antibody has not been determined.

Cell-mediated immunity

Evidence is accumulating that, in some patients with pernicious anaemia, peripheral blood lymphocytes may be sensitized to a variety of gastric antigens. Tai and McGuigan[42] using the lymphocyte transformation test showed that the lymphocytes from six patients out of a total of 16 patients with pernicious anaemia underwent blast transformation in the presence of concentrated gastric juice. In a rather smaller proportion of patients, the lymphocytes responded to a partly purified preparation of human intrinsic factor. However, since the intrinsic factor preparation was not pure, the authors are right to caution the conclusion that intrinsic factor is the antigen responsible for the blast transformation. Similar experiments were unsuccessful in the hands of Fixa *et al.*[43], but they were able to show that commercial hog intrinsic factor inhibited the migration of leukocytes from patients with pernicious anaemia to a significantly greater extent than leukocytes from control subjects[44]. Another study showed that the migration of leukocytes could be inhibited by human gastric intrinsic factor in 40% of patients with pernicious anaemia[45] and, more recently, James *et al.* have reported similar findings[46]. These latter authors, using both the leukocyte migration inhibition test and lymphocyte transformation, found evicence of cell-mediated immunity to intiinsic factor in 86% of patients with pernicious anaemia.

Unfortunately, a critical assessment of the data reveals many inadequacies: the reproducibility of the methods used is not discussed, some studies do not mention whether single or multiple cultures were set up, and the details of the intrinsic factor preparation are not always stated. A more serious objection is the conclusion that intrinsic factor is the antigen responsible for the observed effect when gastric juice or only a partially purified intrinsic factor is used as antigen. The essential control, namely, culture of lymphocytes in gastric juice not containing intrinsic factor, was not included in the studies mentioned so far. The presence of antigens in gastric juice other than intrinsic factor has been shown by Finlayson *et al.*[47]. They found that human gastric juice inhibited the migration of leukocytes in nine out of 12 patients with pernicious anaemia and in one out of seven controls. However, following the filtration of gastric juice on Sephadex G200, they were able to show that fractions which did not contain B_{12}-binding substances were still able to inhibit leukocyte migration in some of the patients.

The presence of circulating sensitized lymphocytes to intrinsic factor is therefore probable, although not proven. However, the significance of cell-mediated immunity in the pathogenesis of pernicious anaemia is largely speculative. Intrinsic factor is certainly not the only gastric antigen which may elicit a cellular immune response. Cellular immunity to gastric mitochondria, gastric microsomes and liver mitochondria has been demonstrated in patients with pernicious anaemia using the leukocyte migration inhibition test[43,49], and evidence for cellular hypersensitivity to non-B_{12}-binding antigens in gastric juice has alreadv been cited. It is interesting that Goldstone *et al.*[49] were unable to demonstrate migration inhibition to a human intrinsic factor preparation although a crude extract of human gastric mucosa inhibited leukocyte migration in 50% of their patients with pernicious anaemia.

Finally, there appears to be no relation between a cell-mediated response to intrinsic factor and the presence of circulating antibody[44,45,47]. Tai and McGuigan[42] found an inverse relationship in so far as blocking (Type I) antibody was absent in the sera of all the patients whose lymphocytes transformed in response to gastric antigens. Binding (Type II) antibody was detected in the serum of one patient whose lymphocytes responded to concentrated gastric juice.

Immunological mechanisms of tissue damage

The available evidence which has been summarized so far is suggestive that an immune response is mounted to self-antigens in patients with pernicious anaemia and that a variety of immunological effector mechanisms may be involved in the pathogenesis of the disease. However, conclusive evidence that such mechanisms are operating is still lacking and it can be reasonably doubted whether any of the immunological phenomena described are of primary aetiological significance. The histological lesion of pernicious anaemia shows features compatible with immunologically-mediated tissue damage but it is indistinguishable from atrophic gastritis found in patients without pernicious anaemia. The situation is further complicated by the fact that atrophic gastritis without pernicious anaemia may be associated with some of the immunological findings found in pernicious anaemia. Certain differences do emerge, however. Table 6.1 shows that only about 40% of these patients have the canalicular antibody in their sera and, in contrast to pernicious anaemia, antibody to intrinsic factor is rarely present. Goldstone *et al.*[49], during their study of the cell-mediated responses to gastric antigens in pernicious anaemia, found that the results obtained using leukocytes from patients with atrophic gastritis without pernicious anaemia did not differ significantly from control data. The number of patients tested was small but, nevertheless, certain patients did show evidence of cellular hypersensitivity to liver mitochondria and one patient's cells appeared to be sensitized to gastric mitochondria.

In a recent review of the problem, Strickland and MacKay[50] have divided atrophic gastritis into two groups. Type A is described as an autoimmune gastritis which characteristically occurs in patients with pernicious anaemia. It affects only the mucosa of the body of the stomach so that the antrum is histologically normal. There is a very high frequency of gastric autoantibodies and the majority of the patients have raised fasting levels of gastrin and an increased G cell mass in the antrum[51]. Type B, on the other hand, is an atrophic gastritis affecting both body and antral mucosa. This group has a low frequency of gastric autoantibodies (10%) and does not have the hypergastrinaemia of Type A, the decreased G cell mass presumably being secondary to the antritis. The aetiology of this group is probably multiple and might include non-specific mucosal irritants. This is an attractive classification and may serve to delineate different aetiologies but it relies mainly on the criterion of a normal antrum. In the authors' experience, antral biopsies taken at endoscopy from patients with pernicious anaemia frequently show some histological abnormality which therefore casts doubt upon the view that the antrum is spared in the atrophic gastritis associated with pernicious anaemia. A systematic study of the antrum in these patients, using fibreoptic endoscopy, will be needed before this point can be solved.

The role of gastric antibodies: In common with other autoantibodies, the role of gastric antibodies in producing the mucosal lesion is still largely speculative. The canalicular antibody is rarely found in the absence of gastritis but, on the other hand, it is infrequently present in cases of Type B gastritis and it is not associated with the gastritis found in patients with gastric ulcer, gastric cancer or with post-gastrectomy gastritis[52,53]. Antibody to intrinsic factor is even more specific and rarely occurs in the absence of pernicious anaemia or its latent form. Such specificity argues against these antibodies being epiphenomena secondary to mucosal damage from whatever cause.

However, pernicious anaemia does occur in patients whose serum and gastric juice does not contain antibody to either the canalicular antigen or intrinsic factor and it is now well documented that the disease may occur in patients with hypogammaglobulinaemia[54]. When pernicious anaemia does occur in association with such a humoral immune deficiency state, it tends to differ from the classical disease in a number of respects. It tends to occur at an early age, antibodies to intrinsic factor and the canalicular antigen are absent, and the fasting serum gastrin levels are not elevated[55]. This latter finding suggests that the gastric mucosal lesion affects both body and antral mucosa but, so far, no systematic study of gastric histology has been made. Nevertheless, it shows that atrophic gastritis severe enough to produce pernicious anaemia can occur in the absence of specific antibody or of circulating immunoglobulin although it has not been shown that antibody to the gastric antigens is not produced locally in the gastric mucosa of these patients. It is tempting to speculate that cell-mediated immune responses may therefore be responsible for the mucosal lesion and, indeed, cellular hypersensitivity to gastric antigens has been reported in some of these patients[46]. Since patients with certain types of immune deficiency are known to have bacterial and parasitic overgrowth in the gastrointestinal tract, it is conceivable that the atrophic gastritis observed may be caused by such agents and may not involve a primary immune mechanism at all.

Despite the fact that, at least in some types of pernicious anaemia, autoantibodies may not be involved in the pathogenesis of the disease, there is some evidence that they might have a pathogenic role in those patients in which they occur. As far as intrinsic factor antibody is concerned, Rose and Chanarin[56] have shown that the absorption of vitamin B_{12} can be correlated with the presence of antibody so that absorption is least in those patients with antibody in both gastric juice and serum. Higher levels of absorption are found in patients with antibody in gastric juice only and still greater levels are found in patients with serum antibody but without antibody in their gastric juice. It has already been mentioned that, when Type I antibody occurs, intrinsic factor–antibody complexes are commonly found in gastric juice. In other words, when the output of intrinsic factor falls because of mucosal damage, the absorption of vitamin B_{12} may be compromised even further by the presence of Type I intrinsic factor antibody in the gastric juice. This will prevent vitamin B_{12} combining with the already small quantities of intrinsic factor available and may therefore precipitate a frank B_{12} deficiency state.

Evidence that circulating intrinsic factor antibodies can induce mucosal damage is much less certain. Some patients have been known to have intrinsic factor antibodies in their sera for many years without developing vitamin B_{12} malabsorption[45]. However, they all had an atrophic gastritis and therefore the preservation of vitamin B_{12} absorption may be more related to the absence of antibody in the gastric juice. Fisher and Taylor[57] reported the passive transfer of intrinsic factor antibody across the placenta of mothers with pernicious anaemia and the infants continued to have circulating antibody for many weeks. They did not develop either achlorhydria or antibody in the gastric juice suggesting that the antibody had no direct effect on the gastric mucosa but the precise histology was not available. The only direct evidence that circulating antibodies to intrinsic factor can cause mucosal damage is based on experiments in rats which have been reported in abstract form only[58]. Rats were injected with IgG–intrinsic factor antibody which had been prepared either from the sera of patients with pernicious anaemia or from rabbits immunized with intrinsic factor. Following repeated injections, the gastric mucosa showed an atrophy of the chief cells, which produce intrinsic factor in the rat, but without any inflammatory response.

Similar experiments in rats, using repeated injections of human IgG parietal cell canalicular antibody, have shown changes affecting the parietal cells[59]. The parietal cell mass was reduced with a concomitant reduction in gastric acid secretion but, again, no inflammatory response was provoked.

Inhibition of acid production by the human canalicular antibody has also been shown using bull-frog gastric mucosa in an *in vitro* system[60]. An acute inflammatory lesion of the gastric mucosa induced by antibody has also been reported[61]. Antisera to guinea pig gastric mucosal antigens were first made in rabbits. The globulin, which included antibody to parietal cell canaliculi, was then injected into guinea pigs and resulted in an acute reaction in the gastric mucosa which had the features of an Arthus reaction. The reaction appeared to be specific since injections of antibody to colonic mucosa did not produce a gastric lesion.

In contrast to these passive transfer experiments, attempts to induce gastritis in experimental animals by active immunization with gastric antigens have been less successful and show considerable species specificity. No definitive gastritis has been induced in rats, guinea pigs or rabbits even though immunization has induced the production of autoantibodies to the parietal cell canalicular antigen. However, patchy areas of atrophic gastritis with some inflammatory infiltrate, as well as circulating gastric autoantibodies have been induced in dogs following immunization with either canine gastric juice or gastric mucosal extracts by a number of workers[62–64]. Andrada *et al.*[65] have also induced a multifocal gastritis in Rhesus monkeys by immunizing them with repeated injections of monkey gastric mucosal suspensions in complete Freund's adjuvant. Not only did the animals develop a mucosal lesion, but they developed parietal cell antibodies in the serum and the serum complement levels, measured as CH_{50}, fell progressively during the experiment.

There is good evidence that the antibody to the canalicular antigen is able to fix complement *in vitro* in the presence of antigen and this has formed the basis of the complement-fixation test originally used to detect the antibody in serum. Whether or not complement can be fixed within gastric mucosa *in vivo* is much less certain although te Velde *et al.*[10] have reported some immunofluorescent observations showing that complement can be detected on parietal cells in tissue sections exposed to serum containing the canalicular antibody. Similar studies have been reported by Jacob and Glass[66]. These latter authors also demonstrated lower serum complement levels (CH50) in patients with pernicious anaemia and in patients with atrophic gastritis of varying aetiology. However, no correlation existed between the complement level and the titre of either canalicular or intrinsic factor antibody. Intrinsic factor antibodies have been generally regarded as non-complement fixing, but fluorescent studies suggest that these antibodies can fix complement when they combine with intrinsic factor in the parietal cell[67].

Despite the experimental observations and the evidence suggesting complement fixation within the mucosa, direct evidence that gastric autoantibodies are cytotoxic to parietal cells, whether in the presence of complement or not, is not available at the present time.

The role of cell-mediated responses: Our knowledge of the significance of lymphocytes sensitized to gastric antigens in the pathogenesis of atrophic gastritis is even more speculative than our knowledge of antibody-induced mucosal damage. However, some of the experimental studies which have successfully induced a gastritis in animals have shown that the animals have developed both humoral and cellular immunity to the immunizing gastric antigen. Andrada *et al.*[65] were able to demonstrate delayed skin hypersensitivity to gastric mucosa in their monkeys although the experimental evidence for this is not given. Krohn and Finlayson[64] found that dogs immunized with gastric juice developed positive delayed skin tests and a positive leukocyte migration inhibition test in response to gastric juice antigens. These indices of cellular immunity appeared simultaneously within the first two weeks of the immunization schedule and they appeared earlier than the humoral response. In all the dogs tested, gastritis occurred before antibodies to the parietal cells were detected in the serum suggesting that the cellular mechanisms may have been more important in causing tissue damage than the humoral response. This conclusion is supported by the experiments of Fixa *et al.*[68]. They first immunized dogs with gastric juice and they were then able to induce a gastritis in an unimmunized recipient dog by injecting it with thoracic duct lymphocytes obtained from the immunized animal. Although the gastritis produced is not identical with the mucosal lesion of pernicious anaemia, there was atrophy of the gastric glands, deposition of collagen and a minimal inflammatory infiltrate.

Discussion

Pernicious anaemia is a disease which is characteristically found in the older age groups. It is also true that the frequency of atrophic gastritis and circulatory antibodies to the parietal cell canaliculus increases with age. However, the presence of antibodies to intrinsic factor in either serum or gastric juice remains specific to that group of patients with pernicious anaemia who are also characterized by their apparent genetic predisposition to other putatively autoimmune diseases. Although experimental evidence is accumulating to suggest that both circulating antibodies and sensitized lymphocytes to gastric antigens may cause mucosal damage, the pathogenesis of the disease remains speculative. One possibility, which has not been tested, is that very small quantities of locally produced antibody may mediate K cell cytotoxicity. Another major problem in our understanding of the disease concerns the origin of the gastric autoantibodies. It seems unlikely that they merely represent an immune response secondary to non-specific mucosal injury in so far as they are directed towards only two gastric antigens and that they only occur in certain groups of patients. It may be that the parietal cell shares common determinants with exogenous antigens, such as viruses or bacteria, in a way similar to colonic epithelial cells and *E. coli*. However, in the only study reported which explores this possibility, no cross-reactivity could be found between intrinsic factor and a wide range of bacterial antigens.[69]

Ulcerative colitis

Whilst the aetiology of ulcerative colitis remains obscure, knowledge of the immunological phenomena associated with the condition continues to grow. As with other chronic gastrointestinal diseases, one of the most important unanswered questions is how far these immunological abnormalities are the cause of the disease and how far they are merely secondary to the extensive ulceration and chronic inflammation present in the gut.

THE INFECTIVE THEORIES

Although Wilks differentiated ulcerative colitis from bacillary dysentery in 1859[70], the possibility of a direct infective cause has continued to stimulate research. *Shigella*[71], a diplostreptococcus[72], and *Bacillus necrophorum*[73] have all been suggested as infective agents; Felsen and Wolarsky stated that 10% of their patients hospitalized for acute bacillary dysentery progressed to the clinical picture of ulcerative colitis and that, in 7% of their patients with ulcerative colitis, *Shigella* could be isolated from the faeces[74]. However, although the development of colitis after an episode of apparently infective diarrhea remains a common clinical observation, recent studies have not consistently found pathogenic faecal organisms. Most have found no differences in the species of organisms isolated from patients compared with normal controls, although higher bacterial counts are found in the patients[75]. Interestingly, Cooke found that the strains of *E. coli* she isolated from patients with colitis were more likely to produce haemolysin and necrotoxin and these may reflect enteropathogenic properties[76], but a serial study of patients passing from remission to relapse suggested that such strains were acquired after the onset of symptoms—they may merely, therefore, be more favoured secondary colonizers of damaged mucosa[77].

Early viral investigations, using tissue-culture techniques, and attempts to transfer the condition using cell-free filtrates, were negative[78]. Recently, however, there have been a number of case reports linking cytomegalovirus infection and ulcerative colitis[79]. Farmer and his associates found that high (>1:8) titres of cytomegalovirus antibody were nearly twice as frequent in patients with colitis as in the general population, and, in three patients, tissue culture of colonic cells showed the presence of the virus, as judged by cytopathogenic effects, indirect immunofluorescence and electron microscopy[80]. Other workers have also shown cytopathogenic effects suggesting viral infection in colonic tissue cultures from patients with ulcerative colitis and Crohn's disease[81]. Again it remains uncertain whether this is aetiologically significant or whether cytomegalovirus is mainly a secondary invader—the organism has been shown to have a predilection for ulcerated areas of the gastrointestinal tract[82].

No infecting organism has convincingly been shown to be associated with the majority of cases of ulcerative colitis, and certainly Koch's postulates remain unfulfilled. It was probably this existence of chronic inflammation without obvious infection that led to ulcerative colitis being considered an 'immunological' disease. On the other hand, many of the immunological phenomena to be discussed could be explained on the basis of a primary, as yet unidentified, infection.

THE IMMUNOLOGICAL THEORIES

There is evidence of a genetic predisposition to ulcerative colitis, perhaps reflecting an underlying immunological abnormality. 5–16% of patients have relatives with inflammatory bowel disease, usually ulcerative colitis, but a significant proportion have Crohn's disease[83,84]. However, although there is one reported family with eight affected relatives, in an apparently autosomal dominant distribution[85], there is no simple pattern of inheritance. No linkage with common genetic markers, such as blood groups or secretor status has been found[86]. Studies of histocompatibility antigens have shown no HL-A type to appear in definite excess in patients[87,88], although minor differences from control groups are reported. In one report in which a definite increase in HL-A 11 was claimed[89], the statistical methods have been the subject of controversy[90,91]. The only constant pattern has been the demonstration that, in patients with ulcerative colitis and associated ankylosing spondylitis, there is the same association with HL-A W27 that is seen when the latter disease occurs alone[92].

There are certainly environmental factors in addition to genetic ones. This is well illustrated by studies of the disease in the Jewish race. In Baltimore, USA, the incidence amongst Jews appeared to be thrice that in the general population[93]; the authors comment that this may be an apparent association in view of different standards of medical care and difficulties in defining the total population. However, a similar finding is reported by Acheson and Nefzeger[94], who, in a study of all patients admitted to hospital from the US Army in one year in wartime, with a matched control group, found the rate in Jews to be twice as high. On the other hand, a recent study of the Jewish population of Tel-Aviv showed the incidence and prevalence of the disease to be only half those reported for the general population in Baltimore, although the rates in Jews whose country of birth was in the Western hemisphere were significantly higher than Israeli- or Asian-born Jews[95].

There are reports of ulcerative colitis in association with 'autoimmune' disorders, such as Hashimoto's disease[96], pernicious anaemia[97], systemic lupus erythematosus[98] and autoimmune haemolytic anaemia[99], and this has been thought to be aetiologically significant. However, in recent studies, it does not appear that antinuclear, parietal cell or antithyroid antibodies are any commoner than in controls[100,101]. Atopic disorders, however, may be more common[102].

More formal tests of immunological status do not differ from normal in these patients. Total serum immunoglobulin levels are normal[103], although secretory IgA may be found in the circulation more commonly[104]. The disease may, however, occur in the markedly hypogammaglobulinaemic patient[105]. Most authors have found the cellular arm of the immune response to be normal, as shown by Mantoux testing[106], the ability to become sensitive to dinitrochlorobenzene[106], and the ability of lymphocytes to transform to non-specific mitogens such as phytohaemagglutinin[107,108]. A study of peripheral lymphocytes showed normal proportions of B- and T-cells, although total numbers were depressed due to an overall lymphopenia and the immunoglobulin markers of the B-cells showed fewer IgG bearing and more IgA bearing cells[109].

It appears that, within the limitations of the methods currently available, the basic immune response mechanisms of colitic patients are intact. Whether triggering of these mechanisms can lead to the disease will be discussed in terms of potential antigens—food allergens, bacterial antigens and the colon itself.

Allergy to dietary antigens: Ulcerative colitis has been attributed to food allergens and many foodstuffs have been suggested—eggs, nuts, milk, tomatoes and so on. Therapeutic successes following allergen-free diets have been claimed, but this is obviously difficult to assess in a condition characterized by apparently spontaneous remissions and relapses.

Much attention has been directed to milk. It is the only foodstuff that has been shown in a controlled trial to affect the course of colitis—Wright and Truelove found the incidence of relapses lower in patients on a milk-free diet than on a control diet in which patients were advised to consume milk liberally[110]. It had previously been shown by Taylor and Truelove, using the tanned red cell haemagglutination technique, that patients with colitis have a greater incidence of anti-milk antibodies, which tended to be at higher titre[111]. In the dietary trial, Wright and Truelove found that if initial antibody titres to milk were high, there was a greater chance of relapsing when taking milk, but the response to a milk-free diet in any individual could not be predicted from the antibody titres, and fluctuations in the titres did not mirror clinical progress. Recent studies using a number of different techniques to estimate anti-milk antibodies have not confirmed the rise in antibody titres in ulcerative colitis[112,113].

Some studies have reported that atopic disorders are associated with ulcerative colitis[102], although others have not found this[84]. If this is so, it might be reasonable to seek for a reaginic, IgE mediated, immediate hypersensitivity response to food allergens. Although an immediate response to intrarectal injections of foodstuffs in colitis patients and not in controls has been described[114], there is no long-term follow-up of these studies, and their interpretation is difficult as the colitic mucosa may be non-specifically more sensitive[115]. As far as IgE mediated response to milk antigens is concerned, Jewell and Truelove could find no evidence of this[116].

Anti-colon antibodies and bacterial antigens: The search for circulating antibodies reacting with the colon has proved a fruitful approach to the immunology of this disease. Whilst there is little support for the concept that 'autoantibodies' are directly pathogenic, the demonstration of cross-reactivity between colonic and bacterial antigens has yielded valuable hypotheses concerning the aetiology of ulcerative colitis.

In 1959, Broberger and Perlmann demonstrated anti-colon antibodies in the sera of children with active colitis by gel precipitation and passive haemagglutination techniques[117]. The antigen used was a phenol–water extract of colonic tissue from neonates who died, unfed, on the first day of life—this tissue being used to minimize the bacterial contamination invariably associated with adult tissue. By the haemagglutination technique 28 out of 30 children had anti-colon antibodies. Broberger and Asherson found similar results in children, but could only demonstrate such antibodies in the sera of about 50% of adults with colitis; antibodies were also found in a minority of patients with systemic lupus erythematosus and rheumatoid arthritis[118].

As the human antigen is scarce, the value of colonic tissue from rats raised in a germ-free environment was investigated[119]. One difficulty was the presence of rat antigens apparently similar to human blood group A antigen[120]. Even after test sera were absorbed with group A red cells, most normal sera caused haemagglutination at low titre. Lagerkrantz *et al.* took a haemagglutination titre of greater than 1 : 16 as significant and found elevated titres in 56% of a group of colitic patients of all ages, compared with 15% of controls[121]. The antigen detected in this way was fairly organ-specific, being found in abundance only in colonic mucus and colonic wall tissue, although in small amounts in stomach, small intestine and kidney[119]. It has also been found in extracts of germ-free rat faeces[120].

Whilst the results of haemagglutination tests for anti-colon antibodies have shown similar results in different series, the incidence of antibodies detected by immunofluorescence has varied widely. With germ-free rat colon Lagerkrantz *et al.* found that about half the patients with elevated haemagglutination titres had autoantibodies, the immunofluorescence being localized to the mucosal epithelium and surface mucus[121]. Zeromski *et al.* showed that these autoantibodies could be of any of the three major immunoglobulin classes[122]. Wright and Truelove found specific colonic epithelial cell fluorescence in 15% of their patients[123] and in other series up to 50% of patients' sera have proved positive[124]. On the other hand, some authors have not detected antibodies in this way[125]. Kraft and Kirsner have reviewed the difficulties of the experimental technique and suggested that other than immunological factors may lead to localization of fluorescent staining[125].

In the haemagglutination tests, the importance of germ-free tissue was emphasized. If adult, non-sterile human colon is used as the source of antigen, no difference in agglutinating titres is found between normal people and colitic patients[119]. This is presumably due to the presence of microbial antigens in this tissue and it is known that, for example, almost all human sera contain antibodies to bacterial lipopolysaccharides.

Perlmann *et al.* made the interesting observation that the haemagglutination reaction of sera from patients with ulcerative colitis with the extract of germ-free rat colon could be inhibited by lipopolysaccharide antigen of *E. coli* 014[119]. This antigen is present at high concentration in extracts of this strain. It is probably a family antigen, the Kunin antigen, which is found throughout the strains of *E. coli* in varying concentration[126]. Subsequently it has been shown that patients with ulcerative colitis commonly have significant titres of anti-*E. coli* 014 antibody, but this is rare in control sera[127,128]. The implication that this and maybe other bacterial antigens have common antigenic determinants with colonic tissue, and that antibodies against the colon may arise from an immune response to bacteria, has subsequently gained wide acceptance.

A direct demonstration of this phenomena was given by Asherson and Holborow[129]. Injection of an *E. coli* strain in complete Freund's adjuvant in rabbits led to the development of anti-colon antibodies, demonstrated by immunofluorescence. The antigen appeared localized to the superficial mucosa, mainly the goblet cells, and to the mucus secretory cells lying deeper. Perlmann *et al.* provided further support for cross-reactivity between *E. coli* 014 and colonic antigens[130]. When anti-colon antibodies were raised in rats by injection of germ-free rat or rabbit colon, the haemagglutination reaction of these antibodies with extracts of rat colon was easily inhibited by extracts of *E. coli* 014, but not by extracts from a number of other strains.

An antibody response against bacterial or faecal antigens subsequently acting against the colon makes an attractive hypothesis for the aetiology of ulcerative colitis, but there is not the correlation between anti-colon antibodies and disease activity that would be expected were they primarily pathogenic. Their presence, and the titres to which they are detectable, do not correlate with the clinical status of the patient[121] nor the duration of the disease, and they have been detected in healthy relatives of patients and in some normal people[131]. Also, they are not directly cytotoxic—Broberger and Perlmann showed that fluorescent-labelled antibody from patients with active colitis became bound to human colonic cells in tissue culture, but no damage was observed[132]. Theoretically, anti-colon antibodies may mediate lymphocyte cytotoxicity when combined with colonic epithelium, and this action would not have been seen in tissue culture. Although this particular possibility has not been explored, the direct action of lymphocytes upon colonic epithelial cells has received much attention.

Lymphocyte-induced cytotoxicity: Perlmann and Broberger demonstrated that white cells from the peripheral blood of patients with ulcerative colitis were cytotoxic for human fetal colonic cells in tissue culture as shown by an increased rate of release of isotope from the labelled colonic cells[133]. This event occurred within an hour of adding the leukocytes and was not seen if small intestine, liver or kidney provided the target cells. Watson *et al.* confirmed this, implicating the lymphocyte as the effector cell and demonstrating the effect upon adult human colonic cells[134]. The sera of patients with colitis had no effect upon colonic cells, although cell-free extracts of patients' lymphocytes had the same effect as the lymphocytes themselves. Subsequently, Shorter and his colleagues have shown that this property is present universally in patients with inflammatory bowel disease[135], that it can be inhibited by horse anti-human thymus serum[136], and that the effect disappears within ten days of colectomy[135].

Lymphocyte cytotoxicity towards colonic epithelial cells has been shown to be a much more complex phenomenon by subsequent work. Shorter *et al.* have shown that this cytotoxic capacity is inhibited by incubating the lymphocytes from patients with serum from other patients with ulcerative colitis or Crohn's disease, an effect which is not seen if the lymphocytes are incubated with autologous or normal serum[137]. The cytotoxic effect of patients' lymphocytes could also be inhibited by treating the cells with goat anti-human IgM serum[138]. Furthermore, they have shown that normal lymphocytes may become cytotoxic to colonic epithelial cells. They were able to induce cytotoxicity by incubating lymphocytes from healthy subjects with sera from patients with inflammatory bowel disease for a period of four days; the effect was not seen after 24 hours of incubation[137]. By fractionating patients' sera, it was found that the factor which induced cytotoxicity in normal lymphocytes resided in the high molecular weight fractions and could not be found in those fractions containing monomeric IgG[138].

Shorter has suggested that normal lymphocytes are rendered cytotoxic by 'cytophilic' antibody, but this raises considerable questions in terms of precise immunological mechanisms. The action of other patients' sera in reducing cytotoxicity is also obscure and although the presence of a blocking antibody or an antigen–antibody complex occupying receptors on the lymphocyte surface may be postulated, there is no evidence on this point. There is the interesting possibility that K cell cytotoxicity may be involved and it would be of great interest to know whether sera containing anti-colon antibodies are more effective in inducing cytotoxicity in normal lymphocytes than sera without these antibodies. Although lymphocyte-mediated cytotoxicity, of whatever type, may be the method of tissue damage in ulcerative colitis, the degree of cytotoxicity manifested by all patients' cells is very similar and no correlation between the magnitude of the *in vitro* effect and clinical state has been reported. It is also possible that this phenomenon is secondary to mucosal inflammation.

E. coli lipopolysaccharide extracts have significant effects upon lymphocyte cytotoxicity. Shorter *et al.* showed that pre-incubation of patients' lymphocytes with a lipopolysaccharide extract from *E. coli* O 119:B14 strain leads to a loss of cytotoxicity, suggesting the presence of common determinants between this strain and colonic epithelial cells[139]. Furthermore, normal lymphocytes incubated *in vitro* for four days with this lipopolysaccharide extract became cytotoxic for colonic epithelial cells[140]. Whatever the mechanism, this result, if confirmed and extended, provides the first direct evidence of a link between a response to a bacterial antigen and colonic cell damage.

In addition to lymphocyte-mediated cytotoxicity, which may depend upon serum factors, there is also evidence of classical cellular immunity to colonic and bacterial antigens. Using leukocyte migration inhibition as an index of cellular immunity, Bull and Ignazack showed that peripheral lymphocytes from patients with ulcerative colitis appear to be sensitized to the Kunin common enterobacterial antigen[141]. Bartnik *et al.* confirmed this, and the degree of inhibition appeared to correlate to some extent with disease activity[142]. Lymphocyte sensitivity to colonic antigens has been reported using both the leukocyte migration inhibition and lymphocyte transformation techniques[143,144]. However, Stefani and Fink were unable to show a cellular immune response to either colonic extracts or a lipopolysaccharide extract of *E. coli* 014, but they did find that the ability of patients' lymphocytes to transform in response to other *E. coli* antigens diminished as their clinical state became worse[145,108]. Hinz *et al.* confirmed the fact that patients' lymphocytes did not differ from normal lymphocytes in their response to *E. coli* 014 lipopolysaccharide but were unable to show the reduced reactivity during a relapse[107].

Fink *et al.*[146], using skin tests as an indicator of cellular hypersensitivity, have suggested that a cellular response may be directed towards a determinant which is only revealed following bacterial action on colonic mucosa. They found that patients showed a positive skin test at 48 hours to colonic tissue only when it had previously been incubated with *E. coli*.

THE PATHOGENESIS OF THE DISEASE

1. *Experimental colitis:* Experimentally, colitis has been induced in a number of animal species by immunological procedures. None has produced a colitis which is totally comparable to the human disease, but they illustrate the diversity of responses that the colon may show to exogenous antigens.

Kirsner and his colleagues have induced a colitis in rabbits sensitized to foreign protein. In rabbits sensitized to egg albumen, they reproduced the Arthus phenomenon by multiple subserosal injections of the antigen at operation which produced a necrotizing haemorrhagic lesion spreading from the injection site[147]. The initial lesion was a perivascular inflammation which was followed by a polymorphonuclear and lymphocytic cell infiltration and finally produced giant cell and granuloma formation. The colon also took part in a Schwartzmann reaction to lysed *Serratia marcescens* as a source of bacterial endotoxin, given initially subserosally and, 24 hours later, intravenously. Again, a haemorrhagic necrotizing lesion developed which was associated with vascular thromboses and which led to the involvement of the whole bowel wall.

A less dramatic reaction, more akin macroscopically and histologically to chronic ulcerative colitis in man, was achieved by the Auer reaction[148]. Auer demonstrated that a non-specific irritant (originally xylol stroked on a rabbit's ear) could lead to a localized hypersensivity response when a sensitized animal was rechallenged systemically. Kirsner *et al.* produced an 'Auer colitis' in egg albumen sensitized rabbits by local colonic instillation of dilute formalin, followed by a challenging intravenous or intraperitoneal dose of egg albumen. With a few hours inflammation, haemorrhage and erosions resulted, with a histological picture of edema, inflammation and disappearance of the glandular layer. With repeated challenge, the mucosa became atrophic. Immunohistochemical studies showed antigen and antibody localized in the perivascular areas[147].

A presumably delayed hypersensitivity reaction has been demonstrated in the guinea pig colon[149]. Animals were sensitized to 2:4 dinitrochlorobenzene (DNCB) applied to the neck area and then challenged rectally with DNCB. In 24 hours, the challenged area was congested with perivascular cuffing and destruction of glandular crypts histologically. Another primarily cellular response, runt disease caused by injection of adult spleen cells into newborn mice, has also caused colitis[150].

The response to injection of colonic extracts and killed bacteria are obviously of great interest. Callahan *et al.* caused a colitis in mice following sensitization with normal or inflamed mouse colon, but their method involved an Auer-type local irritation induced by warm rectal saline and this effect, rather than the specificity of the antigen, may have led to the localization of inflammation within the colon[151]. Perlmann *et al.*, when raising anti-rat and anti-rabbit colon antibodies in rats by intradermal injections of colonic tissue in adjuvant, found severe microscopic damage to the colon, but this was also seen in some animals injected with adjuvant alone[130]. In some reports of colitis induced by colonic extracts, it appears that salmonella contamination was present[152,153]. Passive injection into dogs of anti-dog colon antisera raised in rabbits has been reported to give rise to colitis, but, in some cases, this appears to have been part of a terminal anaphylactic response[154] and in others rectal infusions of formalin were given, which may have localized the response to the colon[155].

Injection of killed coliform bacteria has been reported to cause colitis, but again there was evidence of salmonella contamination[156,153]. Cooke *et al.* found no evidence of morphological change when *E. coli* extracts from the faeces of patients caused production of anti-colon antibodies in rabbits, although there were some increases in enzyme concentrations histochemically detected within the mucosa[157].

The shortcomings of most of the experimental models of colitis lie in their severity and the acuteness of onset. A more chronic ulcerative disease has been induced in animals by long-term feeding with carrageenan, a high molecular weight sulphated polysaccharide derived from seaweed[158]. The mode of action of this is uncertain, although it is of interest that it is a powerful inhibitor of complement activation[159]. The disease induced, however, is primarily caecal and shows no pattern of remission and exacerbation. As spontaneous ulcerative colitis appears to be restricted to man, failure to create a satisfactory animal model is hardly surprising.

2. *Intramucosal immune reactions in man:* The evidence already discussed indicates that the basic immune responses in patients with ulcerative colitis are intact. However, some of these patients possess

circulating antibodies to colonic and bacterial antigens and their lymphocytes also appear to be sensitized to similar, though not necessarily identical, antigens on the basis of *in vitro* testing. It is also clear that, at the present time, the role of these effector mechanisms in the pathogenesis of ulcerative colitis remains entirely speculative. In addition to these systemic immune responses, locally produced antibody and the production of antigen–antibody complexes within the mucosa may contribute to tissue damage.

Immunohistochemical studies on rectal or colonic mucosa have been controversial. Some techniques, adequate for showing the distribution of immunoglobulin containing cells in normal tissues, seem to be inadequate for inflamed tissues, as Brandtzaeg *et al.* have discussed[160]. These authors used a technique comparing directly alcohol-fixed tissues, which retain their total immunoglobulin content, with tissues washed in cold saline for 48 hours to remove extracellular immunoglobulins, and they double-stained with multiple pairs of antibody conjugates allowing a direct comparison of the numbers of cells containing each of the major immunoglobulin classes. In the normal rectal mucosa, there is a predominance of IgA cells which form 90% of the immunoglobulin-containing cells. Although the numbers of IgA cells were doubled, the striking increase was in IgG cells which were present in 30 times their normal numbers. IgM cells were increased five times. The submucosa, normally devoid of such cells, contained a dense population of immunoglobulin-containing cells, predominantly IgG. Within the extracellular fluid of both normal and colitic patients' tissues, the predominant immunoglobulin was IgG, although there was some IgA.

Knowledge of the antigens against which the immune response in the colon is directed would clearly be of considerable importance. The inflamed tissues contain more immunoglobulin than normal, though it is uncertain whether this is a specific response to particular antigens or whether it is due to non-specific invasion of inflamed tissue by plasma cells and extravasation of immunoglobulin from the circulation. In experiments in the mouth, Brandtzaeg has shown that, even when inflammation is due to a specific antigen, less than half the immunoglobulin produced appears to be directed against that antigen[161].

Monteiro *et al.*, by an immunofluorescent technique, sought antibodies against faecal bacteria within the colonic mucosa of patients and controls. They found no antibodies against aerobic organisms, but the mucosa of patients with colitis tended to contain antibodies against anaerobes[162]. These antibodies could not be detected in the sera and so, although predominantly of IgG class, were thought to be locally produced. Clearly the local production of antibodies against faecal anaerobes may be no more than a secondary phenomenon following mucosal damage. Monteiro *et al.* suggest that, even if this is so, antibody production could be a factor in perpetuating inflammation by the formation of antigen–antibody complexes.

The role of immune complexes in ulcerative colitis remains undefined although they may be implicated not only in the mucosal lesion, but also in the aetiology of some of the extra-colonic manifestations. Complexes which can fix $C1_q$, the first component of complement, have been found in the serum of about 30% of these patients[163]. Jewell and MacLennan[164] reported the presence of small immune complexes, containing less than five molecules of IgG, in the serum and were able to show a positive correlation between the presence of complexes and the activity of the disease whether assessed clinically, sigmoidoscopically or histologically. The existence of small antigen–antibody complexes in the circulation probably indicates that complexes of all sizes are being formed within the mucosa. Larger complexes, unlike the smaller ones, are readily phagocytosed and therefore would not be expected in the circulation[165]. Although it is conceivable that small complexes may compromise certain cellular effector mechanisms, by combining with receptors for IgG on the surface of lymphocytes, neutrophils and macrophages, it may be the larger, complement-fixing complexes that are more important in producing mucosal inflammation.

Evidence for the presence of immune complexes in inflamed rectal mucosa has been presented on the basis of immunofluorescent observations[166]. However, it has been argued that, whilst immunoglobulin and C3 may be present in inflamed tissue as part of an immune complex, current immunohistochemical techniques are inadequate to prove this[167]. Another indicator of antigen–antibody reactions is the alteration of serum complement activity. When measured as total haemolytic activity, complement levels have been either normal or raised[168,169] and, in one study, raised levels of C3 and C4 were found[170]. However, the serum level of any individual component is the product of a number of variables; preliminary data show that patients with active disease have an increased fractional catabolic rate of C3 and that it is being selectively deposited in the extravascular compartment.[171].

Crohn's disease

Crohn's disease differs from ulcerative colitis in so far as it typically causes a transmural inflammation which may affect any part of the gastrointestinal tract from the mouth to the anus. The clinical manifestations of the disease are protean but, when it is confined to the colon, it can be difficult to distinguish from classical ulcerative colitis. The hallmark of the disease is the presence of non-caseating epithelioid granulomata with Langhan's type giant cells. These are present in about 60% of cases, a feature which has suggested parallels with tuberculosis and sarcoid and which has coloured much of the approach to the immunology of the disease.

The infective theories

The granulomata of Crohn's disease suggested a mycobacterial infection even though caseation is absent. Tuberculous enteritis commonly involves the terminal ileum and remains an important differential diagnosis of Crohn's disease, especially in those parts of the world where tuberculosis is prevalent. Although in particular patients the distinction may not be straightforward, it may usually be made on the presence of acid-fast bacilli, the nature of the granulomata, and often the presence of tuberculosis elsewhere. The response of exacerbations of Crohn's disease to corticosteroid therapy, and of tuberculous enteritis to specific antibiotic therapy, emphasize the basic differences between the two conditions. Attempts have been made to culture tubercle bacilli from Crohn's tissue but they have been unsucessful[172].

It has been suggested that other mycobacteria may be involved. In ruminants, *Mycobacterium paratuberculosis* causes a chronic hyperplastic enteritis (Johne's disease) with a prediliction for the ileum but often affecting other areas of the gut. Although epithelioid cell collections and a lymphocytic infiltrate are present, ulceration of the mucosa does not occur and the bacilli are readily visible in tissue sections. This organism has not been cultured in cases of Crohn's disease[173]. Following reports that atypical mycobacteria infected with mycobacteriophage might be present in tissues of patients with sarcoidosis, evidence for hypersensitivity to atypical mycobacterial antigens in patients with Crohn's disease was sought but not found[174].

Bacterial cultures of intestinal contents, with particular attention to anaerobic organisms, has shown a similar spectrum of organisms to those found in other bowel diseases with comparable anatomical and functional disturbances[175,176]. No common pathogen has been isolated. A causative organism has been shown in many cases of acute ileitis, for which *Yersinia enterocolitica* (formerly *Pasteurella pseudotuberculosis*) is often responsible. Although at operation this appears like acute Crohn's disease, the natural history of the condition is different[177].

Recent reports of a transmissible agent in Crohn's disease have rejuvenated the infective theories. The initial observations were made in sarcoidosis[178]. Tissue from sarcoid lymph nodes was inoculated into mouse footpads, and caused the development of epithelioid cell granulomata in nearly half the injected animals at that site—furthermore one in ten of the mice developed a positive Kveim reaction at a distant site. Control tissues led only to non-specific inflammatory reactions. Mitchell and Rees performed analagous experiments using tissues from a patient with Crohn's disease[179]. These were particularly pertinent as the same authors had found positive Kveim tests in 51% of patients with Crohn's disease, as will be discussed below. Tissues from an affected ileum and lymph node were injected into mouse footpads, and a control tissue of normal lymph node alone was used. After 3 weeks, five footpads from eight mice given Crohn's tissue showed granulomata and occasional giant cells compared with one footpad from 58 mice given control tissue. Biopsies at 7 months showed granulomata in eight out of 48 footpads injected with Crohn's tissue but no positives were found in the controls. Furthermore, one-third of the mice given Crohn's tissue developed a positive Kveim test but none of the controls, and some mice given Crohn's tissue into the footpad developed granulomata in the ileum. Similar results were obtained by Taub and Siltzbach[180].

In further experiments, ileal tissue from Crohn's patients, or from a patient with colonic carcinoma as a control, were injected after homogenization directly into the wall of the distal ileum of New Zealand rabbits[181]. Rabbits injected with Crohn's tissue developed granulomata, whilst control tissues gave non-specific inflammatory responses or foreign-body reactions. The transmissible agent passed a 100 μ filter and has been passaged.

Unfortunately these results have not always been confirmed. Bolton *et al.*[182] performed serial biopsies up to one year following injection of

Crohn's tissue into multiple sites of guinea pigs, rats and mice, using 295 animals in all. No granulomata were found, nor any lesion which was not also found using control tissue.

The phenomenon of a transmissible agent thus remains *sub judice*. Granulomata may be caused by many factors, not all of which are infective or immunological. If clearance of a non-infective agent from the tissues is slow, passage from one animal to another could occur. Transmissibility, therefore, does not necessarily imply infectivity.

Nonetheless, the descriptions of a transmissible agent have reawakened interest in a possible viral origin for the disease. Early attempts to isolate a virus were negative but, recently, improved techniques have shown the presence of viruses in some cases of Crohn's disease. Although Farmer *et al.* did not find any increase in viral antibody titres in patients with Crohn's disease to parallel the increase in cytomegalovirus titres they reported in ulcerative colitis, these authors did isolate this virus from the tissues of one patient with Crohn's disease[80]. Beeken *et al.* have shown the presence of a virus in tissues and intestinal fluid of 10 out of 18 patients with Crohn's disease by cytopathogenic effects in tissue culture[81]. However, similar effects were found in a number of other intestinal disorders, such as diverticulitis and carcinoma of the colon. The presence of viruses when there is altered intestinal anatomy seems reasonable, but there is little to indicate that those reported to date are primarily pathogenic.

The immunological theories

Studies of relatives of patients with Crohn's disease show that certain families have a tendency to develop inflammatory bowel disease, which may be either Crohn's disease or ulcerative colitis; up to 17% of patients may have a positive family history[83]. There are no known genetic markers to identify persons at risk. Studies of HL-A status show no link with the disease[87], and there is a suggestion, though the number of patients is small, that the link between HL-AW27 and spondylitis may be less marked in patients with Crohn's disease than in those with ulcerative colitis[183].

The humoral antibody system seems unimpaired. Serum immunoglobulin levels are usually normal but may show some elevation of IgA[184,185]; some of this is probably secretory IgA[184]. The turnover of IgG is increased[186], as is IgM turnover if intra-abdominal abscesses are present[187]. The ability to mount primary and secondary antibody responses to an injected antigen (bacteriophage ϕX 174) is normal[188]. The disease has been reported in a patient with sex-linked agammaglobulinaemia, in whose lymph nodes neither germinal centres nor plasma cells were present.[189]

There has however been much controversy on the existence of depressed cellular immunity in the disease. This has been investigated at various levels, from skin tests for common antigens to direct assessment of lymphocyte reactivity.

In a number of uncontrolled series, the incidence of positive Mantoux tests appeared to be strikingly lower than that taken to be normal for the population at large[190,191]. However, using hospital patients as controls, Fletcher and Hinton[192], and subsequently a number of other investigators[193] have found no difference in the degree of tuberculin sensitivity. Delayed skin hypersensitivity to other common antigens (mumps, candida, and trichophyton) has also been found to be normal[194].

Jones *et al.* reported that, as in sarcoidosis, the ability to develop cutaneous hypersensitivity to 2-4 dinitrochlorobenzene was impaired in Crohn's disease, 15 out of 26 patients failing to become sensitive[195]. Normal healthy people were used as controls. Bolton *et al.* used patients as controls, with particular attention to the 'degree of illness'; they found DNCB responses to be depressed in Crohn's patients and control patients if ill, and to be intact in both groups if well[106].

A similar situation exists if direct lymphocyte responses elecited as correlates of cellular immunity are considered. Reduced transformation responses to phytohaemagglutinin (PHA) were reported by Walker and Greaves[196]. Brown *et al.* also found reduced responses to PHA and Concanavalin A (Con A), but responses to pokeweed mitogen were normal[197]. On this basis they suggested that only certain subpopulations of lymphocytes showed reduced function. Asquith *et al.* found reduced PHA responses in a few patients only, and no significant fall in response to Con A or pokeweed mitogen[198]. Responses were markedly depressed in patients on corticosteroid therapy. Further evidence for reduced cellular immunity was the demonstration of a reduced mixed lymphocyte reaction in patients with Crohn's disease[199]. In all these studies normal patients were used as controls, although in some the responses were depressed even when compared with ulcerative colitis.

On the other hand, Ropke[200], and Aas *et al.*[201] found no difference in the response of lymphocytes to non-specific mitogens, although Aas *et al.* reported a high basal uptake of thymidine in patients with Crohn's disease, suggesting that these lymphocytes were already stimulated. In two series in which sick patients with other diseases have been used as controls there was no evidence of decreased lymphocyte reactivity[202,106].

The choice of controls and the many variations of methodology may explain many of the discrepancies in the results reported from different laboratories. In general, it appears that there is probably no gross impairment of cellular immunity in Crohn's disease. Quantification of sub-populations of peripheral blood lymphocytes, again by comparison with normal control subjects, has suggested a slight decrease in the percentage of T-cells, whilst B-cell counts are normal or increased, with a rise in the IgA bearing cells[109]. Nevertheless, it is pertinent to consider whether cellular hypersensitivity occurs towards particular antigens.

Kveim antigens: Mitchell *et al.* reported that 50% of their patients with Crohn's disease had positive Kveim tests[203]. Whilst others confirmed this incidence[204], Siltzbach *et al.* found no positive tests in 23 patients[205]. It appears that these discrepancies have been resolved on the basis of the nature of the sarcoid spleen suspensions. Kveim positivity in Crohn's disease, and subsequently in ulcerative colitis and celiac disease, was reported with a small number of preparations most of which have now been withdrawn[206]. This is probably also the explanation for the reports of leucocyte migration inhibition by sarcoid suspension in Crohn's disease, celiac disease and dermatitis herpetiformis[207,208].

Gut-associated antigens: Either gut contents or the gut itself might initiate an immune response, and there is suggestive evidence for this largely developed from work on ulcerative colitis. Although early studies were unable to demonstrate the anti-colon antibodies found in ulcerative colitis, Lagerkrantz *et al.* reported them in a series of patients with Crohn's disease, most of whom had colonic involvement[121]. They used germ-free rat colon as antigen in both the haemagglutination and immunofluorescent techniques. Deodhar *et al.* found these antibodies in 70% of their patients—the same proportion that they reported in ulcerative colitis[184]. It appears that when only small bowel is involved, the incidence of anti-colon antibodies is lower, though still significant[128].

As in ulcerative colitis, the incidence and titres of antibodies does not correlate well with disease extent or activity. Antibodies to dietary proteins do not occur more commonly in these patients when compared with control subjects[112].

Antibodies to *E. coli* 014 occur commonly at high titre in patients with Crohn's disease, compatible with the concept that *E. coli* lipopolysaccharide may stimulate an antibody response which cross-reacts with the colon[128].

Reports of cell-mediated immunity against gut-associated antigens are discrepant. Dykes reported that small intestinal contents inhibited the migration of leukocytes from patients with Crohn's disease[209], a phenomenon which would correlate well with the clinical observation that surgical bypass of diseased bowel is frequently beneficial. Using similar techniques, inhibition of leucocyte migration has been observed using diseased colonic tissue as antigen[210] but no effect on migration was seen when fetal colon or ileum was used[143]. Lymphocyte transformation has also been employed as an indicator of cellular hypersensitivity. Parent *et al.* found that the lymphocytes from some patients with Crohn's disease were stimulated by certain fractions of intestinal contents but that some normal lymphocytes were also stimulated[211]. Rectal epithelial cells have been found not to stimulate blast transformation in autologous lymphocytes from patients with this disease[144].

The observations of Shorter and his colleagues on the cytotoxicity of lymphocytes for colonic epithelial cells apply to both ulcerative colitis and Crohn's disease[135]. The majority of the patients with Crohn's disease had colonic involvement, but some with disease apparently confined to the small bowel showed this phenomenon[135]. However, it is very interesting that no patient's lymphocytes, not even from those with small bowel involvement, showed cytotoxicity for ileal cells[135]. This fact is a serious challenge to the view that lymphocyte cytotoxicity is an essential part of the pathogenesis of inflammatory bowel disease, as it seems difficult to conceive that patients with Crohn's disease have different methods of tissue damage in adjacent portions of gut.

Pathogenesis of intestinal inflammation

As with ulcerative colitis, the precise immunological mechanisms occurring within the bowel mucosa which ultimately induce the inflammatory response typical of Crohn's disease are quite unknown. Granulomata are usually recognized as hallmarks of cell-mediated immune reactions and there is much experimental evidence to support this. The nature and distribution of immunologically competent cells in diseased human intestine has barely been studied, but a preliminary report suggests that lymphocytes extracted from Crohn's tissues have a diminished PHA response compared with lymphocytes extracted from normal intestine[212]. Such data must be regarded with some caution in view of the data published on the PHA responses of peripheral blood lymphocytes in this disease, but it would be of great interest to study how the subpopulations of lymphocytes alter when the intestine becomes the site of inflammatory disease.

Immunofluorescent staining of plasma cells in the uninvolved gut of patients with Crohn's disease has shown an increased number of cells, particularly of IgA- and IgM-producing cells[213]. In addition, there was marked epithelial fluorescence which was specific for IgM. In other areas of intestine which were histologically diseased, but without ulceration, there was a gross diminution of IgA-containing cells. Green and Fox have suggested that, whatever the mechanism of this phenomenon, the result will be an impairment of locally produced antibody which may facilitate the entry of antigens into the mucosa[213].

The evidence supporting the existence of circulating immune complexes in ulcerative colitis also applies to patients with Crohn's disease[164]. Likewise, their role in their pathogenesis of either the intestinal inflammation or the extra-colonic manifestations remains undefined. The fractional catabolic rate of C3 appears to be increased in patients with Crohn's disease[171].

General discussion

The debate concerning the relation between ulcerative colitis and Crohn's disease continues without being resolved. There are many pointers to suggest that they form part of a spectrum of a single disease process. Patients with either disease have a similar age and sex distribution and they have an increased familial incidence of both diseases. The two diseases share similar extra-intestinal manifestations and they share similar immunological phenomena. From a clinical point of view, there are considerable difficulties in classifying certain patients with colonic disease and some patients, who by all currently accepted criteria have ulcerative colitis, may subsequently show the features of Crohn's disease.

In terms of pathogenesis, an analogy may be drawn from the work of Spector and Heesom[214], who injected preformed antigen–antibody complexes intradermally into rats. Complexes formed at equivalence lead to the formation of granulomata, whereas those formed in antigen excess gave only a non-specific inflammatory response. Ulcerative colitis and Crohn's disease may therefore represent differing responses to an antigenic stimulus. There is no necessity to postulate a unique antigen in these diseases. The primary factor in these conditions may be specific or the disease may merely develop from an incidental insult to the mucosa. In either case, it seems likely that local immune responses will be stimulated once the mucosa becomes inflamed, since the mucosa is in contact with numerous antigens contained within the intestinal stream. The humoral and cellular responses to bacterial antigens, which have been discussed, would support this concept. Local immune complex formation, complement activation, antibodies and lymphocyte hypersensitivity to bacteria which cross-react with colonic antigens, are all mechanisms whereby the inflammatory process may become chronic.

However, a taxonomic analysis has suggested that whereas patients with ulcerative colitis cluster as a fairly distinct population, patients with Crohn's colitis cluster quite separately and would appear to be a much more heterogeneous group[215]. This might suggest a variety of aetiologies. Furthermore, none of the immunological data adequately explain the anatomical distribution of the two diseases, although this could conceivably reflect the distribution of a given antigen or a specific host factor, such as a defect in mucus, which may affect the gastrointestinal tract to a varying extent. One factor which any aetiological theory must explain is the increase in Crohn's disease in the last two decades. This has been reported in several European countries and the rate of admission to British hospitals has increased threefold over the last 12 years[216]. Although the recognition of colonic involvement in Crohn's disease in 1960 may play a part in this increase, as patients previously diagnosed as ulcerative colitis may now be called Crohn's disease, the increase is seen even if only small bowel disease is considered.

REFERENCES

1. MacDonald, W. C., Trier, J. S. and Everett, N. B. (1964). Cell proliferation and migration in the stomach, duodenum and rectum of man: radioautographic studies. *Gastroenterology*, **46**, 405.
2. de Boer, W. G. R. M., Forsyth, A. and Nairn, R. C. (1969). Gastric antigens in health and disease. Behaviour in early development, senescence, metaplasia, and cancer. *Br. Med. J.*, **ii**, 93.
3. Samloff, I. M. and Liebman, W. M. (1973). Cellular localisation of the Group II pepsinogens in human stomach and duodenum by immunofluorescence. *Gastroenterology*, **65**, 36
4. Jewell, D. P., Katiyar, V. N., Rees, C., Wright, J. and Taylor, K. B. (1975). Isolation of parietal cells from guinea pig gastric mucose and the immunological characterization of their antigenic structure. *Gut*, **16**, 603
5. Callender, S. T. and Denborough, M. A. (1957). A family study of pernicious anaemia. *Br. J. Haematol.*, **3**, 88
6. Ardeman, S. and Chanarin, I. (1963). A method for the assay of human gastric intrinsic factor and for the detection and titration of antibodies against intrinsic factor. *Lancet*, **ii**, 1350
7. Wangel, A. G., Callender, S. T., Spray, G. H. and Wright R. (1968). A family study of pernicious anaemia. I. Autoantibodies, achlorhydria, serum pepsinogen and vitamin B_{12}. *Br. J. Haematol.*, **14**, 161
8. Wangel, A. G., Callender, S. T., Spray, G. H. and Wright, R. (1968b). A family study of pernicious anaemia, II. Intrinsic factor secretion, vitamin B_{12} absorption and genetic aspects of gastric autoimmunity. *Br. J. Haematol.*, **14**, 183
9. Doniach, D. and Roitt, I. M. (1966). Family studies on gastric autoimmunity. *Proc. Roy. Soc. Med.*, **59**, 691
10. te Velde, K., Hoedemaeker, P. J., Anders, G. J. P. A., Arends, A. and Nieweg, H. O. (1966). A comparative morphological and functional study of gastritis with and without autoantibodies. *Gastroenterology*, **51**, 138
11. Doniach, D., Roitt, I. M. and Taylor, K. B. (1963). Autoimmune phenomena in pernicious anaemia. Serological overlap with thyroiditis, thyrotoxicosis and systemic lupus erythematosus. *Br. Med. J.*, **i**, 1374
12. Grasbeck, R., Simons, K. and Siukkonen, I. (1966). Isolation of intrinsic factor and its probable degradation product as their vitamin B_{12} complexes from human gastric juice. *Biochem. Biophys. Acta*, **127**, 47
13. Hoedemaeker, P. J., Abels, J., Wachters, J. J., Arends, A. and Nieweg, H. O. (1964). Investigations upon the site of production of Castle's gastric intrinsic factor. *Lab. Invest.*, **13**, 1394
14. Fisher, J. M. and Taylor, K. B. (1969). The intracellular localization of Castle's intrinsic factor by an immunofluorescent technique using autoantibodies. *Immunology*, **16**, 779
15. Rødbro, P., Christiansen, P. M. and Schwartz, M. (1965). Intrinsic factor secretion in stomach diseases. *Lancet*, **ii**, 1200

16. Bardhan, K. D., Wangel, A. G., Whitehead, R., Wright, R., Spray, G. H., Warner, G. T. and Callender, S. T. E. (1969). The relation between the histology of the gastric mucosa, secretion of intrinsic factor, autoimmunity and the absorption of vitamin B_{12}. In *Protides of the biological fluids*. H. Preeters (ed.), p. 393. *Proceedings of the 16th Colloquium, Bruges, Belgium.* (Oxford: Pergamon Press)
17. Taylor, K. B. (1959). Inhibition of intrinsic factor by pernicious anaemia sera. *Lancet*, **ii**, 106
18. Schwartz, M. (1960). Intrinsic factor antibody in serum from patients with pernicious anaemia. *Lancet*, **ii**, 1263
19. Jeffries, G. H., Hoskins, D. W. and Sleisenger, M. H. (1962). Antibody to intrinsic factor in serum from patients with pernicious anaemia. *J. Clin. Invest.*, **41**, 1106
20. Samloff, I. M. and Turner, M. D. (1968). Rabbit blocking and binding antibodies to human intrinsic factor and intrinsic factor–B_{12} complex. *J. Immunol.*, **101**, 578
21. Taylor, K. B., Roitt, I. M., Doniach, D., Couchman, K. G. and Shapland, C. (1962). Autoimmune phenomena in pernicious anaemia: gastric antibodies. *Brit. Med. J.*, **ii**, 1347
22. Samloff, I. M. and Barnett, E. V. (1965). Identification of intrinsic factor autoantibody and intrinsic factor in man by radio-immunodiffusion and radioimmunoelectrophoresis. *J. Immunol.*, **95**, 536
23. Samloff, I. M., Kleinman, M. S., Turner, M. D., Sobel, M. V. and Jeffries, G. H. (1968). Blocking and binding antibodies to intrinsic factor and parietal cell antibody in pernicious anaemia. *Gastroenterology*, **55**, 575
24. Ungar, B., Whittingham, S. and Francis, C. M. (1967). Pernicious anaemia: incidence and significance of circulating antibodies to intrinsic factor and parietal cells. *Austral. Ann. Med.*, **16**, 226
25. Desai, H. G., Dighe, P. K. and Borkar, A. V. (1968). Parietal cell and intrinsic factor antibodies in Indian subjects. *Scand. J. Gastroent.*, **3**, 321
26. Ashworth, L. A. E., England, J. M., Fisher, J. M. and Taylor, K. B. (1967). A new method for detection and measurement of intrinsic factor antibodies. *Lancet*, **ii**, 1160
27. Strickland, R. G., Baur, S., Ashworth, L. A. E. and Taylor, K. B. (1971). A correlative study of immunological phenomena in pernicious anaemia. *Clin. Exp. Immunol.*, **8**, 25
28. Bernier, G. M., and Hines, J. D. (1968). Immunologic heterogeneity of autoantibodies in patients with pernicious anaemia. *New Eng. J. Med.*, **277**, 1386
29. Fisher, J. M., Rees, G. and Taylor, K. B. (1966). Intrinsic factor antibodies in gastric juice of pernicious anaemia patients. *Lancet*, **ii**, 88
30. Schade, S. G., Feick, P. C., Muckerheide, M. and Schilling, R. F. (1966). Occurrence in gastric juice of antibody to a complex of intrinsic factor and vitamin B_{12}. *New Eng. J. Med.*, **275**, 528

31. Rose, M. S. and Chanarin, I. (1969). Dissociation of intrinsic factor from its antibody: Application to study of pernicious anaemia gastric juice specimens. *Brit. Med. J.*, **i**, 468
32. Goldberg, L. S. and Bluestone, R. (1970). Hidden gastric autoantibodies to intrinsic factor in pernicious anaemia. *J. Lab. Clin. Med.*, **45**, 449
33. Goldberg, L. S., Shuster, J. and Fudenberg, H. H. (1969). Gastric autoimmunity in pernicious anaemia. *J. Lab. Clin. Med.*, **73**, 249
34. Baur, S., Koo, N. and Taylor, K. B. (1970). The immunoglobulin class of autoantibody containing cells in the gastric mucosa. *Immunology*, **19**, 891
35. Irvine, W. J., Davies, S. H., Delamore, I. W. and Wynn Williams, A. (1962). Immunological relationship between pernicious anaemia and thyroid disease. *Brit. Med. J.*, **ii**, 454
36. Nairn, R. C. and de Boer, W. G. R. M. (1966). Species distribution of gastrointestinal antigens. *Nature (Lond.)*, **210**, 960
37. Baur, S., Roitt, I. M. and Doniach, D. (1965). Characterisation of the human gastric parietal cell auto-antigen. *Immunology*, **8**, 62
38. Ward, H. A. and Nairn, R. C. (1972). Gastric parietal cell autoantigen. Physical, chemical, and biological properties. *Clin. Exp. Immunol.*, **10**, 435
39. Hoedemaeker, P. J. and Ito, S. (1970). Ultrastructural localisation of gastric parietal cell antigen with peroxidase-coupled antibody. *Lab. Invest.*, **22**, 184
40. Roitt, I. M., Doniach, D. and Shapland, C. (1965). Autoimmunity in pernicious anaemia and atrophic gastritis. *Ann. N.Y. Acad. Sci.*, **124**, 644
41. Baur, S., Fisher, J. M., Strickland, R. G. and Taylor, K. B. (1968). The autoantibody-containing cells in the gastric mucosa in pernicious anaemia. *Lancet*, **ii**, 887
42. Tai, C. and McGuigan, J. E. (1969). Immunologic studies in pernicious anaemia. *Blood*, **34**, 63
43. Fixa, B. and Theiele, H. G. (1969). Delayed hypersensitivity to intrinsic factor in patients with pernicious anaemia. A preliminary report. *Med. Exp. (Basel)*, **19**, 231
44. Fixa, B., Theiele, H. G., Komárkóva, O. and Nožička, Z. (1972). Gastric autoantibodies and cell-mediated immunity in pernicious anaemia—a comparative study. *Scand. J. Gastroent.*, **7**, 237
45. Rose, M. S., Chanarin, I., Doniach, D., Brostoff, J. and Ardeman, S. (1970). Intrinsic-factor antibodies in absence of pernicious anaemia. *Lancet*, **ii**, 9
46. James, D., Asherson, G., Chanarin, I., Coghill, N., Hamilton, S., Himsworth, R. L. and Webster, D. (1974). Cell-mediated immunity to intrinsic factor in autoimmune disorders. *Brit. Med. J.*, **4**, 494
47. Finlayson, N. D. C., Fauconnet, M. H. and Krohn, K. (1972). *In vitro* demonstration of delayed hypersensitivity to gastric antigens in pernicious anaemia. *Am. J. Dig. Dis.*, **17**, 631

48. Brostoff, J. (1970). Migration inhibition studies in human disease. *Proc. Roy. Soc. Med.*, **63**, 905
49. Goldstone, A. H., Calder, E. A., Barnes, E. W. and Irvine, W. J. (1973). The effect of gastric antigens on the *in vitro* migration of leucocytes from patients with atrophic gastritis and pernicious anaemia. *Clin. Exp. Immunol.*, **14**, 501
50. Strickland, R. G. and Mackay, I. R. (1973). A reappraisal of the nature and significance of chronic atrophic gastritis. *Am. J. Dig. Dis.*, **18**, 426
51. Polak, J. M., Coulling, I., Doe, W. and Pearse, A. G. E. (1971). The G cells in pernicious anaemia. *Gut*, **12**, 319
52. Fisher, J. M., Mackay, I. R., Taylor, K. B. and Ungar, B. (1967). An immunological study of categories of gastritis. *Lancet*, **i**, 176
53. Ungar, B., Strickland, R. G. and Francis, C. M. (1971). The prevalence and significance of circulating antibodies to gastric intrinsic factor and parietal cells in gastric carcinoma. *Gut*, **12**, 903
54. Twomey, J. J., Jordan, P. H., Jarrold, T., Trubowitz, S., Ritz, N. D. and Conn, H. O. (1969). The syndrome of immunoglobulin deficiency and pernicious anaemia. *Am. J. Med.*, **47**, 340
55. Hughes, W. S., Brooks, F. P. and Conn, H. O. (1972). Serum gastrin levels in primary hypogammaglobulinaemia and pernicious anaemia. *Ann. Intern. Med.*, **77**, 746
56. Rose, M. S. and Chanarin, I. (1971). Intrinsic factor antibody and absorption of vitamin B_{12} in pernicious anaemia. *Brit. Med. J.*, **1**, 25
57. Fisher, J. M. and Taylor, K. B. (1967). Placental transfer of gastric antibodies. *Lancet*, **i**, 695
58. Inada, M. and Glass, G. B. J. (1972). Effects of prolonged administration of intrinsic factor antibodies on gastric morphology and secretion in rats. *Fed. Proc.*, **31**, 299
59. Tanaka, N. and Glass, G. B. J. (1970). Effect of prolonged administration of parietal cell antibodies from patients with atrophic gastritis and pernicious anaemia on the parietal cell mass and hydrochloric acid output in rats. *Gastroenterology*, **58**, 482
60. Hausamen, T-U, Brus, I., Fisher, J. M. and Taylor, K. B. (1969). Inhibition of production of gastric acid by gastric antibodies. *Clin. Res.*, **17**, 594
61. Hausamen, T-U., Halcrow, D. A. and Taylor, K. B. (1969). Biological effects of gastrointestinal antibodies. II Histological changes in the stomach induced by injection of specific heterologous antibodies. *Gastroenterology*, **56**, 1062
62. Hennes, A. R., Sevelius, H., Lewellyn, T., Joel, W., Woods, A. H. and Wolf, S. (1962). Atrophic gastritis in dogs. *Arch. Path.*, **73**, 281
63. Fixa, B., Vejbora, O., Komárkóva, O., Langr, F. and Parizek, J. (1964). On immunologically induced gastric atrophy in dogs. *Gastroenterologia, Basel*, **102**, 331
64. Krohn, K. J. E. and Finlayson, N. D. C. (1973). Interrelations of humoral and cellular immune responses in experimental canine gastritis. *Clin. Exp. Immunol.*, **14**, 237

65. Andrada, J. A., Rose, N. R. and Andrada, E. C. (1969). Experimental autoimmune gastritis in the Rhesus monkey. *Clin. Exp. Immunol.*, **4**, 293
66. Jacob, E. and Glass, G. B. J. (1969). The participation of complement in the parietal cell antigen–antibody reaction in pernicious anaemia and atrophic gastritis. *Clin. Exp. Immunol.*, **5**, 141
67. Jacob, E. and Glass, G. B. J. (1971). Localisation of intrinsic factor and complement fixing intrinsic factor antibody complex in parietal cell of man. *Clin. Exp. Immunol.*, **8**, 517
68. Fixa, B., Komárkóva, O., Vejbora, O. and Langr, F. (1970). Transfer of experimental gastric lesions in dogs by means of thoracic duct cells. *Suppl. Sbor. Ved. Praci, LFKU SV 13*, **4**, 169
69. Fixa, B., Komárkóva, O., Prixová, J. and Nožička, Z. (1970). On the cross-reactivity between antigens of *E. coli* and of gastric parietal cells in man. *Folia Microbiol. (Praha)*, **15**, 503
70. Wilks, S. (1859). *Lectures on pathological anatomy*. (London: Longman, Brown, Green, Longmans and Roberts)
71. Felsen, J. (1936). The relation of bacillary dysentery to distal ileitis, chronic ulcerative colitis and non-specific intestinal granuloma. *Ann. Intern. Med.*, **10**, 645
72. Bargen, J. A. (1924). Experimental studies on the etiology of chronic ulcerative colitis. *J. Am. Med. Ass.*, **83**, 332
73. Dack, G. M., Dragstedt, L. R. and Heinz, T. F. (1936). *Bacterium necrophorum* in chronic ulcerative colitis. *J. Am. Med. Ass.*, **106**, 7
74. Felsen, J. and Wolarsky, W. (1953). Acute and chronic bacillary dysentery and chronic ulcerative colitis. *J. Am. Med. Ass.*, **153**, 1069
75. Gorbach, S. L., Nahas, L., Plaut, A. G., Weinstein, L., Patterson, J. F. and Levitan, R. (1968). Studies of intestinal microflora. V. Faecal microbial ecology in ulcerative colitis and regional enteritis: relationship to severity of disease and chemotherapy. *Gastroenterology*, **54**, 575
76. Cooke, E. M. (1968). Properties of strains of *Escherichia coli* isolated from the faeces of patients with ulcerative colitis, patients with acute diarrhoea and normal persons. *J. Path. Bact.*, **95**, 101
77. Cooke, E. M., Ewins, S. P., Hywel-Jones, J. and Lennard-Jones, J. E. (1974). Properties of strains of *E. coli* carried in different phases of ulcerative colitis. *Gut*, **15**, 143
78. Schreierson, S. S., Garlock, J. H., Shore, B., Stuart, W. D., Steinglass, M. and Aronson, B. (1962). Studies on the viral etiology of regional enteritis and ulcerative colitis. A negative report. *Amer. J. Dig. Dis.*, **7**, 839
79. Tamura, H. (1973). Acute ulcerative colitis associated with cytomegalic inclusion virus. *Arch. Pathol.*, **96**, 164
80. Farmer, G. W., Vincent, M. M., Fucillo, D. A., Horta-Barbosa, L., Ritman, S., Sever, J. L. and Gitnick, G. L. (1973). Viral investigations in ulcerative colitis and regional enteritis. *Gastroenterology*, **65**, 8
81. Aronson, M. D., Phillips, C. A. and Beeken, W. L. (1974). Isolation of a viral agent from intestinal tissue of patients with Crohn's disease and other intestinal disorders. *Gastroenterology*, **66**, 661

82. Rosen, P., Armstrong, D. and Rice, N. (1973) Gastrointestinal cytomegalovirus infection. *Arch. Intern. Med.*, **132**, 274
83. Singer, H. C., Anderson, J. G. D., Frischer, H. and Kirsner, J. B. (1971). Familial aspects of inflammatory bowel disease. *Gastroenterology*, **61**, 423
84. Binder, V., Weeke, E. and Olsen, J. H. (1966). A genetic study of ulcerative colitis. *Scand. J. Gastroent.*, **1**, 49
85. Morris, P. J. (1965). Familial ulcerative colitis. *Gut*, **6**, 176
86. Winstone, N. E., Henderson, A. J. and Brooke, B. N. (1960). Blood groups and secretor status in ulcerative colitis. *Lancet*, **ii**, 64
87. Gleeson, M. H., Walker, J. S., Wentzel, J., Chapman, J. A. and Harris, R. (1972). Human leucocyte antigen in Crohn's disease and ulcerative colitis. *Gut*, **13**, 438
88. Thorsby, E. and Lie, S. O. (1971). Relationship between the HLA system and susceptibility to disease. *Transpl. Proc.*, **3**, 1305
89. Asquith, P., Mackintosh, P., Stokes, P. L., Holmes, G. K. T. and Cooke, W. T. (1974). Histocompatibility antigens in patients with inflammatory bowel disease. *Lancet*, **i**, 113
90. Russell, A. S. and Schlaut, J. W. (1974). HL–A antigens in inflammatory bowel disease. *Lancet*, **i**, 451
91. Lewkonia, R. M., Woodrow, J. C., McConnell, R. B. and Price Evans, D. A. (1974). HL-A antigens in inflammatory bowel disease. *Lancet*, **i**, 574
92. Brewerton, D. A., Caffrey, M., Nicholls, A., Walters, D. and James, D. C. O. (1974). HL-A 27 and arthropathies associated with ulcerative colitis and psoriasis. *Lancet*, **i**, 956
93. Monk, M., Mendeloff, A. I., Siegel, C. I. and Lilienfeld, A. (1967). An epidemiological study of ulcerative colitis and regional enteritis among adults in Baltimore. I. Hospital incidence and prevalence, 1960–1963. *Gastroenterology*, **53**, 198
94. Acheson, E. D. and Nefzger, M. D. (1963). Ulcerative colitis in the United States Army in 1944. *Gastroenterology*, **44**, 7
95. Gilat, T., Zemishlany, Z., Ribak, J., Benarova, Y. and Lilos, P. (1974). Ulcerative colitis in the Jewish population of Tel Aviv Yafo. II. The rarity of malignant degeneration. *Gastroenterology*, **67**, 933
96. White, R. G., Bass, B. H. and Williams, E. (1961). Lymphadenoid goitre and the syndrome of systemic lupus erythematosus. *Lancet*, **i**, 368
97. Edwards, F. C. and Truelove, S. C. (1964). The course and prognosis of ulcerative colitis. *Gut*, **5**, 1
98. Alarcon-Segovia, D., Herskovic, T., Dearing, W. H., Bartholomew, L. G., Cain, J. C. and Shorter, R. G. (1965). Lupus erythematosus cell phenomenon in patients with chronic ulcerative colitis. *Gut*, **6**, 39
99. Lorber, M., Schwartz, J. I. and Wasserman, L. R. (1955). Association of antibody-coated red blood cells with ulcerative colitis. *Amer. J. Med.*, **19**, 889

100. Harrison, W. J. (1965). Thyroid, gastric (parietal cell) and nuclear antibodies in ulcerative colitis. *Lancet*, **i**, 1350
101. Pulimood, E. M. and Holborow, E. J. (1963). Cited by Glynn, L. E. and Holborow, E. J. in *Auto-immunity and Disease* (1965) (Oxford: Blackwell Scientific Publications)
102. Hammer, B., Ashurst, P. and Naish, J. (1968). Diseases associated with ulcerative colitis and Crohn's disease. *Gut*, **9**, 17
103. Kraft, S. C., Ford, H. E., McCleery, J. L. and Kirsner, J. B. (1968). Serum immunoglobulin levels in ulcerative colitis and Crohn's disease. *Gastroenterology*, **54**, 1251
104. Thompson, R. A., Asquith, P. and Cooke, W. T. (1969). Secretory IgA in the serum. *Lancet*, **ii**, 517
105. Kirk, B. W. and Freedman, S. O. (1967). Hypogammaglobulinaemia, thymoma and ulcerative colitis. *Canad. Med. Ass. J.*, **96**, 1272
106. Bolton, P. M., James, S. L., Newcombe, R. G., Whitehead, R. H. and Hughes, L. E. (1974). The immune competence of patients with inflammatory bowel disease. *Gut*, **15**, 213
107. Hinz, C. F., Perlmann, P. and Hammarstrom, S. (1967). Reactivity *in vitro* of lymphocytes from patients with ulcerative colitis. *J. Lab. Clin. Med.*, **70**, 752
108. Stefani, S. and Fink, S. (1967). Effect of *E. coli* antigens, tuberculin and phytohaemagglutinin upon ulcerative colitis lymphocytes. *Gut*, **8**, 249
109. Strickland, R. G., Korsmeyer, S., Soltis, R. D., Wilson, I. D. and Williams, R. C. (1974). Peripheral blood T and B cells in chronic inflammatory bowel disease. *Gastroenterology*, **67**, 569
110. Wright, R. and Truelove, S. C. (1965). A controlled therapeutic trial of various diets in ulcerative colitis. *Brit. Med. J.*, **ii**, 138
111. Taylor, K. B. and Truelove, S. C. (1961). Circulating antibodies to milk proteins in ulcerative colitis. *Brit. Med. J.*, **ii**, 924
112. McCaffery, T. D., Kraft, S. C. and Rothberg, R. M. (1972). The influence of different techniques in characterising human antibodies to cow's milk proteins. *Clin. Exp. Med.*, **11**, 225
113. Jewell, D. P. and Truelove, S. C. (1972a). Circulating antibodies to cow's milk proteins in ulcerative colitis. *Gut*, **13**, 796
114. Rider, J. A., Moeller, H. C., Devereaux, R. G. and Wright, R. R. (1960). The use of an intramucosal test to demonstrate food hypersensitivity in ulcerative colitis. *Acta Allerg. (Kbh)*, **15, suppl. 7**, 486
115. Mirvish, L. (1960). The mucosa of the recto-sigmoid in ulcerative colitis. *S. Afr. Med. J.*, **34**, 732
116. Jewell, D. P. and Truelove, S. C. (1972b). Reaginic hypersensitivity in ulcerative colitis. *Gut*, **13**, 903
117. Broberger, O. and Perlmann, P. (1959). Autoantibodies in human ulcerative colitis. *J. Exp. Med.*, **110**, 657
118. Asherson, G. L. and Broberger, O. (1961). Incidence of haemagglutinating and complement-fixing antibodies. *Brit. Med. J.*, **i**, 1429

119. Perlmann, P., Hammarstrom, S., Lagercrantz, R. and Gustafsson, B. E. (1965). Antigen from colon of germfree rats and antibodies in human ulcerative colitis. *Ann. N.Y. Acad. Sci.*, **124**, 377
120. Hammarstrom, S., Lagercrantz, R., Perlmann, P. and Gustafsson, B. E. (1965). Immunological studies in ulcerative colitis. II. 'Colon' antigen and human blood group A- and H-like antigens in germ free rats. *J. Exp. Med.*, **122**, 1075
121. Lagercrantz, R., Hammarstrom, S., Perlmann, P. and Gustafsson, B. E. (1966). Immunological studies in ulcerative colitis. III. Incidence of antibodies to colon-antigen in ulcerative colitis and other gastro-intestinal diseases. *Clin. Exp. Immunol.*, **1**, 263
122. Zeromski, J., Perlmann, P., Lagercrantz, R., Hammarstrom, S. and Gustafsson, B. E. (1971). Immunological studies in ulcerative colitis. VII. Anti-colon antibodies of different immunoglobulin classes. *Clin. Exp. Immunol.*, **7**, 469
123. Wright, R. and Truelove, S. C. (1966). Auto-immune reactions in ulcerative colitis. *Gut*, **7**, 32
124. Broberger, O. and Perlmann, P. (1962). Demonstration of an epithelial antigen in colon by means of fluorescent antibodies from children with ulcerative colitis. *J. Exp. Med.*, **115**, 13
125. Kraft, S. C., Rimpila, J. J., Fitch, F. W. and Kirsner, J. B. (1966). Immunohistochemical studies of the colon in ulcerative colitis. *Arch. Path. (Chicago)*, **82**, 369
126. Kunin, C. M. (1963). Separation, characterization and biological significance of a common antigen in Enterobacteriaceae. *J. Exp. Med.*, **118**, 565
127. Lagercrantz, R., Hammarstrom, S., Perlmann, P. and Gustafsson, B. E. (1968). Immunological studies in ulcerative colitis. IV. Origin of autoantibodies. *J. Exp. Med.*, **128**, 1339
128. Thayer, W. R., Brown, M., Sangree, M. H., Katz, J. and Hersh, T. (1969). *Escherichia coli* 0:14 and colon haemagglutinating antibodies in inflammatory bowel disease. *Gastroenterology*, **57**, 311
129. Asherson, G. L. and Holborow, E. J. (1966). Autoantibody production in rabbits. VII. Autoantibodies to gut produced by the injection of bacteria. *Immunology*, **10**, 161
130. Perlmann, P., Hammarstrom, S., Lagercrantz, R. and Campbell, D. (1967). Autoantibodies to colon in rats and human ulcerative colitis: cross-reactivity with *Escherichia coli* 014 antigen. *Proc. Soc. exp. Biol (N.Y.)*, **125**, 975
131. McGiven, A. R., Ghose, T. and Nairn, R. C. (1967). Autoantibodies in ulcerative colitis. *Brit. Med. J.*, **2**, 19
132. Broberger, O. and Perlmann, P. (1963). *In vitro* studies of ulcerative colitis. I. Reactions of patients' serum with human foetal colon cells in tissue cultures. *J. Exp. Med.*, **117**, 705
133. Perlmann, P. and Broberger, O. (1963). *In vitro* studies of ulcerative colitis: II. Cytotoxic action of white blood cells from patients on human foetal colon cells. *J. Exp. Med.*, **117**, 717

134. Watson, D. W., Quigley, A. and Bolt, R. J. (1966). Effect of lymphocytes from patients with ulcerative colitis on human adult colon epithelial cells. *Gastroenterology*, **51**, 985
135. Shorter, R. G., Cardoza, M., Spencer, R. J. and Huizenga, K. A. (1969). Further studies of *in vitro* cytotoxicity of lymphocytes from patients with ulcerative and granulomatous colitis for allogeneic colonic epithelial cells, including the effects of colectomy. *Gastroenterology*, **56**, 304
136. Shorter, R. G., Spencer, R. J., Huizenga, K. A. and Hallenbeck, G. A. (1968). Inhibition of *in vitro* cytotoxicity of lymphocytes from patients with ulcerative colitis and granulomatous colitis for allogeneic colonic epithelial cells using horse anti-human thymus serum. *Gastroenterology*, **54**, 227
137. Shorter, R. G., Huizenga, K. A., ReMine, S. G. and Spencer, R. J. (1970). Effects of preliminary incubation of lymphocytes with serum on their cytotoxicity for colonic epithelial cells. *Gastroenterology*, **58**, 843
138. Shorter, R. G., Huizenga, K. A., Spencer, R. J., Aas, J. and Guy, S. K. (1972). Inflammatory bowel disease. Cytophilic antibody and the cytotoxicity of lymphocytes for colonic cells *in vitro*. *Amer. J. Dig. Dis.*, **16**, 673
139. Shorter, R. G., Cardoza, M. R., ReMine, S. G., Spencer, J. R. and Huizenga, K. A. (1970). Modification of *in vitro* cytotoxicity of lymphocytes from patients with chronic ulcerative colitis or granulomatous colitis for allogeneic colonic epithelial cells. *Gastroenterology*, **58**, 692
140. Shorter, R. G., Cardoza, M., Huizenga, K. A., ReMine, S. G. and Spencer, R. J. (1969). Further studies of *in vitro* cytotoxicity of lymphocytes for colonic epithelial cells. *Gastroenterology*, **57**, 30
141. Bull, D. M. and Ignaczak, T. F. (1973). Enterobacterial common antigen-induced lymphocyte reactivity in inflammatory bowel disease. *Gastroenterology*, **64**, 43
142. Bartnik, W., Swarbrick, E. T. and Williams, C. (1974). A study of peripheral leucocyte migration in agarose-medium in inflammatory bowel disease. *Gut*, **15**, 294
143. Bendixen, G. (1969). Cellular hypersensitivity to components of intestinal mucosa in ulcerative colitis and Crohn's disease. *Gut*, **10**, 631
144. Hunt, P. S. and Trotter, S. (1973). Lymphoblastic response to autologous colon epithelial cells in ulcerative colitis *in vitro*. *Gut*, **14**, 875
145. Stefani, S. and Fink, S. (1969). The ulcerative colitis lymphocyte: reaction to *E. coli* 0.14 and colon antigen. *Scand. J. Gastroenterol.*, **2**, 333
146. Fink, S. and Mais, R. F. (1968). Cell-mediated immune reaction to colon altered by bacteria. *Gut*, **9**, 629
147. Kirsner, J. B. (1965). The immunologic response of the colon. *J. Am. Med. Ass.*, **191**, 809
148. Auer, J. (1920). Local autoinoculation of the sensitized organism with foreign protein as a cause of abnormal reactions. *J. Exp. Med.*, **32**, 427

149. Bicks, R. O. and Rosenberg, E. W. (1964). A chronic delayed hypersensitivity reaction in the guinea pig colon. *Gastroenterology*, **46**, 543
150. Suizer, J. B., Spiro, H. M. and Thayer, W. R. (1966). Colonic manifestations of runt disease. *Yale J. Biol. Med.*, **39**, 106
151. Callahan, W. C., Goldman, R. G. and Vial, A. B. (1963). Auer phenomenon in colon-sensitized mice. *J. Surg. Res.*, **3**, 395
152. Palov, R. O., Halpern, B. and Zweibaum, A. (1967). Experimental production of haemorrhagic ulcerative colitis with autoantibodies. *Med. Hyg.* (Geneva), **25**, 62
153. Kraft, S. C. and Kirsner, J. B. (1971). Immunological apparatus of the gut and inflammatory bowel disease. *Gastroenterology*, **60**, 922
154. Shean, F. C., Barker, W. F. and Fonkalsrud, E. W. (1964). Studies on active and passive antibody induced colitis in the dog. *Am. J. Surg.*, **107**, 337
155. Bicks, R. O. and Walker, R. H. (1962). Immunologic 'colitis' in dogs. *Amer. J. Dig. Dis (n.s.)*, **7**, 574
156. Zweibaum, A., Morard, J. C. and Halpern, B. (1968). Realisation d'une colite ulcero-haemorrhagique experimentale par immunisation bacterienne. *Path. Biol.*, **16**, 813
157. Cooke, E. M., Filipe, M. I. and Dawson, I. M. P. (1968). The production of colonic autoantibodies in rabbits by immunization with *Escherichia coli*. *J. Path. Bact.*, **96**, 125
158. Watt, J. and Marcus, R. (1971). Carrageenan-induced ulceration of the large intestine in the guinea pig. *Gut*, **12**, 164
159. Davies, G. E. (1963). Inhibition of guinea pig complement *in vitro* and *in vivo* by carrageenin. *Immunology*, **6**, 561
160. Brandtzaeg, P., Baklien, K., Fausa, O. and Hoel, P. S. (1974). Immunochemical characterisation of local immunoglobulin formation in ulcerative colitis. *Gastroenterology*, **66**, 1123
161. Brandtzaeg, P. (1972). Local formation and transport of immunoglobulins related to the oral cavity. In *Host resistance to commensal bacteria*. T. Macphee (ed.) 116. (Edinburgh: Churchill, Livingstone)
162. Monteiro, E., Fossey, J., Shiner, M., Drasar, B. S. and Allison, A. C. (1971). Antibacterial antibodies in rectal and colonic mucosa in ulcerative colitis. *Lancet*, **i**, 249
163. Doe, W. F., Booth, C. C. and Brown, D. L. (1973). Evidence for complement-binding immune complexes in adult coeliac disease, Crohn's disease and ulcerative colitis. *Lancet*, **i**, 402
164. Jewell, D. P. and MacLennan, I. C. M. (1973). Circulating immune complexes in inflammatory bowel disease. *Clin. Exp. Immunol.*, **14**, 219
165. Mannik, M. and Arend, W. P. (1971). Fate of preformed immune complexes in rabbits and rhesus monkeys. *J. Exp. Med.*, **134**, 19s
166. Ballard, J. and Shiner, M. (1974). Evidence of cytotoxicity in ulcerative colitis from immunofluorescent staining of the rectal mucosa. *Lancet*, **i**, 1014

167. Baklien, K. and Brandtzaeg, P. (1974). Immunohistochemical localisation of complement in intestinal mucosa. *Lancet*, **ii**, 1087
168. Thayer, W. R. and Spiro, H. M. (1963). Persistence of serum complement in sera of patients with ulcerative colitis. *J. Lab. Clin. Med.*, **62**, 24
169. Fletcher, J. (1965). Serum complement levels in active ulcerative colitis. *Gut*, **6**, 172
170. Ward, M. and Eastwood, M. A. (1974). Serum complement components C3 and C4 in inflammatory bowel disease. *Gut*, **15**, 835
171. Hodgson, H. J. F., Potter, B. J. and Jewell, D. P. (1975). C3 metabolism in inflammatory bowel disease. *Gut*, **16**, 833.
172. Moschcowitz, E. and Wilensky, A. O. (1923). Non-specific granulomata of the intestine. *Amer. J., Med. Sci.*, **166**, 48
173. Van Patter, W., Bargen, J., Dockerty, N., Feldman, W., Mayo, C. and Waugh, J. (1954). Regional enteritis. *Gastroenterology*, **26**, 347
174. Parent, K. and Wilson, I. D. (1971). Mycobacteriophage in Crohn's disease. *Gut*. **12**, 1019
175. Gorbach, S. L. and Tabaqchali, S. (1969). Bacteria, bile and the small bowel. *Gut*, **10**, 963
176. Beeken, W. L. and Kanigh, R. E. (1973). Microbial flora of the upper small bowel in Crohn's disease. *Gastroenterology*, **65**, 390
177. Winblad, S., Nilehn, B. and Sternby, N. (1966). *Yersinia enterocolitica* (*Pasteurella X*) in human enteric infections. *Lancet*, **ii**, 1363
178. Mitchell, D. N. and Rees, R. J. W. (1969). A transmissible agent from sarcoid tissue. *Lancet*, **ii**, 81
179. Mitchell, D. N. and Rees, R. J. W. (1970). Agent transmissible from Crohn's disease tissue. *Lancet*, **ii**, 168
180. Taub, R. N. and Siltszbach, L. E. (1972). In *VIth International Conference Sarcoidosis*. p. 5. (Tokyo: University of Tokyo Press).
181. Cave, D. R., Mitchell, D. N., Kane, S. P. and Brooke, B. R. (1973). Further animal evidence of a transmissible agent in Crohn's disease. *Lancet*, **ii**, 1120
182. Bolton, P. M., Owen, E., Heatley, R. V., Jones Williams, W. and Hughes, L. E. (1973). Negative findings in laboratory animals for a transmissible agent in Crohn's disease. *Lancet*, **ii**, 1122
183. de Deuxchaisnes, C. N., Huaux, J. P., Fiasse, E. and Bruyere, M. de. (1974). Ankylosing spondylitis, sacroileitis, regional enteritis and HL-A 27. *Lancet*, **i**, 1238
184. Deodhar, S. D., Michener, W. M. and Farmer, R. G. (1969). A study of the immunologic aspects of chronic ulcerative colitis and transmural colitis. *Am. J. Clin. Path* **51**, 591
185. Perrett, A. D., Higgins, G., Johnston, H. H., Massarella, G. R., Truelove, S. C. and Wright, R. (1971). The liver in Crohn's disease. *Quart. J. Med.*, **40**, 187
186. Bendixen, G., Jarnum, S., Soltoft, J., Westergaard, H., Weeke, B. and Yssing, M. (1968). IgG and albumen turnover in Crohn's disease. *Scand. J. Gastroenterol.*, **3**, 481

187. Jensen, K. B., Goltermann, N., Jarnum, S., Weeke, B. and Westergaard, H. (1970). IgM turnover in Crohn's disease. *Gut*, **11**, 223
188. Bucknall, R. C., Verrier-Jones, J. and Peacock, D. B. (1974). Antibody production to the bacteriophage ϕx 174 in patients with Crohn's disease. *Gut*, **15**, 345
189. Eggert, R. C., Wilson, I. D. and Good, R. A. (1969). Agammaglobulinaemia and regional enteritis. *Ann. Intern. Med.*, **71**, 581
190. Blackburn, G., Hadfield, G. and Hunt, A. H. (1939). Regional ileitis. *St. Bart. Hosp. Rep.*, **72**, 181
191. Phear, D. (1958). The relation between regional ileitis and sarcoidosis. *Lancet*, **ii**, 1250
192. Fletcher, J. and Hinton, J. M. (1967). Tuberculin sensitivity in Crohn's disease. *Lancet*, **ii**, 753
193. Geffroy, Y., Colin, R., Hecketsweiler, P. H. and Segrestin, M. (1971). Traitement de la maladie de Crohn par le B.C.G. *Arch. Fr. Mal. Appar. Dig.*, **60**, 299
194. Binder, H. J., Spiro, H. M. and Thayer, W. R. (1966). Delayed hypersensitivity in regional enteritis and ulcerative colitis. *Am. J. Dig. Dis.*, **11**, 572
195. Verrier-Jones, J., Housley, J., Ashurst, P. M. and Hawkins, C. F. (1969). Development of delayed hypersensitivity to DNCB in patients with Crohn's disease. *Gut*, **10**, 52
196. Walker, J. G. and Greaves, M. F. (1969). Delayed hypersensitivity and lymphocyte transformation in Crohn's disease and proctocolitis. *Gut*, **10**, 414
197. Brown, S. M., Taub, R. N., Present, D. H. and Janowitz, H. D. (1970). Short-term lymphocyte cultures in regional enteritis. *Lancet*, **i**, 1112
198. Asquith, P., Kraft, S. C. and Rothberg, R. M. (1973). Lymphocyte responses to non-specific mitogens in inflammatory bowel disease. *Gastroenterology*, **65**, 1
199. Richens, E. R., Williams, M. J., Gough, K. R. and Ancill, R. J. (1974). Mixed lymphocyte reaction as a measure of immunological competence of lymphocytes from patients with Crohn's disease. *Gut*, **15**, 24
200. Ropke, C. (1972). Lymphocyte transformation and delayed hypersensitivity in Crohn's disease. *Scand. J. Gastroenterol.*, **7**, 671
201. Aas, J., Huizenga, K. A., Newcomer, A. D. and Shorter, R. G. (1972). Inflammatory bowel disease: lymphocyte responses to non-specific simulation *in vitro*. *Scand. J. Gastroenterol.*, **7**, 299
202. Bird, A. G. and Britton, S. (1974). No evidence for decreased lymphocyte reactivity in Crohn's disease. *Gastroenterology*, **67**, 926
203. Mitchell, D. N., Cannon, P., Dyer, N. H., Hinson, K. F. W. and Willoughby, J. M. T. (1969). The Kveim test in Crohn's disease. *Lancet*, **ii**, 571
204. Karlish, A. J., Cox, E. V., Hampson, F. and Hemsted, E. H. (1970). Kveim test in Crohn's disease. *Lancet*, **ii**, 977

205. Siltzbach, L. E., Vieira, L. O. B. D., Topilsky, M. and Janowitz, H. D. (1971). Is there Kveim responsiveness in Crohn's disease? *Lancet*, **ii**, 634

206. James, D. G. (1975). Kveim revisted, reassessed. *New Eng. J. Med.*, **292**, 859

207. Willoughby, J. M. T. and Mitchell, D. N. (1971). *In vitro* inhibition of leucocyte migration in Crohn's disease by a sarcoid spleen suspension. *Brit. Med. J.*, **3**, 155

208. Pagaltsos, A. S., Kumar, P. J., Willoughby, J. M. T. and Dawson, A. M. (1971). *In vitro* inhibition of leucocyte migration by sarcoid spleen suspension in coeliac disease and dermatitis herpetiformis. *Lancet*, **ii**, 1179

209. Dykes, P. W. (1970). Delayed hypersensitivity in Crohn's disease. *Proc. Roy. Soc. Med.*, **63**, 906

210. Richens, E. R., Williams, M. J., Gough, K. R. and Ancill, R. J. (1974). Leucocyte migration studies in Crohn's disease using Crohn's colon homogenate and mitochondrial and microsomal fractions. *Gut*, **15**, 19

211. Parent, K., Barrett, J. and Dodd Wilson, I. (1971). Investigation of the pathogenic mechanisms in regional enteritis with *in vitro* lymphocyte cultures. *Gastroenterology*, **61**, 431

212. Breucha, G. and Riethmuller, G. (1975). Intestinal lymphocytes in Crohn's disease. *Lancet*, **i**, 976

213. Green, F. H. Y. and Fox, H. (1975). The distribution of mucosal antibodies in the bowel of patients with Crohn's disease. *Gut*, **16**, 125

214. Spector, W. G. and Heesom, N. (1969). The production of granulomata by antibody–antigen complexes. *J. Path.*, **98**, 31

215. Hywel-Jones, J., Lennard-Jones, J. E., Morson, B. C., Chapman, M., Sackin, M. J., Sneath, P. H. A., Spicer, C. C. and Card, W. I. (1973). Numerical taxonomy and discriminant analysis applied to non-specific colitis. *Quart. J. Med.*, **42**, 715

216. Miller, D. S., Keighley, A. C. and Langman, M. J. S. (1974). Changing pattern in epidemiology of Crohn's disease. *Lancet*, **ii**, 691

217. Hooper, B., Whittingham, S., Matthews, J. D., Mackay, I. R. and Curnow, D. H. (1972). Autoimmunity in a rural community. *Clin. Exp. Immunol.*, **12**, 79

218. Isokoski, M., Krohn, K., Varis, K. and Siurala, M. (1969). Parietal cell and intrinsic factor antibodies in a Finnish rural population sample. *Scand, J. Gastroent.*, **4**, 521

219. Coghill, N. F., Doniach, D., Roitt, I. M., Mollin, D. L. and Williams, A. W. (1965). Autoantibodies in simple atrophic gastritis. *Gut*, **6**, 48

220. Schiller, K. F. R., Spray, G. H., Wangel, A. G. and Wright, R. (1968). Clinical and precursor forms of pernicious anaemia in hyperthyroidism. *Quart. J. Med.*, **37**, 451

221. Irvine, W. J., Davies, S. H., Teitelbaum, S., Delamore, I. W. and Wyn Williams (1965). The clinical and pathological significance of gastric parietal cell antibody. *Ann. N.Y. Acad. Sci.*, **124**, 657

222. Ungar, B., Stocks, A. E., Martin, F. I. R., Whittingham, S. and Mackay, I. R. (1968). Intrinsic factor antibody, parietal cell antibody and latent pernicious anaemia in diabetes mellitus. *Lancet*, **ii**, 415
223. Dagg, J. H., Goldberg, A., Anderson, J. R., Beck, J. S. and Gray, K. G. (1965). Autoimmunity in iron-deficiency anaemia. *Ann. N.Y. Acad. Sci.*, **124**, 692
224. Irvine, W. J., Clarke, B. F., Scarth, L., Cullen, D. R. and Duncan, L. J. P. (1970). Thyroid and gastric autoimmunity in patients with diabetes mellitus. *Lancet*, **ii**, 163
225. Irvine, W. J., Stewart, A. G. and Scarth, L. (1967). A clinical and immunological study of adrenocortical insufficiency (Addison's Disease). *Clin. Exp. Immunol.*, **2**, 31
226. Blizzard, R. M., Chee, D. nad Davis, W. (1967). The incidence of adrenal and other antibodies in the sera of patients with idiopathic adrenal insufficiency (Addison's Disease). *Clin. Exp. Immunol.*, **2**, 19
227. Blizzard, R. M., Chee, D. and Davis, W. (1966). The incidence of parathyroid and other antibodies in the sera of patients with idiopathic hypoparathyroidism. *Clin. Exp. Immunol.*, **1**, 119

CHAPTER 7

The mononuclear phagocytic functions of the liver

M. Bjørneboe and Hanne Prytz

Introduction

The reticuloendothelial system was the name originally proposed by Aschoff for a system of cells of great morphological diversity linked together by the property of phagocytosis[1]. This cell system comprises endothelial cells, fibrocytes, reticular cells of spleen and lymph nodes, reticuloendothelial cells of lymph and blood sinuses including Kupffer cells, histiocytes, splenocytes and monocytes. Several attempts have been made through the years to find a better descriptive term than the reticuloendothelial system. The most recent proposal, and generally an acceptable one, has been the introduction of the term mononuclear phagocyte system, 'comprising a group of cells that are related by similarities of morphology, function and origin'[2]. This mononuclear phagocyte system (MPS) comprises precursor cells (in the bone marrow), promonocytes (in the bone marrow), monocytes (in the bone marrow and in the blood) and macrophages in connective tissue (histiocytes), liver (Kupffer cells), lung (alveolar macrophages), spleen (free and fixed macrophages), lymph nodes (free and fixed macrophages), bone marrow (macrophages), serous cavities (pleural and peritoneal macrophages), bone tissue (osteoclasts), and nervous system (microglial cells). The part of the mononuclear phagocytic system to be described here is the system of macrophages in the liver, the Kupffer cells. Most studies concerned with the MPS have not made a distinction between Kupffer cells and other macrophages but described the system as a whole. However, the fact that the Kupffer cells comprise by far the greatest part of the MPS, together with their strategic localization in relation to the blood flow from the gastrointestinal tract, justifies discussing them as a special entity. In recent years the idea has repeatedly been put forward that the function of these cells is different from other phagocytic cells, especially with regard to immune phenomena. In this chapter we wish to describe the functions of the Kupffer cells with special emphasis on their role in immune processes.

Morphology

The cells lining the sinusoids of the liver, the endothelial or littoral cells, comprise in the rat about one-third of the total number of cells in the liver[3–5], but less than 3% of the volume of the liver[5]. In humans, however, it has been found that the endothelial cells comprise 15% of the total number of liver cells[6]. 'Some of the lining endothelial cells are potentially phagocytic and known as the stellate cells of Kupffer[7].' These cells bulge into the lumina of the sinusoids and may have prominent cytoplasmic processes. The opinion that the Kupffer cells in the liver are sitting across the lumina of the sinusoids may be a neglect of three dimensional analysis of histological sections[8], though other authors still favour the description of Kupffer cells as stellate cells attached to the walls of the sinusoids by long processes[9]. These cells can be recognized among the endothelial cells by their low nuclear/

cytoplasmic ratio, their irregular shape, the presence of granules varying in shape and density, and the occurrence of worm like bodies at the cell surface[10]. They have a filamentous and fuzzy cell coat[11]. This division into lining endothelial cells and phagocytic endothelial or Kupffer cells is still a controversial subject[12–14]. A third kind of cell connected with the sinusoids are the perisinusoidal cells, also called fat storage cells. These cells are of interest because it has been claimed that they are the source of collagen production in liver cell injury[15]. The origin of the Kupffer cells is not settled. They may come from the mononuclear cells of the blood but other possibilities are that they are derived from cells already present in the sinusoids or originate in the spleen[9]. They can probably migrate within the liver and, via the blood stream, to other organs.[9]

Kupffer cells can be isolated by different methods: a pronase digestion followed by differential centrifugation[16]; or iron loading with intravenous iron, and enzyme digestion following which iron containing and non-iron containing cells are separated by a magnetic technique[17]. The isolated Kupffer cells retain their phagocytic properties, and may be maintained in cell culture[18]. Enzyme studies[19,20] and immunochemical characterization[21] of the cell isolates have been described.

Phagocytosis

Phagocytosis in general

Phagocytosis is the process by which phagocytic cells engulf particulate matter. The particles become attached to the surface of the cell, the cell membrane folds and the so-called phagosomes, vacuoles containing the phagocytized material, are formed. This process can be closely followed in experimental animals in isolated perfused livers[22,23], in tissue slices[24,25] and in isolated Kupffer cells[18]. In experimental animals the process has most frequently been studied using colloid carbon[26]. These particles, when injected intravenously, cannot leave the circulation unless they are phagocytized by the cells of the MPS, and therefore their disappearance rate will be an expression of the function of these cells. The concentration in the serum is determined photometrically. After injection into an experimental animal, most of the carbon will be fixed in the Kupffer cells in the liver, smaller amounts being fixed in the spleen and in the bone marrow. The clearance curve in the blood can be analysed mathematically. It can be demonstrated that particles are phagocytized according to an exponential function of their concentration in relation to time:

$$C = C_o \times 10^{kt} \text{ or } k = \frac{\log C - \log C_o}{t}$$

where t is the time interval between the measurements of the concentrations C and C_0. The constant k in the equation, the phagocytic index, measures the rate of phagocytosis. Below a certain critical concentration of the colloid practically all colloid is cleared in the liver during one passage. This very efficient extraction in the liver can be used to calculate the liver blood flow[26]. When the injected dose is increased the phagocytic index decreases and at the same time more and more carbon is taken up by the spleen. The absolute amount of carbon phagocytized is, however, increased with the dose of carbon injected and approaches asymptotically a maximal value that can be calculated. It is also possible to calculate the phagocytic activity per unit weight of liver + spleen[26] and to estimate an index of individual cellular phagocytic activity independent of perfusion[27]. Such studies of the kinetics of phagocytosis have most often, in experimental animals, been performed with unphysiological substances such as colloid carbon or radioactive gold. The dynamics of phagocytosis seem, however, to be the same for other substances used and to be the same in many animal species.

For investigations in humans radioisotopically labelled human serum albumin[28,29] or artificial MPS test lipid emulsions[30] have been employed. Radiocolloidal gold and a colloidal sulphide of ^{99m}Tc have also been used, but mainly for hepatic scintillography[31].

These experimental assessments of phagocytic functions, measure the function not only of the Kupffer cells but also of phagocytic cells in other organs such as spleen and bone marrow. The Kupffer cells, however, play by far the largest role. It has also to be stressed that these equations calculated for inert substances such as colloidal carbon or gold may not be directly applicable to the phagocytosis of complex chemical compounds which are broken down in the phagocytic cells, or of microbial organisms. However, these experimental studies have contributed much to our knowledge of phagocytosis and of the various factors that modify the functions of phagocytic cells.

Phagocytosis of bacteria: The phagocytic clearance of bacteria by the

MPS follows an exponential pattern in only the first few minutes[32]. Thereafter the clearance rate becomes slower, probably due to the presence of bacteria highly resistant to phagocytosis. No inverse relationship can be demonstrated between dose and rate of clearance of bacteria. Maximum extraction during passage through the liver and spleen is lower than for colloids. Nevertheless the capacity of the MPS to continue to phagocytize bacteria is very great. Stimulation and depression of the MPS do not necessarily influence resistance to infection[33]. The phagocytosis of bacteria is much increased by specific antibody and also by a non-specific factor in normal serum which enhance phagocytosis by exerting an opsonin-like effect[34].

The fate of phagocytized bacteria varies. Some are killed rapidly, but others are resistant to the bactericidal activity of phagocytic cells and are capable of multiplication within the cells. Phagocytosis and intracellular killing are not necessarily interdependent processes. Careful early studies by blood cultures in bacterial endocarditis demonstrated that the lowest bacterial concentration in the blood was found in the hepatic vein, and that the liver thus had an important filter effect for microbes[35]. Intracellular parasitization of the MPS with one microbe may enhance the resistance of the body to infection with another microbe[36].

Phagocytosis of viruses: Many viruses are phagocytized by the MPS, e.g. bacteriophages, tobacco mosaic virus, Newcastle disease virus, Riley virus, ectromelia virus, canine hepatitis virus and murine hepatitis virus. It has been shown that specific antibody increases the rate of viral phagocytosis. Some viruses that initiate an infectious process in the host are also phagocytized and some of these viruses seem to be able to replicate in the phagocytic cells. Murine hepatitis virus enters the Kupffer cells before it appears in the liver parenchymal cells. Resistance to this virus, genetically determined, can be demonstrated to correlate with failure of viral infection to produce cytopathic effects in cultures of macrophages[37]. The role of the MPS in the pathogenesis of experimental viral hepatitis has recently been reviewed[38]. Since relatively few of the viruses discussed are hepatotropic it is likely that the Kupffer cells may determine whether or not liver parenchymal cells become infected. Most of the viruses are phagocytized by the Kupffer cells, although there are known exceptions, e.g. poliovirus Type I. There they may be inactivated (influenza and vaccinia), may be passed through to the hepatocytes (Rift valley fever), or may replicate (ectromelia or mouse pox, yellow fever, infectious canine hepatitis and possibly murine hepatitis virus). In human viral hepatitis, enlarged prominent Kupffer cells are a characteristic feature. Hepatitis B antigen–antibody complexes are found in occasional Kupffer cells and phagocytosis of the hepatitis virus may be involved in the pathogenesis of the disease.

Phagocytosis of proteins: Phagocytosis is most often discussed in relation to particulate matter. Soluble proteins, however, are also phagocytized and this is a crucial step in the induction of the primary immune response[39]. It has been shown that all the molecules in a solution of a 'foreign' protein are not homogenous with respect to their ability either to induce tolerance or provoke antibody production[39]. Aggregated molecules are more easily phagocytized and so are heat or otherwise denatured proteins[40,41]. Soluble antigen-antibody complexes are also phagocytized and this is dependent on the antigen-antibody ratio, being maximal when they are mixed in optimal proportions[42,43].

Factors that influence phagocytosis

The 'blockade' phenomenon: Repeated injections of colloidal carbon will decrease the rate of blood clearance of this colloid because of saturation or so-called 'blockade' of the MPS. Phagocytosis will, however, never be completely suppressed and the 'blockade' will be of short duration because saturated cells are replaced by new proliferating cells.

In man, 'blockade' of the MPS has been described using radio isotopically labelled aggregated human serum albumin particles [^{131}I]-AA. The effect of the 'blockade' was measured with radioactive gold, radioactive chromic phosphate and [^{131}I]-AA. 'Blockade' was shown to be specific, clearance of similar particles being more inhibited than clearance of dissimilar particles[44].

'Blockade' may cause a change in organ distribution of other substances injected. It was shown that radiolabelled sheep red blood cells (SRBC) given intravenously to mice, after an intravenous dose of colloidal carbon, were taken up less in the liver and more in the spleen. In the same experiments it was demonstrated that the immune response was higher in the mice given colloid carbon[45]. An inverse correlation between uptake of SRBC in liver and spleen was, however, not found in another study[46]. Saturation, 'blockade', of the hepatic MPS can also be brought about by immune complexes. In mice soluble human serum albumin (HSA)/anti HSA immune complexes are preferentially cleared by the hepatic MPS, when the molecular composition exceeds Ag_2Ab_2. Due to the saturation of the MPS, complexes of this size may persist in the circulation and may be deposited in non-heptic tissue[42,43].

Depression of phagocytosis: The phagocytic capacity decreases slightly but significantly with age in man[48], and a similar depression in rats may be accompanied by morphological changes in the liver MPS[47]. Surgical trauma induces a transient depression due to a decrease in Kupffer cell phagocytosis[49–51], and in dietary protein deficiency there is also phagocytic depression[52]. Chemical depressants are lead acetate[53,54], ethyl palmitate[9], cyclophosphamide[55,56] (azathioprine in contrast is without effect[57,58]) halothane, morphine and pentobarbital[59]. Corticosteroids also depress; this phenomenon was more marked in germ-free mice, holoxenic mice being more resistant to this effect[60]. With small doses, however, phagocytic activity was increased. These differences in the corticosteroid studies could be due to infections induced by their administration in non-sterile animals, the depressing action of the steroids being counterbalanced by the stimulation of the MPS caused by the infections[60]. Alcohol stimulates in low doses, but depresses after a single high dose[59,61]. In severely intoxicated mice phagocytosis and killing of bacteria by peritoneal macrophages was decreased[62]. In pregnancy phagocytic function is depressed during the first two trimesters, and enhanced during the last trimester principally due to increased Kupffer cell activity[63]. Whereas anti-lymphocytic serum depresses after one injection, a transient stimulation occurs when more injections are given[64].

Liver, spleen and other parts of the MPS are target organs of endotoxin (the lipopolysaccharide fraction of Gram-negative bacilli). [^{131}I]-labelled endotoxin is specifically concentrated in the liver. The effect on the phagocytic activity of the MPS is a depression, sometimes, but not always, followed by stimulation[65–67]. Animals can be protected against the lethal effect of endotoxin by prophylactic corticosteroid treatment[68].

Stimulation of phagocytosis: Intravenously injected colloids in a concentration below a certain critical level are, as already mentioned, removed at rates proportional to portal blood flow. At concentrations above this critical level increased phagocytic clearance and increased blood flow may occur together, but clearance rates need not be statistically dependent upon blood flow[69]. In experimental rats phagocytosis is markedly depressed after partial hepatectomy. However, on a weight basis enhanced phagocytosis is found due to increased perfusion of the residual liver mass[70]. Lung and spleen phagocytosis, however, is increased due to increased availability of injected particles to extrahepatic macrophages[70]. Stimulation of the MPS has been reported following transplantation of small skin grafts[71].

The effect of infections on the MPS varies. They have no effect if they are rapidly fatal. In more protracted infections transient stimulation, and in mild infections stronger stimulation, are seen[26]. Observations indicate that bacterial infections stimulate[72], whereas viral infections inhibit non-specific phagocytosis[73].

Chemical stimulants include zymosan, a yeast extract[74,75], brewer's yeast [76], glucan[77], glyceryl ester of oleic acid[24], *Corynebacterium parvum* vaccine[78], a lipid fraction of *Mycobacterium tuberculosis*[79,80] and estrogens[81–83]. Whole body radiation has given conflicting results in animal studies[84]. When stimulation is found this is probably confined to the Kupffer cells[85].

METABOLIC FUNCTIONS OF THE HEPATIC MPS

Aged, incompatible and abnormal red cells are taken up by the MPS and broken down there. About a quarter of the phagocytic cells in the liver are 'erythrophagocytic' and these cells play an important role in bilirubin formation[86]. 'Blockade' of the MPS with thorotrast has been shown to inhibit bilirubin production[87]. The iron released from the heme of phagocytized red cells is either returned to the plasma or stored in the form of haemosiderin granules[88,89].

The MPS is a major site for the removal of coagulation and fibrinolytic products from the circulation and the Kupffer cells play a major role in this removal[90]. Overloading the liver macrophages with denatured albumin impairs the capacity of these cells to remove subsequently infused fibrinolytic products[91]. Whereas intravenously injected denatured albumin is rapidly removed from the circulation by the MPS, predominantly by Kupffer cells, and catabolized, native albumin is catabolized there only to a small extent[92–94].

Kupffer cells probably play a significant role in the uptake and metabolism of fatty acids[95,96]. Intravenously injected colloidal suspensions of cholesterol are removed by macrophages, primarily by the Kupffer cells, and probably again delivered to lipoproteins in serum[97,98]. Normal chylomicrons containing cholesterol or triglyceride are removed essentially by the liver parenchymal cells[99].

Studies on isolated Kupffer cells have shown that they are important in biotransformation of steroids essential for many biological processes particularly those concerned with inflammation[100], and also that of all macrophage cell types they have the greatest endotoxin-detoxifying activity[101].

Alterations in the phagocytic activity of the MPS occur in patients with malignant neoplasms, and in experimental animals stimulation of the MPS has been shown to inhibit tumour spread[102,103].

Acute and chronic liver disease and hepatic MPS functions

Animal experiments

In studies in rats using colloidal carbon and measuring total body MPS activity, acute carbon tetrachloride injury[104], tannic acid induced necrosis[105], and fatty liver produced by a choline deficient diet[106], all resulted in increased phagocytic activity. Rats with an inactive cirrhosis after chronic carbon tetrachloride exposure showed only a small increase in phagocytosis[104]. The increase in phagocytosis in choline deficiency occurred only when linoleic acid was present in the diet[106], and is perhaps related to the stimulating effect of linoleic acid on phagocytosis[24].

In more recent studies in which liver phagocytic activity *per se* was assessed in a rat/carbon tetrachloride cirrhosis model, the ability of the Kupffer cells to sequester immune complexes of bovine serum albumin (BSA)/anti-BSA and of *Salmonella adelaide* was impaired, the degree of impairment increasing with the severity of the cirrhotic process[107]. In rats MPS 'blockade' increased and MPS stimulation reduced the susceptibility to galactosamine induced liver damage[108].

Human liver disease

Histological changes in Kupffer cells are regularly observed in acute and chronic liver disease and, on light microscopy, comprise hypertrophy and hyperplasia of these cells.

Using [^{125}I]-labelled microaggregated human serum albumin ([^{125}I]-MAA) a significant decrease in total MPS activity was demonstrated in patients with alcoholic cirrhosis, many of whom had clinical or radiographic evidence of portal systemic shunting[27]. In other forms of cirrhosis normal results were obtained. In alcoholics with mild hepatic abnormalities but without cirrhosis and again using [^{125}I]-MAA total body MPS activity was depressed, probably due to alcohol *per se*[109]. Using radioactive colloidal gold and hepatic scintigraphy in patients with alcoholic cirrhosis, the extrahepatic uptake was shown to have a negative correlation with hepatic parenchymal function and a positive correlation to portal pressure[110].

Using [^{131}I]-labelled heat aggregated human serum albumin, the extraction rate in a single passage through the liver was 89% in a normal person and 62% in a patient with cirrhosis[111]. Similar results were found with radiolabelled colloid chromic phosphate[112]. In these investigations extraction by the liver was studied using catheterization of the portal and hepatic veins or by study of tissue distribution of the colloid, and therefore they reveal changes or Kupffer cell functions. Changes in liver blood flow will also affect liver MPS function, but such an effect is to be expected only when the substance to be phagocytized is present in the blood below a certain 'critical' concentration and only when total hepatic blood flow is reduced. The contribution of portal blood to total hepatic blood flow is decreased in cirrhosis[113], but total hepatic blood flow is not always decreased[114,115]. In patients with a portacaval shunt the total hepatic blood flow is usually lower than normal[116].

In summary, therefore, experimental and clinical studies demonstrate a decrease in the phagocytic function of the Kupffer cells in cirrhosis. The total phagocytic capacity of the body may be normal or even increased.

Antibody production and hepatic MPS function

Immunologically, macrophages have two main functions: (1) Catabolism and elimination of potentially immunogenic molecules, (2) Concentration and retention of a small amount of immunogen. The first function has not been sufficiently stressed[117]. The decreased function of the Kupffer cells in respect of the elimination of immunogens is now regarded as the main cause of the increased antibody production in diseases of the liver, a postulate which was advanced several years ago.

Intracardiac injection of neoarsphenamine inhibited sensitization to this substance on skin challenge shortly afterwards[118]. Feeding of certain substances prevented skin sensitization to the same haptens later applied to the skin[119]. Injection of an antigen into the portal vein could inhibit delayed contact sensitivity to the same antigen[120]. The special role of the liver was first pointed out in studies on the production of antibodies against l-chloro-2,4-dinitrobenzene (DNCB) in dogs[121]. Feeding with DNCB for 20 days inhibited the production of antibodies to DNCB given subcutaneously 14 days later. The inhibition was abolished if portacaval transposition was performed in the dogs before feeding. It was concluded from these experiments that if the antigen was carried to the liver before entry into the lymphatics and into the general circulation, the ability of the organism to recognize and react to the antigen on later contact was decreased. A kind of tolerance was established. The strategic interposition of the liver between the gastro-intestinal tract and the general circulation insured against sensitization of the organism to simple antigens absorbed via the portal blood from the intestinal contents. The increased serum immunoglobulin concentrations in diseases of the liver could result from impairment of this hepatic function.

Two possible explanations for these observations could be made: (1) the immunogenic property of antigens is destroyed in the liver, and (2) antigens sequestered in the liver produce a tolerogenic effect, so that sensitization against them is prevented for some time. Evidence in support of the second concept has recently been produced[122]. A state of partial specific immunological tolerance to a soluble high molecular weight food protein, bovine serum albumin, was achieved in rats by oral administration of the antigen. The antigen was absorbed in the native form and was found in minute concentrations in serum. The form of tolerance induced had features in common with the state of tolerance induced by parenteral administration of small amounts of the same antigen. We shall now examine the evidence in favour of the first concept, i.e. the destruction of the immunogenicity of antigens by the liver.

Immunogenicity of antigens phagocytized in the Kupffer cells

Proteins are, as already mentioned, broken down in Kupffer cells probably by enzymes in the phagolysosomes. A small part of the phagocytized antigen may be passed on to immunocytes in a more immunogenic form. It appears that antigen-charged Kupffer cells are ineffective in transferring an immunogenic stimulus to lymphocytes circulating through the liver sinusoids.[123] A further possibility is that Kupffer cells are more efficient than other phagocytes in breaking down antigens.

The fate of bacteriophage in mammalian tissue has been investigated by measuring the ability of subcellular fractions from cells which had ingested phage to induce antibody production[124]. Although the immunogenicity of certain subcellular fractions was increased during the first 48 hours the total immunogenicity rapidly disappeared in liver tissue. Isolated Kupffer cells from mice containing T_4 bacteriophage transferred to normal animals provoked little or no antibody production[125]. It was suggested that Kupffer cells destroyed antigens and did not cooperate in antibody synthesis.

Liver and spleen have been shown to differ greatly in their handling of sheep erythrocytes[126]. Examination of the immunogenicity of this antigen in mice showed that subcellular fractions prepared from liver tissue had lost their antigenic property completely in 12 hours whereas fractions prepared from the spleen retained their antigenicity for several days. Using the same antigen it has been shown that the immunogenic potential of low molecular weight RNA extracted from rat peritoneal exudate cells was about 10 times higher than that extracted from Kupffer cells[127]. In non-immune germ-free mice in whom bacteriophage Lambda was injected the bacteriophage disappeared rapidly from the liver as measured by a plaque forming technique, whereas the bacteriophage was retained much longer in the spleen[128].

If it is accepted that the main function of the Kupffer cells in relation to antigens is to destroy them, then a decrease in the function of the Kupffer cells will result in an increased antigenic load, and consequently increased antibody production. This phenomenon will be especially pronounced for those organisms against which phagocytosis is the most important defence mechanism[129].

Humoral antibody production in liver disease

Evidence that patients with hepatic cirrhosis produce increased antibody responses was first shown in 1951[130]. A significantly greater antibody production to diphtheria toxoid was observed in Schick-negative cirrhotic patients as compared with Schick-negative controls. However, other workers, using tetanus toxoid and brucella antigen found no differences in antibody response[131–133]. In primary biliary cirrhosis a decreased antibody response to primary immunization with haemocyanin was reported; the response in cryptogenic cirrhosis was also depressed but to a lesser extent[134]. Following immunization with blood group A and B isoantigens, patients with acute or chronic hepatitis produced a greater antibody response than normal controls, the responses being greatest in the chronic hepatitis group[135].

The results obtained are thus conflicting. It is possible that immunization with subcutaneous injection of antigen is a situation in which it is difficult to demonstrate the influence of the liver on antibody production. Antigens absorbed from subcutaneous tissue into the blood will presumably have already initiated antibody production locally before they reach the liver. In the evaluation of the results, attention should also be paid to the type of antigen used (soluble or particulate), the requirement of thymus-derived and bursa-equivalent cell co-operation for humoral antibody production and the type of immune response (primary or secondary) measured.

In 1971, we suggested that an increased load of antigen rather than an increased ability to produce antibody was the cause of the high immunoglobulin level in cirrhosis[138]. This hypothesis presumes that most of the normal immunoglobulins in the blood are antibodies to antigens of intestinal microbial flora. Since most of the blood from the intestinal tract is drained by the portal vein, intestinal microbial antigens pass through the liver sinusoids. If it is assumed that the normal liver neutralizes the antigenic effect of these substances, abnormalities in the hepatic circulation (either intra- or extra-hepatic shunting) could result in an increased antigenic challenge. In support of this hypothesis it had been shown that serum immunoglobulin levels were increased after portacaval shunting[139]. It was therefore proposed that antibodies to common intestinal bacteria should be studied in patients with cirrhosis. An increase in these antibodies should be expected if the hypothesis was correct. Such an increase in anti-*Salmonella* agglutinins in patients with chronic active liver diseases had been reported and was further evidence in favour of the hypothesis[140].

A study of the frequency of antibodies to common O types of *Escherichia coli* (*E. coli*) in patients with cirrhosis and normal controls was then undertaken[141]. Such antibodies are known to be thymus-independent[142]. Using the 10 most common O group *E. coli* antigens found in Denmark, and with a classical agglutination method, there was a much higher frequency of antibodies against these antigens in the cirrhosis patients.

Furthermore, the highest incidence of positive reactions was found in patients with cirrhosis who had had a portacaval shunt[141]. Simultaneously with these observations, and using bentonite particles coated with lipopolysaccharide antigens prepared from *E. coli*, increased antibody titres in patients with liver disease, particularly in chronic active hepatitis were shown[143]. Increased antibody titres against bacteroides, rat-colon antigen and dietary proteins were also found[143]. It seemed therefore that impaired Kupffer cell function in liver disease might result in an inability to sequester antigens absorbed from the gastrointestinal tract, and thus lead to increased antibody formation.

However, other observations were not consistent with this simple idea. High titres of antibody to rubella and measles virus in patients with chronic liver disease were demonstrated[144,145]. Rising titres of these viral antibodies were demonstrated in a patient with ulcerative colitis in whom chronic active hepatitis developed and in association with the development of the liver disease[145]. Consequently, it was postulated that either damaged Kupffer cells were not able to regulate the amount of circulating viral antigen, or that they released antigen temporarily sequestered within them.

In 1972 we proposed a modified form of the original hypothesis[146]. Control of immunoglobulin production is an important physiological effect of the liver, exercised not only on portal blood but on all blood perfusing liver sinusoids. Antigen absorbed via the portal blood stream comes into immediate contact with the liver MPS, whereas antigen passing into the systemic blood stream will come into contact perhaps simultaneously with the liver MPS and other component cells of the MPS. Thus simple chemical compounds absorbed into the intestinal capillaries will enter the portal blood stream, whereas larger molecules (lipids, proteins and microbes) pass through the intestinal lymphatic system and reach the systemic circulation via the thoracic duct. The strategic position of the liver between the intestinal tract and the systemic circulation may not thus be so important. What is decisive, however, is that the Kupffer cells constitute by far the largest part of the body's MPS. We must now examine several observations in human liver disease and in experimental cirrhosis in animals, and see how they fit in with this hypothesis.

Clinical studies: The reported increased incidence of antibodies to microbial antigens in various liver diseases is summarized in Table

7.1 [140,141,143–145,147–154]. The cirrhosis group is considered as a whole in the table, but it is of interest that increased titres of viral antibodies have not been demonstrated in alcoholic cirrhosis[145,149]. There is no evidence of a viral antigenaemia in these liver diseases, nor is there evidence that the viruses persist in Kupffer cells[147]. However, it seems likely that there is continuous release of viral antigen from some source[145]. A common feature of those viruses to which increased antibody titres in liver disease have been demonstrated is that they are associated with viraemia during the acute infection[150]. Increased antistreptolysin[155,156] and antistaphylolysin[155] have also been reported in cirrhosis.

Table 7.1 MICROBIAL ANTIBODIES IN SERUM IN LIVER DISEASES

	Acute hepatitis	*Chronic active hepatitis*	*Cirrhosis*	*Fatty liver*
Escherichia coli	+	+	+	+
Salmonellae		+	+ / — } (a)	—
Bacteroides	+	+	+	
Haemophilus influenza B	—	—	—	
Mycoplasma pneumonial		—	—	
Rubella		+	+ / — } (b)	
Measles		+	+ (c)	
Parainfluenza I		—	—	
Herpes simplex		—	—	
Varicella/zoster		—	—	
Cytomegalovirus	+	+	+	
Coxackie B		—	—	
Toxoplasma gondii			+ (c)	
Adenovirus	+			

(a) See references 140, 141 and 157
(b) See references 145, 147 and 150
(c) Primary biliary cirrhosis (154)

In extended studies on antibodies to *E. coli* in hepatic cirrhosis, we showed that increased antibody titres were apparent in all types of cirrhosis, but were most frequently found in alcoholic cirrhosis. Furthermore, patients with fatty liver had more *E. coli* antibodies than controls, but with a lower titre than in cirrhosis; a higher incidence of positive results was noted in alcoholic fatty liver as compared with non-alcoholic fatty liver. Chronic alcoholics without demonstrable liver disease on liver biopsy were no different from controls[157]. The total phagocytic function of the MPS in man is depressed by alcohol[109], and in experimental animals alcohol causes depression of white-cell mobilization and inhibits phagocytosis and intracellular destruction of organisms by macrophage[158]. Thus a functional defect of the MPS of the liver due to alcohol induced disturbance of liver structure could be further aggravated by the direct effect of alcohol on the MPS, and thereby contribute further to the development of high titre *E. coli* antibodies.

Distortion of the liver structure influences the microcirculation and presumably thereby reduces the phagocytic function of the MPS of the liver. Therefore a correlation between the degree of hepatic morphological alterations and serum immunoglobulin levels should be expected, and was sought in cirrhosis[159]. The morphological changes evaluated on liver biopsies comprised distortion of the lobular architecture, fibrosis, fatty change, 'activity' and proliferation and ceroid content of the Kupffer cells. Positive correlations between the degree of fibrosis and distorted lobular architecture and serum IgA levels were found. Furthermore, positive correlations between the degrees of fibrosis, ceroid + fibrosis and proliferation of Kupffer cells and serum IgG levels were demonstrated[159].

Portasystemic shunt operations have been shown to influence the serum levels of immunoglobulins and *E. coli* antibodies in patients with cirrhosis. In 107 patients an average increase in serum gammaglobulin from 1·83 g/100 ml before operation to 2·24 g/100 ml 4 weeks after operation was found[139]. These findings were confirmed in 54 patients with cirrhosis of the liver subjected to a portacaval shunt operation[160]. The increase shown was from 1·86 g/100 ml to 2·30 g/100 ml 7–9 weeks after operation[160]. Careful study of the different sources of error, i.e. infectious complications, patency of the shunt, change of blood volume and especially the large amounts of blood and plasma adminisered, led to the conclusion that the gammaglobulin increase observed was related to the change in liver circulation established by the portacaval shunt. Thirty-one patients with cirrhosis and a portacaval shunt were subsequently compared with 128 cirrhotics without a shunt. Patients with cirrhosis and a portacaval shunt had higher serum IgG levels and more *E. coli* O group antibodies than patients with cirrhosis but without a shunt.

These observations can be explained as follows: (1) antigens absorbed in the portal blood bypass the liver in the shunt, thus gaining direct access to antibody producing sites in spleen and lymph nodes, and provoking an increase in antibody production, (2) because of low liver blood flow in patients with portacaval shunts[116,161,162], and because Kupffer cell function is depressed by low hepatic blood flow[111], the controlling effect of the liver MPS on the immunogenicity of antigens is decreased and antibody production is enhanced. This will also affect antibody production to gut-derived microbial antigens absorbed in the intestinal lymphatics. It is of note that the titres of *E. coli* antibodies in alcoholic cirrhosis patients with a shunt were no higher than in non-alcoholics with a shunt. The effects of the changes on hepatic circulation thus eclipsed the smaller effect of alcohol on phagocytic activity.

Animal experimental studies: There are a number of experimental studies on the relationship between liver injury and serum immunoglobulin levels. Partial hepatectomy leads to increased antibody productions[136]. Enhanced antibody production has been demonstrated against sheep erythrocytes given intraperitoneally in experimental acute and chronic liver injury in rats produced by carbon tetrachloride or allyl alcohol[137]. In rats dietetic liver damage[163] and azo dye ('butter yellow') induced liver damage[164], produced a reversible increase in serum immunoglobulin levels. Conflicting reports have appeared on the influence of the rat microbial flora on the development of liver injury. The development of cirrhosis in rats fed on necrogenic or choline-deficient diet was delayed or prevented by antibiotic treatment[165,166]. However, in another study, chronic liver injury was induced in both germ-free and conventional rats treated with azo dye[167]. In this study lower levels of immunoglobulin were found in the germ-free animals as compared with conventional animals, but the increase in immunoglobulin during the experiment was of the same order in the two groups[167]. Thus the microflora was not essential for the developing hypergammaglobulinemia, and hepatocyte breakdown products were the presumed antigens responsible.

The influence of the route of administration of antigen has been investigated in a number of studies. Repeated injections of small amounts of sheep red blood cells via the portal vein in the rat induced a lower antibody response than immunization via the inferior vena cava. The decreased response was associated with a higher hepatic uptake of the red blood cells[168]. Following injury with carbon tetrachloride there was a higher primary antibody response, a decreased hepatic uptake of antigen, and no difference in the antibody response dependent on portal vein or inferior vena caval injections[46]. Using a soluble antigen, bovine serum albumin, it was shown that in non-immune rats hepatic uptake was minimal and independent of the route of administration[42,107]. However, after immunization, hepatic uptake was greater following mesenteric vein administration as compared with femoral vein injection. When preformed BSA/anti-BSA immune complexes were injected, greater amounts were sequestered in the liver following mesenteric vein injection, and the greatest amount was sequestered when these complexes were formed in optimal proportions. In the cirrhotic rats the ability of the liver to trap such complexes and also to trap particulate antigen like *Salmonella adelaide* was significantly impaired; the loss of function was related to the severity of the cirrhotic process[107].

A proposal that antibodies to soluble proteins (absorbed from the gut) form part of a physiological mechanism for preventing the proteins from entering the systemic circulation was also made in these studies[42]. These antibodies, derived from the spleen, form complexes in the portal circulation, with the absorbed antigen, and those complexes are then sequestered in the liver. Inefficient trapping of such complexes may result in some of the extra-hepatic manifestations associated with liver damage, e.g. arthritis and glomerulonephritis.

Following portacaval anastomosis in rats the serum immunoglobulin levels rise[169–171]. In one study the serum immunoglobulin levels in shunted animals observed over a 12-week period was four times higher than pre-operatively when compared with sham-operated controls[172]. In neomycin treated shunted animals the immunoglobulin levels rose only transiently, returning to pre-operative levels by the twelfth week. This suggested that most of the rise in immunoglobulins was due to a rise in bacterial antibodies. It was confirmed in these same studies that antibodies to rat *E. coli* lipopolysaccharide rose in the portacaval shunted group to a maximum value after 6 weeks, but dropped thereafter to a titre which at 12 weeks however was six times higher than the pre-operative value[172]. Insofar as bacterial antigens are absorbed via the mesenteric lymphatic system, it has to be postulated from these studies that the increased antibody production is related to a defective phagocytic function of the Kupffer cells due to reduced hepatic blood flow.

In summary, therefore, the Kupffer cells constitute the largest part of the mononuclear phagocytic system of the body. Normal Kupffer cells do not process phagocytized antigens for an antibody response but, on the contrary, destroy their immunogenicity. The phagocytic capacity of the liver is reduced by decreased liver blood flow, changes in the hepatic microcirculation, and damage to Kupffer cells. Antigens are diverted from the liver to antibody producing sites, and increased immunoglobulin production results.

Bacterial infections in liver disease

An increased incidence of infection in hepatic cirrhosis has been recognized for a long time. Bacteraemia in these patients and a possible explanation for this phenomenon was discussed in 1954[173]. This bacteraemia may be due to Gram-negative or Gram-positive organisms, and a review of the literature suggests a frequency of occurrence of 3–6% in cirrhotic patients[174–188]. Spontaneous peritonitis with few clinical symptoms, often caused by Gram-negative bacilli but with no evident point of entry has also been described in patients with cirrhosis[189–194].

A decreased 'filtering' of the organisms by the diseased liver, shunting of blood past the liver and decreased local resistance of the intestinal mucosa have been postulated as mechanisms for these complications. Of these mechanisms only the third one has not previously been discussed in this chapter.

Studies in germ-free animals in recent years have shown that the normal serum immunoglobulins of mice, rats, guinea pigs, rabbits, goats, sheep and piglets are antibodies to the intestinal microbial flora[195,196]. Serum immunoglobulin levels in germ-free animals are very low, but following infection of their intestinal tract immunoglobulin values increase to normal levels. It has been proposed that in man also normal serum immunoglobulins, or so-called 'natural antibodies', consist mainly of antibodies to intestinal organisms[138]. This hypothesis is supported by the observations of Kunin[197] that antibodies to common *E. coli* O antigens, demonstrable by the sensitive haemagglutination test, could be demonstrated in almost all subjects over the age of 2 years. Before that age these antibodies were undetectable or present in low titres. Studies in a single adult were reported where antibodies could be found to almost all of 145 different *E. coli* antigens studied. In an investigation of *E. coli* antibodies[198], the occurrence of antibodies against six different serotypes of commensal *E. coli* has been reported in all members of the normal control group (38 adults). It would thus seem reasonable to assume that all normal humans have had subclinical infections by microbes from the gut. The question is how these infections take place.

It was observed early that salmonellae pass from the gut to the blood via the intestinal lymphatics[199]. Experiments in which the content of organisms in the cisterna chyli or the thoracic duct have been followed after their instillation in the intestine have shown that only an exceedingly small fraction of these organisms is recovered in the lymph[200-203]. The absorption starts soon after the instillation, increases with the number instilled, is inversely related to the size of the micro-organisms and is without relation to lymph flow. The penetration of the intestinal epithelium by salmonellae and related microbes takes place without much damage to the epithelial lining[204]. The primary site of bacterial penetration probably involves the distal ileum[205]. To follow the exact route of the few penetrating microbes to the draining lymph nodes may be beyond present technical capabilities[206].

Many authors have supposed that intestinal organisms pass into the portal vein via the intestinal capillaries although there is very little support for this point of view. Studies of blood cultures from the human portal vein have been reported several times with conflicting results[207-209]. Blood drawn from a catheter placed during laparotomy in the portal vein through the umbilical vein gave positive cultures in only 2 of 25 patients[210], and the same techniques used by us has consistently given negative cultures[211]. In ulcerative colitis blood cultures from the portal vein immediately after the abdomen was opened and before colectomy showed positive cultures in 24 of 100 patients, *E. coli* being frequently found[212]. It must be concluded from these observations that with the exception of the studies in ulcerative colitis there is little evidence that intestinal microbes pass from the gut to the portal vein.

A very slow continuous small influx of intestinal organisms from the gut via the intestinal lymphatics, the thoracic duct and hence into the systemic circulation, may however occur in the human similar to the previously cited experimental observations in animals. In cirrhosis several studies have shown that the intestinal flora extends higher up in the small intestine than in normal persons[213,214]. This may result in an increased influx of organisms and may be important in the spontaneous development of bacteraemia. Studies in which bacteriological culture of human liver biopsy material has been performed, provide little evidence of any increased 'infection' of the liver in various hepatic diseases.[215-218].

In experimental studies, however, rats with an established cirrhosis, unlike normal animals, were not able to kill *E. coli* injected via the portal vein[219]. In dogs, there is a continual seeding of the liver by bacteria derived from the gut via the portal vein. Pretreatment of dogs with neomycin has been shown to reduce bacteraemia and delay the fatal complications which follow hepatic arterial ligation[220], or hepatectomy[221]. Thus in the dog the liver is of considerable importance in controlling infection derived from the gut.

The occurrence of bacteraemia and spontaneous peritonitis in patients with cirrhosis seems currently therefore to be best explained on the basis of impaired hepatic mononuclear phagocytic function.

The possible role of the hepatic MPS in the pathogenesis of cirrhosis

The aetiology of cirrhosis of the liver remains a highly controversial subject. The most important factors involved are alcohol, viral hepatitis, chronic obstruction and infection of the biliary tract, and autoimmune mechanisms. The first three factors are certainly of importance but the role of autoimmunity is still debatable and is discussed at length elsewhere in this book.

Even if certain factors have been shown to cause liver injury it has been difficult to explain the chronicity of the cirrhotic process. The concept of autoimmunity tries to overcome this difficulty by invoking immune mechanisms in a self-perpetuating process. In this section we will discuss how the MPS of the liver can be of importance for the development of a cirrhotic process. We shall put forward arguments that support the contention that defects of function of liver MPS could be a factor of importance for the development and progression of cirrhosis.

A small but continuous absorption of organisms into the general circulation, mainly from the intestinal tract, is probably a normal occurrence. An indication of the presence of these microbes are the antibodies to common *E. coli* types demonstrated in normal human sera. In the presence of an intact normal defence mechanism in the body this continuous absorption does not lead to bacteraemia. In respect of the *Enterobacteriaceae* phagocytosis is the most important defence mechanism, and this phagocytosis takes place predominantly in the Kupffer cells. If these cells are severely damaged, e.g. by hepatitis virus or alcohol, this might have important consequences for defence against absorbed microbes. We propose that one of these consequences could be inflammation of the liver tissue which, if continued, could result in progression to and the development of cirrhosis[157,222]. In support of this idea are the previously cited observations of increased titres of antibodies against intestinal organisms in cirrhotic patients and the occurrence of septicaemia and asymptomatic peritonitis, often caused by *Enterobacteriaceae*, in 3–6% of hospitalized patients with cirrhosis. Evidence of bacterial infection in the diseased liver has been found by some authors but not by others. This discrepancy might be due to these organisms being present in such small numbers that their demonstration by culture of small amounts of tissue and blood is difficult. The demonstration of specific antibody production however is possible.

We have for some time studied the occurrence of *E. coli* antibodies in disease. So far chronic granulomatous disease of childhood (CGD) is, apart from cirrhosis and fatty liver, the only disease where we have found increased amounts of these antibodies[223]. In CGD, killing of microbes by polymorphonuclear leukocytes is deficient, and probably also killing by fixed macrophages[224]. In CGD, patients suffer from infections, predominantly with the same organisms as cirrhotics[224]. These infections occur with a high frequency and most patients die young. In patients with Kupffer cell damage caused by alcohol or hepatitis virus low grade infections in the liver could presumably occur, with the development of cirrhosis and on occasion this results in the occurrence of septicaemia or peritonitis. The organisms are not, as usual, killed in the Kupffer cells but attack liver tissue. They are not able to multiply excessively however, due to other defence mechanisms, e.g. humoral, and beyond the liver they are controlled by other intact components of the MPS. The difference between CGD and liver cirrhosis could be explained if we assume that the deficient phagocytosis is generalized in CGD but localized to the liver in cirrhosis. This would fit with the clinical course in the two diseases.

A number of other observations in human diseases are compatible with this hypothesis. The increasing levels of *E. coli* antibodies in three groups of patients, alcoholics with normal liver pathology, alcoholic fatty liver, and alcoholic cirrhosis[157], are compatible with the concept that *E. coli* plays a role in the pathogenesis of liver changes in these diseases. The observation that the prognosis improves considerably in patients with alcoholic cirrhosis when they stop drinking[225] is compatible with the concept that alcoholic damage of the Kupffer cells is an important factor in the progression of the disease. It should be stressed that alcohol, due to its relatively higher concentration in the portal blood, will have a greater effect on Kupffer cells than on other parts of the MPS. The effects of corticosteroid treatment in alcoholic and non-alcoholic cirrhosis can be explained by this hypothesis. In alcoholic cirrhosis with especially high levels of *E. coli* antibodies[157] infections presumably play an important, perhaps decisive, role in the development of cirrhosis. Prednisone treatment does not improve, and perhaps even worsens, prognosis in this disease[226-228].This could be due to increased susceptibility to infections caused by further depression of Kupffer cell function by prednisone. Prednisone treatment improves prognosis in non-alcoholic cirrhosis[226,227]. This could be due to autoimmune mechanisms being more important in these in the progression to cirrhosis. The observation that postmenopausal women are more prone to chronic hepatitis and cirrhosis[229] may be related to their low blood estrogen level. It has been shown that estrogens are very strong activators of the MPS[81], and it could well be that damage to Kupffer cells by hepatitis virus together with estrogen lack increases susceptibility to infections in the liver.

There is some experimental support for the hypothesis. Dietary necrosis of the liver cannot be produced in germ-free animals[230] and dietary production of cirrhosis can be prevented by treatment with broad spectrum antibiotics[166]. Rats with normal livers destroy radiolabelled *E. coli* injected into the portal vein, whereas cirrhotic animals are not able to kill these microbes[219]. However, cirrhosis has been produced in germ-free rats with butter yellow derivates[167]. This observation of course argues against our hypothesis, or rather against this hypothesis as the only explanation for the development of cirrhosis of the liver.

Endotoxaemia due to decreased hepatic clearance of endotoxin absorbed from the gut may also be of importance for the initiation and perpetuation of liver damage[61,231,232]. Endotoxaemia in humans has been reported in fulminant hepatic failure[233], but to our knowledge no reports of endotoxaemia in the portal vein or in the general circulation in patients with cirrhosis have been published, although it has been claimed recently that unexplained fever occasionally seen in alcoholic liver disease correlates with endotoxaemia[234].

The hypothesis could be tested by therapeutic trials. Earlier studies of antibiotic treatment of cirrhosis[235,236] should be resumed with newer, better antibiotics. Such trials should be performed during episodes of clinical deterioration. The grave prognosis in viral hepatitis in postmenopausal women has previously been mentioned[229]. Prophylactic treatment with estrogens should be tried with doses of estrogen that have been shown to stimulate human MPS[237]. Other stimulants of the MPS could also be tried in chronic liver diseases.

Conclusions

1. The Kupffer cells of the liver as a unit have a unique role in the mononuclear phagocytic system of the body. This is because they constitute by far the largest component of this system; because of their strategic relationship to the blood flow from the gastrointestinal tract; because of their different relationship with lymphocytes as compared with other macrophages; and because of their special antigen-handling properties.
2. Pathological processes in the liver profoundly affect Kupffer cell functions, partly because of a direct effect on these cells and partly because of changes in hepatic microcirculation secondarily affecting these cells.
3. The Kupffer cells have an important role in controlling the immunogenicity of gut-derived and other antigens in the general circulation. Impaired Kupffer cell function enhances immune response to these antigens.
4. The increased incidence of microbial antibodies and of bacteraemia and asymptomatic peritonitis in patients with cirrhosis is a manifestation of impaired Kupffer cell function in controlling microbial pathogens absorbed from the gut.
5. A comparison is made between chronic granulomatous disease of childhood and hepatic cirrhosis, the defect in phagocytic function being generalized in the former, and localized in the latter. It is postulated that one of the causes of progression of the cirrhotic process could be a low grade chronic inflammatory process in the liver due to impaired Kupffer cell phagocytic activity.

REFERENCES

1. Aschoff, L. (1924). Das reticulo-endotheliale System. *Ergebn. Inn. Med. Kinderheilk.*, **26**, 1
2. Furth, R. van, Cohn, Z. A., Hirsch, J. G., Humphrey, J. H., Spector, W. G. and Langevoort, H. L. (1972). The mononuclear phagocyte system: a new classification of macrophages, monocytes, and their precursor cells. *Bull. Wld. Hlth. Org.*, **46**, 845
3. Jandl, J. H., Files, N. M., Barnett, S. B. and Macdonald, R. A. (1965). Proliferative response of the spleen and liver to hemolysis. *J. Exp. Med.*, **122**, 299
4. Weibel, E. R., Stäubli, W., Gnägi, H. R. and Hess, F. A. (1969). Correlated morphometric and biochemical studies on the liver cell. I. Morphometric model, stereologic methods, and normal morphometric data for rat liver. *J. Cell. Biology*, **42**, 68
5. Greengard, O., Federman, M. and Knox, W. E. (1972). Cytomorphometry of developing rat liver and its application to enzymic differentiation. *J. Cell Biology*, **52**, 261
6. Gates, G. A., Henley, K. S., Pollard, H. M., Schmidt, E. and Schmidt, F. W. (1961). The cell population of human liver. *J. Lab. Clin. Med.*, **57**, 182
7. *Gray's Anatomy* (1973). R. Warwick and P. L. Williams (eds.) p. 1308 (Edinburgh: Longman)
8. Elias, H. (1952). Morphology of the stellate cells of Kupffer. *The Chicago Med. School Quarterly*, **13**, 60
9. Stuart, A. E. (1970). *The reticulo-endothelial system.* (Edinburgh and London: Livingstone)
10. Wisse, E. and Daems, W. T. (1970) Fine structural study on the sinusoidal lining cells of rat liver. In *Mononuclear phagocytes.* R. van Furth (ed). p. 200 (Oxford: Blackwell)
11. Emeis, J. J. and Wisse, E. (1971). Electron microscopic cytochemistry of the cell coat of Kupffer cells in rat liver. In *Adv. Exp. Med. Biol.*, **15**. The reticulo-endothelial system and immune phenomena. N. R. Di Luzio and K. Flemming (eds.) p. 1 (New York: Plenum Press)
12. Aterman, K. (1958). Some observations on the sinusoidal cells of the liver. *Acta Anat. (Basel)*, **32**, 193
13. Carr, I. (1970). The fine structure of the mammalian lymphoreticular system. *Int. Rev. Cytol.*, **27**, 283
14. Wisse, E. (1972). An ultrastructural characterization of the endothelial cell in the rat liver sinusoid under normal and various experimental conditions, as a contribution to the distinction between endothelial and Kupffer cells. *J. Ultrastruct. Res.*, **38**, 528
15. Shaba, J. K., Patrick, R. S. and McGee, J. O'D. (1973). Collagen synthesis by mesenchymal cells isolated from normal and acutely-damaged mouse liver. *Br. J. Exp. Path.*, **54**, 110

16. Roser, B. (1968). The distribution of intravenously injected Kupffer cells in the mouse. *J. Reticuloendothel. Soc.*, **5**, 455
17. Berliner, D. L., Nabors, C. J. Jr. and Dougherty, T. F. (1964). The role of hepatic and adrenal reticuloendothelial cells in steroid biotransformation. *J. Reticuloendothel. Soc.*, **1**, 1
18. Melly, M. A., Duke, L. J. and Koenig, M. G. (1972). Studies on isolated cultured rabbit Kupffer cells. *J. Reticuloendothel. Soc.*, **12**, 1
19. Civen, M. and Brown, C. B. (1973). Distribution of tyrosine alfa-ketoglutarate transaminase activity in Kupffer cell and whole liver fractions of rat liver. *J. Reticuloendothel. Soc.*, **14**, 522
20. Berg, T. and Boman, D. (1973). Distribution of lysosomal enzymes between parenchymal and Kupffer cells of rat liver. *Biochim. Biophys. Acta (Amst.)*, **321**, 585
21. Lundkvist, U., Goeringer, G. C. and Perlmann, P. (1966). Immunochemical characterization of parenchymal and reticuloendothelial cells of rat liver. *Exp. Mol. Path.*, **5**, 427
22. Zimmermann, W. E. and Rehfeld, K. H. (1971). Function and importance of the RES during perfusion of the liver. In *Adv. Exp. Med. Biol.*, **15**, The reticuloendothelial system and immune phenomena. N. R. Di Luzio and K. Flemming (eds.) p. 119 (New York: Plenum Press)
23. Schimassek, H. and Helms, J. (1967). The function of the reticuloendothelial system studied with isolated perfused rat livers. In *Adv. Exp. Med. Biol.*, **1**, The reticuloendothelial system and atherosclerosis. N. R. Di Luzio and R. Paoletti, (eds.) p. 46 (New York: Plenum Press)
24. Di Luzio, N. R. (1972). Employment of lipids in the measurement and modification of cellular, humoral, and immune responses. *Adv. Lipid. Res.*, **10**, 43
25. Kitchen, A. G. and Megiriam, R. (1971). Heparin enhancement of Kupffer cell phagocytosis *in vitro*. *J. Reticuloendothel. Soc.*, **9**, 13
26. Biozzi, G. and Stiffel, C. (1965). The physiopathology of the reticuloendothelial cells of the liver and spleen. In *Progress in liver diseases*, **2**, H. Popper and F. Schaffner (eds.) p. 166 (New York and London: Grune and Stratton)
27. Cooksley, W. G. E., Powell, L. W. and Halliday, J. W. (1973). Reticuloendothelial phagocytic function in human liver disease and its relationship to haemolysis. *Br. J. Haemat.*, **25**, 147
28. Iio, M. and Wagner, H. N. Jr. (1963). Studies of the reticuloendothelial system (RES). I. Measurement of phagocytic capacity of the RES in man and dog. *J. Clin. Invest.*, **42**, 417
29. Wagner, H. N. and Iio, M. (1964). Studies of the reticuloendothelial system (RES). III. Blockade of the RES in man. *J. Clin. Invest.*, **43**, 1525
30. Di Luzio, N. R. and Riggi, S. J. (1964). The development of a lipid emulsion for the measurement of reticuloendothelial function. *J. Reticuloendothel. Soc.*, **1**, 136
31. Jones, E. A. (1967). Hepatic scintillography. *Gut*, **8**, 418

32. Rogers, D. E. (1960). Host mechanisms which act to remove bacteria from the blood stream. *Bact. Rev.*, **24**, 50
33. Biozzi, G., Stiffel, C. and Mouton, D. (1963). Stimulation et dépression de la fonction phagocytaire du système réticuloendothélial par des émulsions de lipides. Relations avec quelques phénomènes immunologiques. *Rev. franç. Étud. Clin. Biol.*, **8** 341
34. Benacerraf, B. (1964). Functions of the Kupffer cells. In *The liver*, **2**, C. Rouiller (ed.) p. 37 (New York and London: Academic Press)
35. Beeson, P. B., Brannon, E. S. and Warren, J. V. (1945). Observations on the sites of removal of bacteria from the blood in patients with bacterial endocarditis. *J. Exp. Med.*, **81**, 9
36. Howard, J. G. (1961). The reticulo-endothelial system and resistance to bacterial infection. *Scot. Med. J.*, **6**, 60
37. Bang, F. B. and Warwick, A. (1959). Macrophages and mouse hepatitis. *Virology*, **9**, 715
38. Sabesin, S. M. and Koff, R. S. (1974). Pathogenesis of experimental viral hepatitis. *New Eng. J. Med.*, **290**, 944 and 996
39. Frei, P. C., Benacerraf, B. and Thorbecke, G. J. (1965). Phagocytosis of the antigen, a crucial step in the induction of the primary response. *Proc. Nat. Acad. Sci. (USA)*, **53**, 20
40. Thorbecke, G. J., Maurer, P. H. and Benacerraf, B. (1960). The affinity of the reticulo-endothelial system for various modified serum proteins. *Br. J. Exp. Path.*, **41**, 190
41. Buys, C. H. C. M., Elferink, G. L., Bouma, J. M. W., Gruber, M. and Nieuwenhuis, P. (1973). Proteolysis of formaldehyde-treated albumin in Kupffer cells and its inhibition by suramin. *J. Reticuloendothel. Soc.*, **14**, 209
42. Thomas, H. C. and Vaez-Zadeh, F. (1974). A homeostatic mechanism for the removal of antigen from the portal circulation. *Immunology*, **26**, 375
43. Haakenstad, A. O. and Mannik, M. (1974). Saturation of the reticulo-endothelial system with soluble immune complexes. *J. Immunol.*, **112**, 1939
44. Wagner, H. N. and Iio, M. (1964). Studies of the reticuloendothelial system (RES). III. Blockade of the RES in man. *J. Clin. Invest.*, **43**, 1525
45. Souhami, R. L. (1972). The effect of colloid carbon on the organ distribution of sheep red cells and the immune response. *Immunology*, **22**, 685
46. Triger, D. R. and Wright, R. (1973). Studies on hepatic uptake of antigen. II. The effect of hepatotoxins on the immune response. *Immunology*, **25**, 951
47. Patek, P. R., de Mignard, V. A. and Bernick, S. (1967). Age changes in structure and responses of reticulo-endothelial cells of rat liver. *J. Reticuloendothel. Soc.*, **4**, 211
48. Wagner, H. N., Migita, T. and Solomon, N. (1966). Effect of age on reticuloendothelial function in man. *J. Geront.*, **21**, 57

49. Saba, T. M. (1970). Mechanism mediating reticuloendothelial system depression after surgery. *Proc. Soc. Exp. Biol. Med.*, **133**, 1132
50. Saba, T. M. (1972). Effect of surgical trauma on the clearance and localization of blood-borne particulate matter. *Surgery*, **71**, 675
51. Scovill, W. A. and Saba, T. M. (1973). Humoral recognition deficiency in the etiology of reticuloendothelial depression induced by surgery. *Ann. Surg.*, **178**, 59
52. Deo, M. G., Bhan, I. and Ramalingaswami, V. (1973). Influence of dietary protein deficiency on phagocytic activity of the reticuloendothelial cells. *J. Pathol.*, **109**, 215
53. Trejo, R. A., Di Luzio, N. R., Loose, L. D. and Hoffman, E. O. (1972). Reticuloendothelial and hepatic functional alterations following lead acetate administration. *Exp. Mol. Pathol.*, **17**, 145
54. Hoffman, E. O. Trejo, R. A., Di Luzio, N. R. and Lamberty, J. (1972). Ultrastructural alterations of liver and spleen following acute lead administration in rats. *Exp. Mol. Pathol.*, **17**, 159
55. Zschiesche, W., Augsten, K., Ozegowski, W. and Krebs, D. (1970). Alkylating anticancer agents and phagocytosis. I. Effects of a homologous series of 1,2-substituted 5-bis (β-chloroethyl)-amino-benzimidazole derivates on carbon clearance. *J. Reticuloendothel. Soc.*, **8**, 538
56. Zschiesche, W. (1972). Alkylating anticancer agents and phagocytosis. II. Effects of alkylating agents on numerical distribution and histochemistry of reticuloendothelial cells. *J. Reticuloendothel. Soc.*, **12**, 16
57. Gotjamanos, T. (1971). The effect of azathioprine on phagocytic activity and morphology of reticuloendothelial organs in mice. *Pathology*, **3**, 171
58. Pisano, J. C., Patterson, J. T. and Di Luzio, N. R. (1972). Reticuloendothelial function in immune-suppressed animals. *J. Reticuloendothel. Soc.*, **12**, 361
59. Lemperle, G., Herdter, F. and Gospos, F. (1971). The stimulating or depressing effect of various drugs on the phagocytic function of the RES. In *Adv. Exp. Med. Biol.*, **15**, The reticuloendothelial system and immune phenomena. N. R. Di Luzio and K. Flemming (eds.) p. 87 (New York: Plenum Press)
60. Benveniste, J., Higounet, F. and Salomon, J.-C. (1970). Effects of various doses of prednisolone on the phagocytic activity in axenic and holoxenic mice. *J. Reticuloendothel. Soc.*, **8**, 499
61. Ali, M. V. and Nolan, J. P. (1967). Alcoholic induced depression of reticuloendothelial function in the rat. *J. Lab. Clin. Med.*, **70**, 295
62. Louria, D. B. (1963). Susceptibility to infection during experimental alcoholic intoxication. *Trans. Ass. Amer. Phycns.*, **76**, 102
63. Graham, C. W. and Saba, T. M. (1973). Opsonin levels in reticuloendothelial regulation during and following pregnancy. *J. Reticuloendothel. Soc.*, **14**, 121
64. Grogan, J. B. (1970). Reticuloendothelial system function after single and multiple injections of antilymphocyte serum. *J. Reticuloendothel. Soc.*, **8**, 561

65. Howard, J. G. (1959). Activation of the reticuloendothelial cells of the mouse liver by bacterial lipopolysaccharide. *J. Path. Bact.*, **78**, 465
66. Friedberg, K. D., Garbe, G. and Westermann, M. (1971). Beeinflussung des reticulo-endothelialen Systems durch Cyclophosphamid, Endotoxin und Polyvinylpyridin-N-oxid. *Naunyn-Schmiedeberg's Arch. exp. Path. Pharmak.*, **269**, 57
67. Carmel, N., Markus, R., Gross, J. and Stern, K. (1972). Reticuloendothelial phagocytosis of ^{51}Cr-labelled sheep red cells in mice. II. Effects of lipopolysaccharide on phagocytosis and hemopexin levels. *Israel J. Med.*, **8**. 1783
68. Agarwal, M. K. (1972). Assessment of the nature of reticuloendothelial contribution during endotoxicosis in mice. *J. Reticuloendothel. Soc.*, **12**, 40
69. Normann, S. J. (1973). Reticuloendothelial system function. VI. Experimental alterations influencing the correlation between portal blood flow and colloid clearance. *J. Reticuloendothel. Soc.*, **13**, 47
70. Saba, T. M. (1970). Liver blood flow and intravascular colloid clearance alterations following partial hepatectomy. *J. Reticuloendothel. Soc.*, **7**, 406
71. Gotjamanos, T. (1971). The response of the reticuloendothelial system to skin transplantation. Phagocytic indices and weights of reticuloendothelial organs of mice bearing primary skin isografts and allografts. *Aust. J. Exp. Biol. Med. Sci.*, **49**, 249
72. Wagner, H. N. Jr., Iio, M. and Hornick, R. B. (1963). Studies of the reticuloendothelial system (RES). II. Changes in the phagocytic capacity of the RES in patients with certain infections. *J. Clin. Invest.*, **42**, 427
73. Wagner, H. N. Jr., Iio, M. and Hornick, R. B. (1963). Inhibition of the phagocytic capacity of the human reticuloendothelial system in viral infections. *J. Clin. Invest.*, **42**, 990
74. Munson, A. E., Regelson, W. and Wooles, W. R. (1970). Tissue localization studies in evaluating the functional role of the RES. *J. Reticuloendothel. Soc.*, **7**, 366
75. Hupka, A. L. and Karler, R. (1973). Biotransformation of ethylmorphine and heme by isolated parenchymal and reticuloendothelial cells of rat liver. *J. Reticuloendothel. Soc.*, **14**, 225
76. Sinar, Y., Kaplun, A., Hai, Y. and Halperin, B. (1974). Enhancement of resistance to infectious diseases by oral administration of brewer's yeast. *Infection Immunol.* **9**, 781
77. Di Luzio, N. R. and Morrow, H. S. III (1971). Comparative behaviour of soluble and particulate antigens and inert colloids in reticuloendothelial-stimulated or depressed mice. *J. Reticuloendothel. Soc.*, **9**, 273
78. Halpern, B. N. Prévot, A. R., Biozzi, G., Stiffel, C., Mouton, D., Morard, J. C., Bouthildier, Y. and Descreusefond, C. (1964). Stimulation de l'activité phagocytaire du système reticuloendothelial provoquée par Corynebacterium parvum. *J. Reticuloendothel. Soc.*, **1**, 77

79. Donald, K. J. and Pound, A. W. (1971). The effect of a tubercle bacillary lipid on the clearance rate of colloidal carbon from the blood of rabbits. *Brit. J. Exp. Path.* **52**, 256
80. Donald, K. J. and Pound, A. W. (1973). Proliferation and migration of reticuloendothelial cells following injection of a tubercle bacillary lipid. *Br. J. Exp. Path.*, **54**, 79
81. Nicol, T., Bilbey, D. L. J., Charles, L. M., Cordingley, J. L. and Vernon-Roberts, B. (1964). Oestrogen: the natural stimulant of body defense. *J. Endocr.*, **30**, 277
82. Grampa, G. (1967). Reticuloendothelial system stimulation by estrogens and thorium dioxide retention in rat liver. In *Adv. Exp. Med. Biol.*, **1**, The reticuloendothelial system and atherosclerosis. N. R. Di Luzio and R. Paoletti (eds.) p. 214 (New York: Plenum Press)
83. Warr, G. W. and Šljivič, V. S. (1973). Activity of the reticuloendothelial system and the antibody response. I. Effect of stilboestrol on RES activity and localization of sheep erythrocytes in the mouse. *Br. J. Exp. Path.*, **54**, 56
84. Flemming, K., Flemming, C. and Nothdurft, W. (1970). The phagocytic activity of the reticuloendothelial system of mice following whole-body X-irradiation. *J. Reticuloendothel. Soc.*, **7**, 1
85. Šljivič, V. (1970). Radiation and the phagocytic function of the reticuloendothelial system. *Br. J. Exp. Path.*, **51**, 130
86. Bissell, M. D., Hammaker, L. and Schmid, R. (1972). Liver sinusoidal cells. Identification of a subpopulation for erythrocyte catabolism. *J. Cell Biology*, **54**, 107
87. Dumont, A. E., Stertzer, S. H. and Mulholland, J. H. (1962). Experimental biliary obstruction: effect of thorotrast on lymph and serum bilirubin levels. *Amer. J. Physiol.*, **202**, 704
88. Vannotti, A. (1957). The role of the reticuloendothelial system in iron metabolism. In *Physiopathology of the reticulo-endothelial system.* B. N. Halpern, B. Benacerraf and J. F. Delafresnaye (eds.) p. 172 (Oxford: Blackwell)
89. Noyes, W. D., Bothwell, T. H. and Finch, C. A. (1960). The role of the reticulo-endothelial cell in iron metabolism. *Brit. J. Haemat.*, **6**, 43
90. Walsh, R. T. and Barnhart, M. I. (1969). Clearance of coagulation and fibrinolysis products by the reticuloendothelial system. *Thrombosis et diathesis haemorrhagica, Suppl.* **36**, 83
91. Barnhart, M. L. and Cress, D. C. (1967). Plasma clearance of products of fibrinolysis. In *Adv. Exp. Med. Biol.*, **1**, The reticuloendothelial system and atherosclerosis. N. R. Di Luzio, and R. Paoletti (eds.) p. 492 (New York: Plenum Press)
92. Freeman, T., Gordon, A. H. and Humphrey, J. H. (1958). Distinction between catabolism of native and denatured proteins by the isolated perfused liver after carbon loading. *Brit. J. Exp. Path.*, **39**, 459
93. Freeman, T. (1959). The biological behaviour of normal and denatured human plasma albumin. *Clin. chim. Acta*, **4**, 788

94. Buys, C. H. C. M., Elferink, G. L., Bouman, J. M. W., Gruber, M. and Nieuwenhuis, P. (1973). Proteolysis of formaldehyde-treated albumin in Kupffer cells and its inhibition by suramin. *J. Reticuloendothel. Soc.*, **14**, 209
95. Di Luzio, N. R. and Saba, T. M. (1971). Liver parenchymal and Kupffer cell metabolism of ^{14}C-labelled acetate, palmitate, and triglyceride. *J. Reticuloendothel. Soc.*, **10**, 392
96. Cornell, R. P. and Saba, T. M. (1971). Vascular clearance and metabolism of lipid by the reticuloendothelial system in dogs. *Amer. J. Physiol.*, **221**, 1511
97. Nilsson, Å. and Zilversmit, D. B. (1972). Fate of intravenously administered particulate and lipoprotein cholesterol in the rat. *J. Lipid. Res.*, **13**, 32
98. Nilsson, Å. and Zilversmit, D. B. (1972). Release of phagocytosed cholesterol by liver macrophages and spleen cells. *Biochim. Biophys. Acta* (*Amst.*), **260**, 479
99. Di Luzio, N. R. and Riggi, S. J. (1967). Participation of hepatic parenchymal and Kupffer cells in chylomicron and cholesterol metabolism. In *Adv. Exp. Med. Biol.*, **1**, The reticuloendothelial system and atherosclerosis. N. R. Di Luzio and R. Paoletti (eds.) p. 382 (New York: Plenum Press)
100. Berliner, D. L., Nabors. C. J. Jr. and Dougherty, T. F. (1964). The role of hepatic and adrenal reticuloendothelial cells in steroid biotransformation. *J. Reticuloendothel. Soc.*, **1**, 1
101. Trejo, R. A. and Di Luzio, N. R. (1973). Comparative evaluation of macrophage inactivation of endotoxin. *Proc. Soc. Exp. Biol. Med.*, **144**, 901
102. Magarey, C. J. (1972). The control of cancer spread by the reticuloendothelial system. *Ann. Roy. Coll. Surg. Engl.*, **50**, 238
103. Woodruff, M. F. A., McBride, W. H. and Dunbar, N. (1974). Tumour growth, phagocytic activity and antibody response in *Corynebacterium parvume*-treated mice. *Clin. Exp. Immunol.*, **17**, 509
104. Paumgartner, G., Longueville, H. and Leevy, C. M. (1967). Determinants of phagocytosis in liver injury. *T. Gastro-ent.*, **10**, 469
105. Mitjavila, M. S., Gaillard, D. and Derache, M. R. (1971). Toxicologie. Activité de système reticulo-endothélial lors d'une intoxication aiguë par l'acide tannique chez le Rat. *C. R. Acad. Sci.* (*Paris*), **272**, 1313, Series D
106. Spratt, M. G. and Kratzing, C. C. (1971). The effect of dietary lipids and α-tocopherol on RES activity in choline deficiency. *J. Reticuloendothel. Soc.*, **10**, 319
107. Thomas, H. C., MacSween, R. N. M. and White, R. G. (1973). Role of the liver in controlling the immunogenicity of commensal bacteria in the gut. *Lancet*, **i**, 1288.
108. Grün, M., Liehr, H., Grün, W., Rasenack, U. and Brunswig, D. (1974). Influence of liver RES on toxic liver damage due to galactosamine. *Acta Hepato-gastroenterol.* (*Stuttg.*), **21**, 5

109. Liu, Y. K. (1973). Phagocytic function of reticuloendothelial system in alcoholics. *Clin. Res.*, **21**, 606

110. Millette, B., Chartrand, R., Lavoie, P. and Viallet, A. (1973). The extra-hepatic uptake of radioactive colloidal gold in cirrhotic patients as an index of liver function and portal hypertension. *Amer. J. Dig. Dis., New Ser.*, **18**, 719

111. Halpern, B. N., Biozzi, F., Pequignot, G., Delaloye, B., Stiffel, C. and Mouton, D. (1959). Mesure de la circulation sanguine du foie et de l'activité phagocytaire du système réticulo-endothelial chez le sujet normal et le sujet cirrhotique. *Path. et Biol.*, **7**, 1637

112. Rankin, J. G. Playuost, M. R. and Beal, R. W. (1961). Significance of alterations in extraction and distribution of colloidal chromic phosphate in patients with liver disease. *J. Lab. Clin. Med.*, **58**, 920

113. Moreno, A. H., Burchell, A. R., Rousselot, L. M., Panke, W. F., Slafsky, S. F. and Burke, J. H. (1967). Portal blood flow in cirrhosis of the liver. *J. Clin. Invest.*, **46**, 436

114. Reynolds, T. B. and Redeker, A. G. (1965). Hepatic hemodynamics and portal hypertension. In *Progress in liver diseases*, **2**. H. Popper and F. Schaffner, (eds.) p. 457 (New York and London: Grune and Stratton)

115. Winkler, K. (1970). The vascular derangement in cirrhosis. A pathophysiologic survey. In *Skandia International Symposia 1969*, Alcoholic cirrhosis and other toxic hepatopathias. A. Engel and T. Larsson (eds.) p. 195 (Stockholm: Nord. Bokhandlens Förlag)

116. Redeker, A. G., Geller, H. M. and Reynolds, T. B. (1958). Hepatic wedge pressure, blood flow, vascular resistance and oxygen consumption in cirrhosis before and after end-to-side portacaval shunt. *J. Clin. Invest.*, **37**, 606

117. Unanue, E. R. and Cerrottini, J.-C. (1970). The function of macrophages in the immune response. *Seminars Haematol.*, **7**, 225

118. Sulzberger, M. B. (1929). Hypersensitiveness to arsphenamine in guinea-pigs. *Arch. Derm. Syph. (Chic.)*, **20**, 669

119. Chase, M. (1946). Inhibition of experimental drug allergy by prior feeding of the sensitizing agent. *Proc. Soc. Exp. Biol. Med.*, **61**, 257

120. Battisto, J. R. and Miller, J. (1962). Immunological unresponsiveness produced in adult guinea pigs by parenteral introduction of minute quantities of hapten or protein antigen. *Proc. Soc. Exp. Biol. Med.*, **111**, 111

121. Cantor, H. M. and Dumont, A. (1969). Hepatic suppression of sensitization to antigen absorbed into the portal system. *Nature (Lond.)*, **215**, 744

122. Thomas, H. C. and Parrott, D. M. V. (1974). The induction of tolerance to a soluble protein antigen by oral administration. *Immunology*, **27**, 631

123. Howard, J. G. (1970). The origin and immunological significance of Kupffer cells. In *Mononuclear phagocytes*. R. van Furth (ed.) p. 178 (Oxford: Blackwell)

124. Uhr, J. W. and Weissmann, G. (1965). Intracellular distribution and

degradation of bacteriophage in mammalian tissues. *J. Immunol.*, **94**, 544

125. Inchley, C. J. (1969). The activity of mouse Kupffer cells following intravenous injection of T_4- bacteriophage. *Clin. Exp. Immunol.*, **5**, 173
126. Franzl, R. E. (1972). The primary immune response in mice. III. Retention of sheep red blood cell immunogens by the spleen and liver. *Infect. Immunity*, **6**, 469
127. Archer, S. and Wust, C. J. (1973). Comparison of immunogenic RNA extracted from peritoneal exudate cells and Kupffer cells of the rat. *Ann. N.Y. Acad. Sci.*, **207**, 241
128. Geier, M. R., Trigg, M. E. and Merril, C. R. (1973). Fate of bacteriophage Lambda in non-immune germ-free mice. *Nature* (*Lond.*), **246**, 221
129. Good, R. A. (1972). Concluding remarks. In *Phagocytic mechanisms in health and disease*. R. C. Williams and H. H. Fudenberg (eds.) p. 190 (Stuttgart: Georg Thieme Verlag)
130. Havens, W. P., Shaffer, J. M. and Hopke, C. J. (1951). The production of antibody by patients with chronic hepatic disease. *J. Immunol.*, **67**, 347
131. Cherrick, G. R., Pothier, L., Dufour, J.-J. and Sherlock, S. (1959). Immunologic response to tetanus toxoid inoculation in patients with hepatic cirrhosis. *New Eng. J. Med.*, **261**, 340
132. Søborg, M. and Tygstrup, N. (1970). Increased cellular immunological response in patients with cirrhosis of the liver. *Scand. J. Gastroent.*, **5**, *Suppl.* **7**, 43
133. Bjørneboe, M., Jensen, K. B., Scheibel, I., Thomsen, Aa. C. and Bentzon, M. W. (1970). Tetanus antitoxin production and gamma globulin levels in patients with cirrhosis of the liver. *Acta Med. Scand.*, **188**, 541
134. Fox, R. A., Dudley, F. J. and Sherlock, S. (1973). The primary immune response to haemocyanin in patients with primary biliary cirrhosis. *Clin. Exp. Immunol.*, **14**, 473
135. Fiaschi, E., Naccarato, R. and Fagiolo, U. (1970). Quelques aspects d'immunité humorale et cellulaire dans l'hepatite virale aiguë. *Rev. Méd. Franc.*, **45**, 215
136. Havens, W. P. Jr., Schlosser, M. E. and Klatchko, J. (1956). The production of antibody by partially hepatectomized rats. *J. Immunol.*, **76**, 46
137. Paronetto, F. and Popper, H. (1964). Enhanced antibody formation in experimental acute and chronic liver injury produced by carbon tetrachloride or allyl alcohol. *Proc. Soc. Exp. Biol.* (*N.Y.*), **116**, 1060
138. Bjørneboe, M. (1971). Anti-*Salmonella* agglutinin in chronic active liver disease. Letter to the editor, *Lancet*, **ii**, 484
139. Esser, G. (1969). Pfortaderhochdruck und Eiweisstoff-wechsel, p. 21 (Berlin: Walter de Gruyter and Co.)
140. Protell, R. L., Soloway, R. D., Martin, W. J., Schoenfield, L. J. and

Summerskill, W. H. J. (1971). Anti-*Salmonella* agglutinins in chronic active liver disease. *Lancet*, **ii**, 330

141. Bjørneboe, M., Prytz, H. and Ørskov, F. (1972). Antibodies to intestinal microbes in serum of patients with cirrhosis of the liver. *Lancet*, **i**, 58
142. Poe, W. J. and Michael, J. G. (1974). The lack of cellular co-operation in the immune response to *E. coli* O127. *J. Immunol.*, **113**, 1033
143. Triger, R. D., Alp, M. H. and Wright, R. (1972). Bacterial and dietary antibodies in liver disease. *Lancet*, **i**, 60
144. Closs, O., Haukenes, G., Gjone, E. and Blomhoff, J. P. (1971). Raised antibody titres in chronic liver disease. Letter to the editor, *Lancet*, **ii**, 1202
145. Triger, D. R., Kurtz, J. B., MacCallum, F. O. and Wright, R. (1972). Raised antibody titres to measles and rubella viruses in chronic active hepatitis. *Lancet*, **i**, 665
146. Bjørneboe, M. and Prytz, H. (1972). Relation between australia antigen and autoimmune hepatitis. Letter to the editor, *Lancet*, **i**, 1335
147. Closs, O., Haukenes, G., Blomhoff, J. P. and Gjone, E. (1973). High titres of antibodies against rubella and morbilli virus in patients with chronic hepatitis. *Scand. J. Gastroent.*, **8**, 523
148. Laitinen, O. and Vaheri, A. (1974). Very high measles and rubella virus antibody titres associated with hepatitis, systemic lupus erythematosus, and infectious mononucleosis. *Lancet*, **i**, 194
149. Thomas, H. C., Holden, R., Ironside, J. and Sommerville, R. G. (1974). Viral and bacterial antibodies in primary biliary cirrhosis and other chronic liver diseases. *Digestion*, **10**, 383
150. Triger, D. R., Kurtz, J. B. and Wright, R. (1974). Viral antibodies and autoantibodies in chronic liver disease. *Gut*, **15**, 94
151. Alwen, J. (1973). Antibodies to adenovirus in patients with infectious hepatitis. Letter to the editor, *Lancet*, **i**, 1452.
152. Almeida, J. D., Gay, F. W. and Wreghitt, T. G. (1974). Pitfalls in the study of hepatitis A. *Lancet*, **ii**, 748
153. Fiala, M., Nelson, R. J., Myhre, B. A., Guze, L. B., Overby, L. R. and Ling, C. M. (1974). Cytomegalovirus in non-B post-transfusion hepatitis. Letter to the editor, *Lancet*, **ii**, 1206.
154. MacSween, R. N. M., Galbraith, I., Thomas, M. A., Watkinson, G., and Ludlam, G. B. (1973). Phytohaemagglutinin (PHA) induced lymphocyte transformation and *Toxoplasma gondii* antibody studies in primary biliary cirrhosis. *Clin. Exp. Immunol.*, **15**, 35
155. Waldenström, J., Winblad, S., Hällén, J., Liungman, S. and Persson, B. (1964). Hypergammaglobulinämie und Ausfall verschiedener serologischer Reaktionen bei alkoholischer und kryptogenetischer Leberzirrhose. *Acta hepato-splenol.* (*Stuttg.*), **11**, 347
156. Blank, H. (1972). *Immunologische Serumuntersuchungen und Hauttestungen nach Splenektomie*. Dissertationsdruck, p. 46 (Augsburg: Blasaditsch)

157. Prytz, H., Bjørneboe, M., Ørskov, F. and Hilden, M. (1973). Antibodies to *Escherichia coli* in alcoholic and non-alcoholic patients with cirrhosis of the liver or fatty liver. *Scand. J. Gastroent.*, **8**, 433
158. Louria, D. B. and Almy, T. P. (1963). Susceptibility to infection during experimental alcohol intoxication. *Trans. Ass. Amer. Phycns.*, **76**, 102
159. Prytz, H., Bjørneboe, M., Poulsen, H., Christoffersen, P. and Ørskov, F. (1974). Hepatic morphology, immunoglobulins and antibodies to *E. coli* in cirrhosis. *Digestion*, **10**, 375
160. Prytz, H., Bjørneboe, M., Johansen, T. S. and Ørskov, F. (1974). The influence of portasystemic shunt operation on immunoglobulins and *Escherichia coli* antibodies in patients with cirrhosis of the liver. *Acta Med. Scand.*, **196**, 109
161. Benhamou, J.-P., Sicot, C. and Erlinger, S. (1971). Exposés de physiologie et de physiopathologie hépatique. I. Le débit sanguin hépatique. *Presse Med.*, **79**, 185
162. Crosti, P. F., Giovanelli, C. A., Bardi, V. and Vigo, P. L. (1971). Hepatic blood flow in cirrhosis. Letter to the editor, *Lancet*, **ii**, 322
163. Zaki, F. G. and Hoffbauer, E. W. (1964). Serum proteins in fatty cirrhosis of the rat. *Arch. Path.*, **77**, 9
164. Cook, H. A., Griffin, A. C. and Luck, J. M. (1949). Tissue proteins and carcinogenesis. II. Electrophoretic studies on serum proteins during carcinogenesis due to azo dyes. *J. Biol. Chem.*, **177**, 373
165. György, P., Stokes, J., Goldblatt, H. and Popper, H. (1951). Antimicrobial agents in the prevention of dietary hepatic injury (necrosis, cirrhosis) in rats. *J. Exp. Med.*, **93**, 513
166. Rutenburg, A. M., Sonnenblick, E., Koven, I., Aprahamian, H. A., Reiner, L. and Fine, J. (1957). The role of intestinal bacteria in the development of dietary cirrhosis in rats. *J. Exp. Med.*, **106**, 1
167. Bauer, H., Paronetto, F., Porro, R. F., Einheber, A. and Popper, H. (1967). The influence of the microbial flora on liver injury and associated serum gamma globulin elevation. *Lab. Invest.*, **16**, 847
168. Triger, D. R., Cynamon, M. H. and Wright, R. (1973). Studies on hepatic uptake of antigen. I. Comparison of inferior vena cava and portal vein routes of immunization. *Immunology*, **25**, 941
169. Kennan, A. L. (1964). Changes in plasma proteins after portacaval shunt in the rat. *Proc. Soc. Exp. Biol. (N.Y.)*, **116**, 543
170. Bismuth, H., Benhamou, J.-P. and Lataste, J. (1963). L'anastomose porto-cave expérimentale chez le rat normal. *Presse Med.*, **71**, 1859
171. Meyers, O. L. and Keraan, M. (1973). Experimental hyperglobulinaemia. In *The Liver (Proc. of the Internat. Liver Conf., Cape Town)*. S. J. Saunders and J. Terblanche (eds.) p. 78 (London: Pitman)
172. Keraan, M., Meyers, O. L., Engelbrecht, G. H. C., Hickman, R., Saunders, S. J. and Terblanche, J. (1974). Increased serum immunoglobulin levels following portacaval shunt in the normal rat. *Gut*, **15**, 468
173. Bennett, I. L. Jr. and Beeson, P. B. (1954). Bacteraemia: A consideration of some experimental and clinical aspects. *Yale J. Biol. Med.*, **26**, 241

174. Caroli, J. and Platteborse, R. (1958). Septicémie porto-cave. Cirrhoses du foie et septicémie a colibacille. *Sem. Hôp. Paris*, **34**, 472/SP, 113
175. Tisdale, W. A. and Klatskin, G. (1960). The fever of Laennec's cirrhosis. *Yale J. Biol. Med.*, **33**, 94
176. Jones, E. A., Crowley, N. and Sherlock, S. (1967). Bacteraemia in association with hepatocellular and hepatobiliary disease. *Postgrad. Med. J., Suppl.* **43**, 7
177. Bergerault, P., LeBodic, Mme M.-F., Lenne, Mme Y., LeBodic, L., Oudea, P. and Miniconi, P. (1973). La fièvre 'cryptogénétique' de la cirrhose alcoolique. Corrélations cliniques, biologiques et anatomo-pathologiques dans 72 cas. *Annales de Gastroenterologie et d'Hépatologie*, **9**, 537
178. Lemierre, A., Augier, P. and Mahoudeau-Campoyer, D. (1932). Sur quelques cas de colibacillémie. *Rév. Med. (Paris)*, **49**, 333
179. Jager, B. V. and Lamb, M. E. (1943). Sporadic infections caused by *Salmonella suipestifer* and *Salmonella oranienburg*. *New Eng. J. Med.*, **228**, 299
180. Angrist, A. and Mollov, M. (1946). Bacteriologic clinical and pathologic experience with 86 sporadic cases of *Salmonella* infection. *Am. J. Med.*, **212**, 336
181. Whipple. R. L. and Harris, J. F. (1950). *B. coli* septicaemia in Laennec's cirrhosis of the liver. *Ann. Intern. Med.*, **33**, 462
182. Martin, W. J., Spittel, J. A., Morlock, C. G. and Baggenstoss, A. H. (1956). Severe liver disease complicated by bacteremia due to gram-negative bacilli. *Arch. Intern. Med.*, **98**, 8
183. Tisdale, W. A. (1961). Spontaneous colon bacillus bacteremia in Laennec's cirrhosis. *Gastroenterology*, **40**, 141
184. Marlon, A., Gentry, L. and Merigan, T. C. (1971). Septicemia with *Pasteurella pseudotuberculosis* and liver disease. *Arch. Intern. Med.*, **127**, 947
185. Abramovitch, H. and Butas, C. A. (1973). Septicemia due to *Yersinia enterocolitica*. *Canad. Med. Ass. J.*, **109**, 1112
186. Defronzo, R. A., Murray, G. F. and Maddrey, W. C. (1973). *Aeromonas* septicaemia from hepatobiliary disease. *Am. J. Dig. Dis., New Ser.*, **18**, 323
187. Palutke, W. A., Boyd, C. B. and Carter, G. R. (1973). *Pasteurella multocida* septicaemia in a patient with cirrhosis. Report of a case. *Am. J. Med. Sci.*, **266**, 305
188. Chow, A. W. and Guze, L. B. (1974). Bacteriodacaea bacteraemia: Clinical experience with 112 patients. *Medicine (Baltimore)*, **53**, 93
189. Kerr, D. N. S., Pearson, D. T. and Read, A. E. (1963). Infection of ascitic fluid in patients with hepatic cirrhosis. *Gut*, **4**, 394
190. Conn, H. O. (1964). Spontaneous peritonitis and bacteraemia in Laennec's cirrhosis caused by enteric organisms. *Ann. Intern. Med.*, **60**, 568
191. Conn, H. O. and Fessel, J. M. (1971). Spontaneous bacterial peritonitis in cirrhosis: Variations on a theme. *Medicine (Baltimore)*, **50**, 161

192. Ansari, A. (1971). Spontaneous acute peritonitis with bacteraemia in patients with decompensated Laennec's cirrhosis. *Am. J. Gastroent*, **55**, 265
193. Curry, N., McCallum, R. W. and Guth, P. H. (1974). Spontaneous peritonitis in cirrhotic ascites. A decade of experience. *Am. J. Dig. Dis., New Ser.*, **19**, 685
194. Epstein, M., Calia, F. M. and Gabuzda, G. J. (1968). Pneumococcal peritonitis in patients with post necrotic cirrhosis. *New Eng. J. Med.*, **278**, 69
195. Sell, S. (1964). Immunoglobulins of the germ free guinea pig. *J. Immunol.*, **93**, 122
196. Sell, S. and Fahey, J. L. (1964). Relationship between gamma globulin metabolism and low serum gamma globulin in germ free mice. *J. Immunol.*, **93**, 81
197. Kunin, C. M. (1962). Antibody distribution against non-enteropathic *E. coli. Arch. Int. Med.*, **110**, 676
198. Webster, A. D. B., Efter, T. and Asherson, G. L. (1974). *Escherichia coli* antibodies: A screening test for immunodeficiency. *Br. Med. J.*, **3**, 16
199. Ørskov, J. and Moltke, O. (1928). Studien über den Infektionsmechanismus bei verschiedenen Paratyphus-Infektionen an weissen Mäusen. *Z. Immun.-Forsch.*, **59**, 24
200. Arnold, L. (1929). Alterations in the endogenous enteric bacterial flora and microbic permeability of the intestinal wall in relation to the nutritional and meteorological changes. *J. Hyg. (London)*, **29**, 82
201. Hildebrand, G. J. and Wolochow, H. (1962). Translocation of bacteriophage across the intestinal wall of the rat. *Proc. Soc. Exp. Biol. (N.Y.)*, **109**, 183
202. Hildebrand, G. J., Lamanna, C., Wolochow, H. and Meyers, C. E. (1963). Passage of microorganisms through the intestinal wall. Effect of surgical stress, hydrocortisone and the impairment of normal defence mechanisms. *Proc. 2nd World Congress Gastroenterol., Munich* 1962, **2**, 752
203. Wolochow, H., Hildebrand, G. J. and Lamanna, C. (1966). Translocation of micro-organisms across the intestinal wall of the rat: Effect of microbial size and concentration. *J. Infect. Dis.*, **116**, 523
204. Takeuchi, A. (1971). Penetration of the intestinal epithelium by various micro-organisms. *Current Topics Pathol.*, **54**, 1
205. Carter, P. B. and Collins, F. M. (1974). The route of enteric infection in normal mice. *J. Exp. Med.*, **139**, 1189
206. Collins, F. M. (1972). Salmonellosis in orally infected specific pathogen-free C57B1 mice. *Infection and Immunity*, **5**, 191
207. Coblentz, A., Kelly, K. H., Fitzpatrick, L. and Bierman, H. R. (1954). Microbiologic studies of the portal and hepatic venous blood in man. *Am. J. Med. Sci., New Ser.*, **228**, 298
208. Schatten, W. E., Desprez, J. D. and Holden, W. D. (1955). A bacteriologic study of portal-vein blood in man. *Arch. Surg.*, **71**, 404

209. Taylor, F. W. (1956). Blood-culture studies of the portal vein. *Arch. Surg.*, **72**, 889
210. Dencker, H., Kamme, C., Norryd, C., Mardh, P. A. and Tylén, U. (1974). Examination for aerobic and anaerobic bacteria in human portal blood collected by transumbilical catheterization. *Scand. J. Gastroent.*, **9**, 367
211. Prytz, H., Christensen, J. H. and Korner, B. To be published
212. Eade, M. N. and Brooke, B. N. (1969). Portal bacteraemia in cases of ulcerative colitis submitted to colectomy. *Lancet*, **i**, 1008
213. Martini, G. A., Phear, E. A., Ruebner, B. and Sherlock, S. (1957). The bacterial content of the small intestine in normal and cirrhotic subjects: Relation to methionine toxicity. *Clin. Sc. i*, **16**, 35
214. Lal, D., Gorbach, S. L. and Levitan, R. (1972). Intestinal microflora in patients with alcoholic cirrhosis: Urea-splitting bacteria and neomycin resistance. *Gastroenterology*, **62**, 275
215. Sborov, V. M., Morse, W. C., Giges, G. and Jahnke, E. J. (1952). Bacteriology of the human liver. *J. Clin. Invest.*, **31**, 986
216. McCloskey, R. V. and Gold, M. (1973). Bacteraemia after liver biopsy. *Arch. Intern. Med.*, **132**, 213
217. Le Frock, J., Ellis, C., Turchik, J. B. and Weinstein, L. (1973). Transient bacteraemia associated with percutaneous liver biopsy. *Clin. Res.*, **21**, 843
218. Rogers, C. A. and Sharp, H. L. (1974). Complications of percutaneous liver biopsy. Letter to the editor, *Lancet*, **i**, 931
219. Rutenberg, A. M., Sonnenblick, E., Koven, I., Schweinburg, F. and Fine, J. (1959). Comparative response of normal and cirrhotic rats to intravenously injected bacteria. *Proc. Soc. Exp. Biol.*, **101**, 279
220. Schatten, W. E. (1954). The role of intestinal bacteria in liver necrosis following experimental excision of the hepatic arterial supply. *Surgery*, **36**, 256
221. Gans, H., Mori, K., Lindsey, E., Kaster, B. L. F., Richter, D., Quinlan, R., Dineen, P. A. and Tan, B. H. (1971). Septicaemia as a manifestation of acute liver failure. *Surg. Gynec. Obstet.*, **132**, 783
222. Bjørneboe, M. and Prytz, H. (1975). Kupffer cells and cirrhosis. Letter to the editor, *Lancet*, **i**, 45
223. Prytz, H., Bjørneboe, M., Koch, C. and Ørskov, F. To be published
224. Johnston, R. B. and Baehner, R. L. (1971). Chronic granulomatous disease: Correlation between pathogenesis and clinical findings. *Pediatrics*, **48**, 730
225. Tygstrup, N., Juhl, E. and the Copenhagen Study Group for Liver Diseases (1971). The treatment of alcoholic cirrhosis. The effect of continued drinking and prednisone on survival. In *Alkohol und Leber* (*Alcohol and Liver*) (Internat. Symposium Oktober 1970, Frieburg). W. Kerok, K. Sickinger and H. H. Hennekeuser (eds.) p. 519 (Stuttgart and New York: Schattauer Verlag)
226. The Copenhagen Study Group for Liver Diseases (1969). Effect of

prednisone on the survival of patients with cirrhosis of the liver. *Lancet*, **i**, 119

227. The Copenhagen Study Group for Liver Diseases (1974). Sex, ascites and alcoholism in survival of patients with cirrhosis. Effect of prednisone. *New Eng. J. Med.*, **291**, 271
228. Campra, J., Hamlin, E. M., Kirschbaum, R. J., Olivier, M., Redeker, A. G. and Reynolds, T. B. (1973). Prednisone therapy of acute alcoholic hepatitis. Report of a controlled trial. *Ann. Int. Med.*, **79**, 625
229. Bjørneboe, M. (1974). Viral hepatitis and cirrhosis. *Clinics in Gastroenterology*, **3**, 409
230. Luckey, T. D., Reyniers, J. A., György, P. and Forbes, M. (1954). Germ free animals and liver necrosis. *Ann. N.Y. Acad. Sci.*, **57**, 932
231. Broitman, S. A., Gottleib, L. S. and Zamcheck, N. (1964). Influence of neomycin and ingested endotoxin in the pathogenesis of choline deficiency cirrhosis in the adult rat. *J. Exp. Med.*, **119**, 633
232. Nolan, J. P. and Ali, M. V. (1968). Endotoxin and the liver. I. Toxicity in rats with choline deficient fatty livers. *Proc. Soc. Exp. Biol. (N.Y.)*, **129**, 29
233. Wilkinson, S. P., Arroyo, V., Gazzard, B. G., Moodie, H. and Williams, R. (1974). Relation of renal impairment and haemorrhagic diathesis to endotoxaemia in fulminant hepatic failure. *Lancet*, **i**, 521
234. Nolan, J. P. and Ali, M. V. (1974). Endotoxaemia in liver disease. Letter to the editor, *Lancet*, **i**, 999
235. Schaffer, J. M., Bluemile, L. W., Sborov, V. M. and Neffe, J. R. (1950). Studies on the use of aureomycin in hepatic disease. IV. Aureomycin therapy in chronic liver disease. With a note on dermal sensitivity. *Am. J. Med. Sci.*, **220**, 173
236. Goldbloom, R. S. and Steigmann, F. (1951). Aureomycin therapy in hepatic insufficiency. *Gastroenterology*, **18**, 93
237. Magarey, C. J. (1972). The control of cancer spread by the reticulo-endothelial system. *Ann. Roy. Coll. Surg. Engl.*, **50**, 238

CHAPTER 8

Aetiological factors in immune-mediated liver disease

A. L. W. F. EDDLESTON

Introduction

Immunological reactions have long been thought to be of importance in the pathogenesis of two main types of chronic liver disease, namely chronic active hepatitis and primary biliary cirrhosis. More recently, however, there has been an increasing awareness of the involvement of immune responses in the production of acute liver injury induced by viruses or drugs. This, in turn, has focused attention on the possible aetiological role of these agents in chronic liver disease. Although the hepatitis B virus appears to play no part in the development of primary biliary cirrhosis there is now considerable evidence to suggest that it may be a common aetiological agent in chronic active hepatitis. The discovery of the hepatitis B antigen greatly facilitated progress in this area. Using sensitive techniques for detecting both the viral product itself and immune responses to it, important links have been established between acute hepatitis and chronic active hepatitis and it is now possible to sketch the outlines of the complex cellular and humoral interactions which determine the clinical expression of hepatitis B virus infection.

The role of the immune system in the pathogenesis of drug-induced hepatic damage is not so clearly defined, partly because it has always been difficult to establish a clear cause and effect relationship in any individual case but mainly because little immunological data has yet been obtained. Nevertheless, a number of drugs are now thought to be capable of inducing chronic liver disease which closely mimics chronic active hepatitis both clinically and pathologically, and it is possible that the immune responses which may underlie these idiosyncratic reactions are very similar to those associated with viral infection.

The hepatitis viruses

Although infectious jaundice had been clearly defined as a distinct clinical entity by the beginning of this century, the existence of two epidemiologically and immunologically distinct forms of viral hepatitis was not clearly established until the 1940s. The names *virus A*, giving rise to infectious hepatitis after a short incubation period, and *virus B*, giving rise to serum hepatitis after a long incubation period, were introduced to replace the old terminology of infective jaundice and homologous serum jaundice respectively. Viral hepatitis is now defined as acute inflammation of the liver caused by either of these two agents[1], and excludes, by common usage, hepatitis caused by well recognized viruses such as yellow fever virus, cytomegalovirus, Epstein–Barr virus, herpes simplex virus and others. Experimental studies, particularly those carried out by Krugman and his colleagues[2], in which serum pools producing short and long incubation hepatitis were obtained and called MS-1 and MS-2, established that serum hepatitis could be transmitted orally, though less readily than infectious hepatitis. On the other hand infectious hepatitis could be transmitted by injection although the attack rate was lower than for serum hepatitis, and up to 20% of cases of hepatitis following blood transfusion are thought to be due to the shorter incubation agent[3].

Attempts to isolate the responsible agents by standard virological techniques were all unsuccessful and further progress was not achieved until the now famous intervention of a geneticist in 1964[4]. Blumberg's fortuitous discovery of an immunologically distinct antigen in the serum of an Australian aborigine, and the subsequent recognition of its close association with serum hepatitis and hepatitis B virus[5] has led to a series of revolutionary advances in understanding of this type of viral hepatitis. The antigen was first named Australia antigen but there is now general support for the term hepatitis B antigen (HBAg) as this allows for the future introduction of as yet undiscovered hepatitis-related antigen–antibody systems as C, D, etc.[6] Examination of HBAg-positive sera by electron-microscopy showed three types of particle; a small spherical one 20 nm in diameter, tubular forms 20 $\times$ 100 nm and a larger, more complex Dane particle with a diameter of 42 nm and having an inner

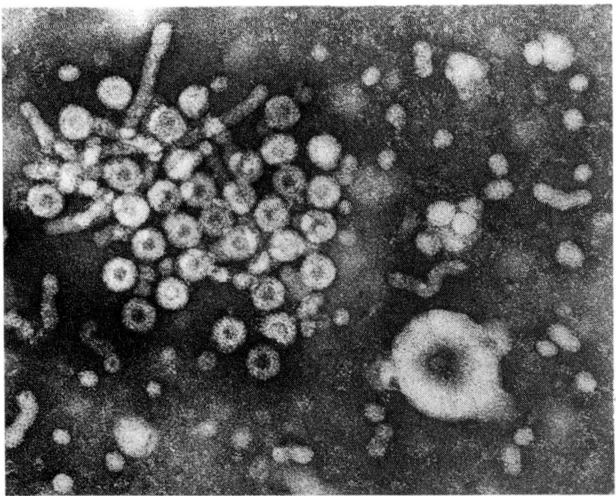

FIGURE 8.1 The morphology of the hepatitis B antigen in serum as seen by electron microscopy. This specimen contains an unusually large number of Dane particles. (By courtesy of Professor A. J. Zuckerman)

core 27 nm in diameter (Figure 8.1). The inner core of the Dane particle has now been shown to contain DNA polymerase and twin stranded DNA, and is probably the nucleo-capsid of the hepatitis B virus. It is referred to as hepatitis B core antigen (HBcAg), in distinction to hepatitis B surface antigen (HBsAg) which comprises the outer coat of the Dane particle and the other small spherical and tubular particles.

HBcAg has resemblances to some rhinoviruses and appears to have a different antigenic composition from HBsAg, being aggregated by sera from patients who have recovered from HBAg-positive acute hepatitis and no longer have demonstrable antibody to HBsAg[7].

Similar advances in the understanding of virus A hepatitis have only recently been forthcoming. Virus-like particles which seem to be specially aggregated by convalescent sera have been observed in the faeces of patients with hepatitis A infection[8], and although caution has been urged when interpreting these results[9] the fact that this material has proved infectious in marmosets suggests that hepatitis-A virus is present[10]. Similar particles are not observed in the serum and the Milan, or epidemic hepatitis associated antigen discovered in the acute phase sera of patients with hepatitis[11] is now known to be a lipoprotein, lacking specificity for hepatitis A or even for liver disease[12].

Chronic liver disease following hepatitis B virus infection

Although cirrhosis as a rare consequence of acute hepatitis had been recognized for many years, the ability to detect HBsAg in serum and thus to infer the continued presence of hepatitis B virus infection has allowed more exact estimates of the frequency of this complication and the acquisition of more detailed clinical and laboratory information during the development of chronic liver injury. The data collected by the Copenhagen Hepatitis Acuta Programme has been particularly valuable. In an initial study of 112 patients with serum hepatitis, HBsAg remained persistently detectable in the serum in 11 and of these, eight developed chronic active hepatitis and two chronic persistent hepatitis[13], diagnoses confirmed pathologically on liver biopsy.

However, only a minority of cases of chronic persistent hepatitis or chronic active hepatitis are associated with persistence of HBsAg in the serum. Chronic persistent hepatitis has been shown to follow antigen-negative acute viral hepatitis[14] and in a series of 100 cases reported from the United States, persistent antigenaemia was present in only 10%[15]. The reported frequency of HBsAg in chronic active hepatitis in temperate countries ranges from 3%[16] to 51%[17] and seems to reflect the frequency of hepatitis B infection in the community. In the USA the frequency is 10–15%[18,19]. One group in the UK found antigen present in 8%[20] although five of the six positive subjects in that series were of foreign origin. In our own series, using a sensitive radioimmunoassay technique, 17 (17%) of 98 cases were found to have HBsAg in the serum[21]. The frequency in males was higher, 13 (36%) of 36 cases, than in females, four (6%) of 62. The clinical picture in HBsAg-positive chronic active hepatitis is said to have certain differences from that described in antigen-negative cases. The patients tend to be male rather than female, autoantibodies are usually absent from the sera and multisystem involvement is not present to the same degree[22]. However, we were unable to confirm these findings apart from the male preponderance in those with persistent antigenaemia[21]. In fact, the other reported differences particularly in the occurrence of autoantibodies may simply be related to the sex difference in the two groups. The course of HBsAg-positive chronic active hepatitis is said to be less rapidly progressive than the antigen-negative disease[17] but again in our own series, the probability of survival at 6 years was not significantly different[21].

In those cases of chronic active hepatitis in which HBsAg persists in the serum there are obviously strong grounds for assuming that persistence of virus B infection is in some way responsible for the chronic liver damage. Recent studies in HBsAg-negative cases have suggested that a previous episode of hepatitis B virus infection may also have been important in initiating the disease in this group[23]. Thus, cellular immunity to HBsAg, as assessed by the leukocyte migration test, was found in 63% of such cases (Figure 8.2) indicating previous exposure to the virus, and in the Copenhagen series of patients with acute hepatitis followed prospectively, three of those in whom HBsAg disappeared from the serum went on to develop antigen-negative chronic active hepatitis[13]. A similar course of events has been recorded in one of our cases[23].

Asymptomatic carriers of hepatitis B surface antigen

Screening of blood samples on a large scale to detect HBsAg soon established the presence of persistent carriers of the antigen in the population. Their prevalence is about 1 in 1000 in North America and the UK but is much higher in some other countries, particularly in tropical Africa, Asia and the Mediterranean littoral. Clinical investigation of these apparently healthy carriers has shown that a proportion of them have asymptomatic liver disease. In one study from Copenhagen[24], liver biopsies were normal in 13 of 24 carriers examined, but showed chronic persistent hepatitis in 10 (41%) and cirrhosis in one (5%). In a similar study in the UK, only 9% had entirely normal liver histology although the changes were very minor in a further 38%[25]. On the other hand, all of 22 young Greek soldiers who were carriers of the antigen had normal liver histology or only mild non-specific changes[26] and there seems little doubt that some individuals with persistent antigenaemia have *no* evidence of liver disease.

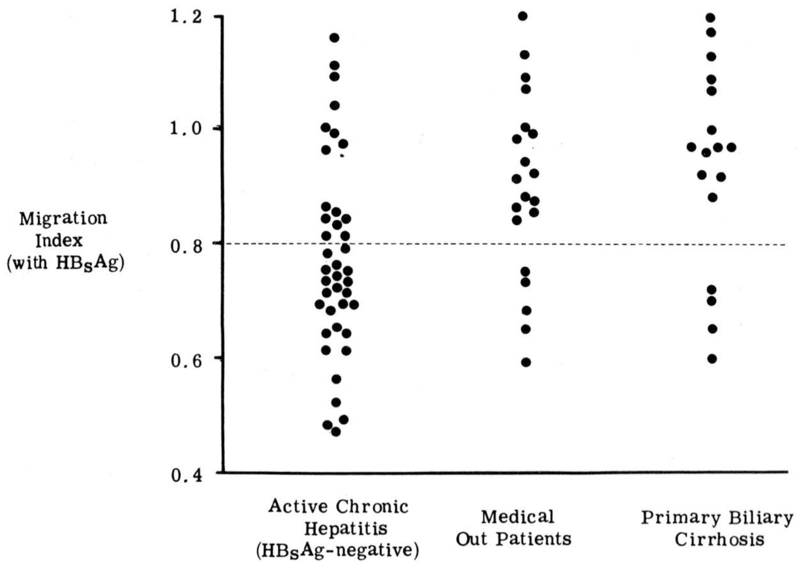

FIGURE 8.2 Results of the leukocyte migration test with HBsAg as antigen in 40 cases of antigen-negative chronic active hepatitis, in 17 with primary biliary cirrhosis and in 20 patients attending a general medical clinic. The dotted line indicates the lower limit of the normal range. The frequency of sensitization in the chronic active hepatitis group (63%) is significantly higher than that in each of the control groups (24% and 25% respectively, $p<0.02$)

There is also an increased frequency of the carrier state in patients with immunodeficiency, usually secondary to some other condition such as Down's syndrome, lepromatous leprosy, diabetes or uraemia, and in patients receiving immunosuppressive or cytotoxic therapy. These carriers differ from the healthy carriers in the population in having a greater incidence of liver disease. Thus, 65% of carriers with Down's syndrome had histological abnormalities on liver biopsy[27] and 75% of carriers with treated Hodgkin's disease had chronic persistent hepatitis[28], while untreated Hodgkin's patients were all antigen-negative.

The pathogenesis of virus-induced liver damage

The extremely variable clinical response to hepatitis B virus infection, ranging from acute hepatitis to chronic active hepatitis, and the finding of carriers who apparently exist in harmless symbiosis with the virus has stimulated a great deal of thought and discussion. What are the viral or host factors which determine the end result?

VIRAL FACTORS

The discovery of antigenic differences between certain HBsAg-positive sera focused attention on the role of different subtypes in pathogenesis. Two major subtypes have been identified in the Western hemisphere. A common antigenic determinant has been designated *a*, and two other mutually exclusive determinants *d* and *y*. Some interesting differences in the distribution of these subtypes are already apparent[29–31]. Most cases of acute hepatitis are due to *ay*. This is the subtype found in Krugman's MS-2 serum pool and was also responsible for the serious outbreak of hepatitis in the Edinburgh renal unit. *Ay* is common in drug addicts. The predominant subtype among blood donors and asymptomatic carriers is *ad*, but it has also been found in acute hepatitis and in some of the outbreaks in renal units. The subtypes breed true in the sense that all cases in an isolated outbreak have been due to the same subtypes, either *ay* or *ad*[29,32] and infection with one subtype does not necessarily confer immunity against subsequent infection with the other[33]. The distribution appears to differ between countries; whereas there was a marked preponderance of subtype *ad* in patients with chronic hepatitis in the United States[30], four out of five carriers with chronic persistent hepatitis examined in Sweden were *ay*[31]. There is also evidence that the dominant subtype associated with clinical hepatitis in a population may change with time. Sera collected in Stockholm in 1953 from patients with acute hepatitis showed predominantly subtype *ad*, while today subtype *ay* is dominant within the same area[34].

The distribution of subtypes seems, therefore, to reflect epidemiological influences rather than inherent differences in the strains of virus and there was, until recently, little evidence that the outcome of virus B infection was dependent on viral factors. However, in 1972 a new group of precipitating antigens in HBsAg-positive sera were described[35] one of which was designated the *e*-antigen. This was quite different from previously described determinants, since it appeared as a precipitin line between two HBsAg-positive sera, and showed a reaction of non-identity with HBsAg using the Ouchterlony technique. The *e*-antigen was present in some HBsAg-positive hepatitis sera, mostly from patients on haemodialysis, and antibody against *e*-antigen was found in serum specimens from healthy carriers of HBsAg. The nature of the new antigen and its relationship to the hepatitis B virus is not yet clear but it does seem to be specific for hepatitis B infection, being absent in 96 normal blood donors and in 365 patients with HBsAg-negative liver diseases[36]. Of considerable interest, is the observation that it may be a prognostic marker of the outcome of HBsAg-positive hepatitis[36]. In 168 patients with HBsAg-positive acute hepatitis, a striking difference in the frequency of the *e*-antigen on initial testing was found between patients who subsequently cleared HBsAg (4% positive) and those in whom HBsAg persisted in the serum (65% positive). This difference was reflected in the results of follow-up biopsies, 11 (58%) of 19 patients who developed chronic hepatitis or cirrhosis being *e*-antigen positive on initial testing compared with only one (2%) of 41 patients with histological resolution. The finding of antibodies against the *e*-antigen in healthy carriers of HBsAg in whom no Dane particles had been demonstrated and the fact that antibodies to HBsAg are also found in such patients suggests that there may be a close relationship between the Dane particle and the *e*-antigen. However, Magnius has clearly shown that the *e*-antigen is not physically part of the Dane particle[37] and it may be that the two are closely associated because the *e*-antigen is produced by infected cells only at a time when they are also making core antigen and complete Dane particles. The presence of Dane particles in the sera is not restricted to patients with HBsAg-positive chronic liver disease and more information is needed before the mechanism linking the *e*-antigen with persistence of hepatitis B virus infection can be understood.

Host factors

Immune-mediated liver injury: The fact that a symbiotic union between virus and host can exist in healthy carriers of HBsAg implies that the virus itself is not damaging to liver cells, and also suggests that the hepatocellular damage in patients with acute or chronic hepatitis is associated with some indirect mechanism triggered by the presence of the virus. In other infections with viruses that are not cytopathic, the immune response to viral antigens has been implicated in the production of tissue damage. Thus, in experimental lymphocytic choriomeningitis in mice, the neurological lesions are thought to be mediated by a cellular immune reaction directed at viral determinants on the surface of infected cells. The disease can be almost completely suppressed by either induction of tolerance to the virus, irradiation or immunosuppression with drugs[38]. Application of such a theory of immunopathology to hepatitis B virus infection could certainly explain the existence of the healthy carrier state, with a total lack of immune response to hepatitis B surface antigen, and also the occurrence of acute hepatitis in those individuals who are able to destroy virus-infected cells by the development of appropriate cellular and humoral immunity. The results of several recent studies strongly support this hypothesis.

Healthy carriers: Examination of liver biopsies from healthy carriers by immunofluorescence for the presence of HBsAg has shown that many hepatocytes contain the antigen in their cytoplasm. This has been confirmed using a new histochemical technique which can reliably detect intracellular material in those hepatocytes which contain HBsAg on immunofluorescence (Figure 8.3). It is likely that these cells also

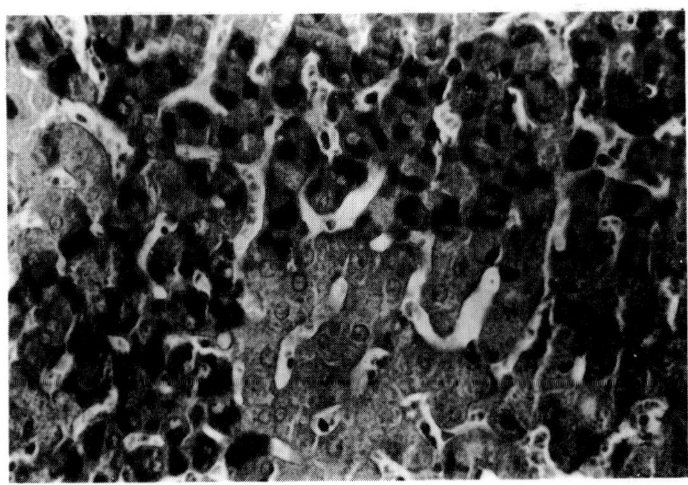

FIGURE 8.3 Section of a liver biopsy from a healthy carrier of HBsAg treated with a modified orcein stain[68]. Hepatocytes containing HBsAg show darkly staining cytoplasmic inclusions. (By courtesy of Dr B. Portmann)

contain complete virions for, although it is possible in theory for HBsAg to be present in the absence of mature virus particles, blood from these carriers is known to be capable of transmitting acute hepatitis. There is no evidence of a generalized defect in cellular immunity in healthy carriers[39] but an increasing number of observations confirm a specific absence of a cell-mediated response to HBsAg in these individuals[40,41]. We have recently investigated 38 blood donors found to be positive for HBsAg on routine screening[42]. Cellular immunity to HBsAg was assessed using the leukocyte migration test and the results were clearly related to the presence or absence of biochemical evidence of liver damage, as judged by serum aspartate aminotransferase levels. Only 13% of those with normal liver function showed inhibition of leukocyte migration in the presence of HBsAg whereas this was observed in 47% of those with elevated enzyme levels (Table 8.1). Most of those

Table 8.1 CELLULAR IMMUNITY TO HEPATITIS B SURFACE ANTIGEN IN 38 ASYMPTOMATIC BLOOD DONORS. RESULTS OF THE LEUCOCYTE MIGRATION TEST WITH HBsAg AS ANTIGEN IN RELATION TO SERUM ASPARTATE AMINOTRANSFERASE LEVELS AND HISTOLOGICAL FINDINGS ON LIVER BIOPSY

	Serum aspartate aminotransferase		*Histological findings*		
	Normal (N = 23)	*Abnormal* (N = 15)	*Normal* (N = 2)	*Minor changes* (N = 7)	*Chronic hepatitis* (N = 7)
Number with migration-inhibition	3 (13%)	7 (47%)	0	1 (14%)	3 (43%)

From Lee, W. M. *et al.* (1975)[41]

with abnormal liver function had the histological changes of chronic active or chronic persistent hepatitis on liver biopsy while minor parenchymal lesions were present in the majority of those with a normal serum aspirate aminotransferase level. Only two patients had normal or unrelated changes on biopsy and in both there was no evidence of cellular immunity to HBsAg. Antibody to HBsAg was not detected by radioimmunoassay in any of these carriers and electron microscopy of serum samples showed only free particles with no aggregates to indicate the presence of immune complexes.

Acute hepatitis: The acquisition of humoral and cellular immunity to HBsAg during acute antigen-positive hepatitis has been well documented in several studies. A humoral antibody response is not usually detectable during the early stages of the illness but this is perhaps not surprising in view of the vast excess of antigen in the serum. Following clearance of HBsAg, specific antibody can be detected in almost every case if a sensitive technique such as radioimmunoassay is used[43]. Cell-mediated immunity to HBsAg seems to follow a similar time course. There is general agreement that cellular responses to the antigen, either lymphocyte transformation[40] or leukocyte migration inhibition[41], are almost always demonstrable during convalescence but investigators differ in their ability to show sensitization early in the course of the disease. This data is particularly important in relation to the hypothesis of immune-mediated liver damage, for if a cellular response to HBsAg is the cause of hepatocyte injury then this immunological reaction should be detectable at the time of presentation. Dr William Lee, in our unit, has studied cellular and humoral immunity to HBsAg in 23 patients with acute type B hepatitis followed serially from the time of admission up to one year later. Of 20 patients who presented within a week of the onset of the disease, 11 (55%) had evidence of cell-mediated immunity to the antigen and at 4 weeks this was present in all those tested (Figure 8.4). Follow-up is, as yet, incomplete but in the majority of patients followed for more than 6 months cellular immunity to HBsAg has remained detectable.

Of the nine patients with negative results on the leukocyte migration test at the onset, six had serum titres of HBsAg higher than that used in the migration test chamber (approximately 1/256 by complement fixation). In contrast, such high HBsAg titres were present in none of those who showed migration inhibition on initial testing and it is possible that high antigen levels *in vivo* might interfere with the demonstration of sensitization *in vitro*. Indeed, in those who were initially unresponsive, inhibition of migration was observed when the level of HBsAg in the serum had fallen. This may be one reason why some investigators have failed to detect cellular immunity to HBsAg at the onset of acute hepatitis but another possibility is the use of suboptimal concentrations of antigen in the test system. For the leukocyte migration test, an antigen is usually used at a concentration which just fails to produce inhibition of migration in non-sensitized individuals. However, when the antigen concerned is a product of a virus to which the general population is exposed, this method is difficult to apply. Cellular immunity to HBsAg has been found in 30% of a healthy population of factory workers and 86% of a group of immunologists who were continually exposed to HBsAg-positive material[44]. If the HBsAg concentration in the test system is reduced to eliminate these positive responses in 'normal' individuals, then the sensitivity of the assay will be considerably

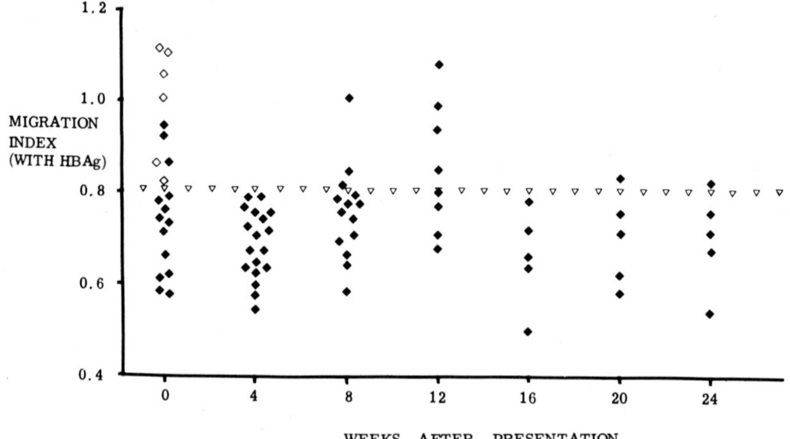

FIGURE 8.4 A serial study of cellular immunity to HBsAg as detected by the leucocyte migration test, in patients with acute type B hepatitis. (From Lee, Wm. *et al.* in preparation.) Open symbols, serum titre of HBsAg >1/256 by complement fixation

diminished. This effect can be clearly shown using suboptimal concentrations of defined antigens such as purified protein derivative (PPD)[45], where an independent assessment of sensitization is possible by intradermal skin tests.

Chronic liver disease: These problems in interpreting the results of assays of cell-mediated immunity are particularly relevant to studies of cellular responses to HBsAg in patients with antigen-positive chronic liver disease. There is general agreement that sensitization to HBsAg is detectable in at least half of these cases and our own studies in the HBsAg positive blood donors referred to earlier showed that 47% of those with a raised Serum Aspartate AminoTransferase (SGOT) level had evidence of cellular immunity to the antigen. Similar results have been obtained in patients with HBsAg positive chronic active hepatitis. Of 12 patients we have studied, eight showed inhibition of leukocyte migration with HBsAg including all of those who were tested before starting on conventional immunosuppressive therapy[23]. Thus from an immunological viewpoint there does seem to be a clear difference in the cellular response to HBsAg between healthy carriers and those with chronic liver disease. In the former group there is no evidence of humoral or cellular immunity to the antigen whereas in the latter cell-mediated immunity is detectable almost as frequently as in patients with acute hepatitis.

These findings certainly support the hypothesis that liver damage in hepatitis B virus infection is due to a cellular immune response directed at viral antigens. However, if virus infected hepatocytes are being destroyed in those patients with HBsAg positive chronic liver disease why does the virus infection persist and why can a few HBsAg containing cells still be detected in liver biopsies from such cases?[26] One possible explanation is that there is a qualitative or quantitative defect in the production of neutralizing antibody, allowing the virus to penetrate previously uninfected hepatocytes which then produce new virions before they acquire viral determinants on their surface and are destroyed by effector lymphocytes. This act of cell lysis would in turn release the newly formed virions to infect other cells and complete the cycle. Dissemination of the vaccinia virus with infection of cells at distant sites is a well known complication of vaccination, and appears to be due to such a failure in the production of neutralizing antibody since further dissemination can be prevented by the administration of immunoglobulin containing high titre antibody to the virus[46].

Autoimmunity in chronic active hepatitis

While the evidence presented so far suggests that the hepatitis B virus is an important aetiological agent in chronic active hepatitis, other studies have implicated autoimmune mechanisms in pathogenesis. The presence of antibodies reacting with a wide variety of tissue antigens in patients and their relatives[47] suggests an inherited predisposition to autoimmunity, although in the absence of organ specificity it is unlikely that these antibodies are directly involved in production of liver damage. Indeed, the internal cell constituents with which they react would be inaccessible to the immune system *in vivo*. Liver-specific antibodies directed at cell surface determinants, which could be more damaging to hepatocytes, have not yet been detected in the serum, but immunoglobulin has been identified on the cell membrane of hepatocytes from patients with active disease[48].

Early studies of cellular immunity to liver homogenates showed a high frequency of positive responses in chronic active hepatitis[49] but reactions to such mixed and ill-defined antigenic material could not easily be related to pathogenesis. The isolation, by Meyer zum Buschenfelde of two human liver-specific antigens was therefore, of considerable importance. One was a lipoprotein which appeared to be a normal constituent of the hepatocyte cell membrane and the other a soluble component of the cytoplasm[50]. Rabbits immunized repeatedly with a mixture of those two antigens developed inflammatory lesions in the liver closely resembling chronic active hepatitis[51] (Figure 8.5) and in

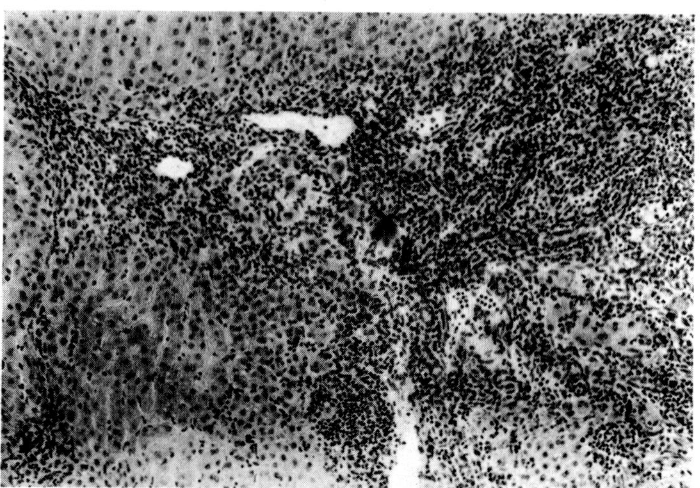

FIGURE 8.5 Histological changes in the liver of a rabbit which had received multiple injections of human liver-specific antigens. The changes are similar to those seen in liver biopsies from patients with chronic active hepatitis. (By courtesy of Dr K. H. Meyer zum Buschendelde)

some animals these progressed to cirrhosis[52]. The cell-surface lipoprotein seemed to be of particular importance in the induction of these lesions[51], and in our own studies of cellular immunity to this antigen using the leucocyte migration test we have been able to demonstrate sensitization in 66% of 58 patients with chronic active hepatitis. The frequency of sensitization to the lipoprotein was highest (93%) in untreated cases and lowest (43%) in those who had shown a good response to immunosuppressive therapy (Table 8.2).

Table 8.2 EFFECT OF IMMUNOSUPPRESSIVE THERAPY IN CHRONIC ACTIVE HEPATITIS ON CELLULAR IMMUNE RESPONSE TO THE LIVER-SPECIFIC LIPOPROTEIN (LSP)

	Number tested	*Inhibition of leucocyte migration with LSP as antigen*
Untreated	14	13 (93%)
Treated: with abnormal serum bilirubin	23	16 (70%)
Treated: with normal serum bilirubin	21	9 (43%)

Sensitization to a surface antigen might be expected to be damaging to hepatocytes and we have recently been able to demonstrate killing of isolated rabbit hepatocytes when incubated with lymphocytes from 20 of 22 patients with chronic active hepatitis[53] (Figure 8.6). Rabbit hepatocytes were chosen since they are easier to maintain in tissue culture than human liver cells and the rabbit lipoprotein is known to share antigenic determinants with the human protein[50]. Other experiments strongly suggest that the cytotoxicity is due to an immunological reaction directed at this cell surface antigen. It is, for instance, considerably reduced by the addition of small amounts of human or rabbit liver-specific lipoprotein but is not blocked by a similar material prepared from human kidney[53].

Although it is impossible to prove that these cellular reactions are primarily responsible for the liver damage in chronic active hepatitis, the similarity of the histological lesions in the rabbits immunized with human liver-specific antigens suggests that the immune response to the hepatocyte-surface lipoprotein in patients with this disease is not just an epiphenomenon but could be of central importance in pathogenesis.

The link between virus-directed responses and autoimmunity

If an autoimmune response to a hepatocyte surface lipoprotein is the pathogenic reaction common to all varieties of chronic active hepatitis, what initiates the self-destructive process? One obvious candidate is the hepatitis B virus which is persistently present in some cases and appears

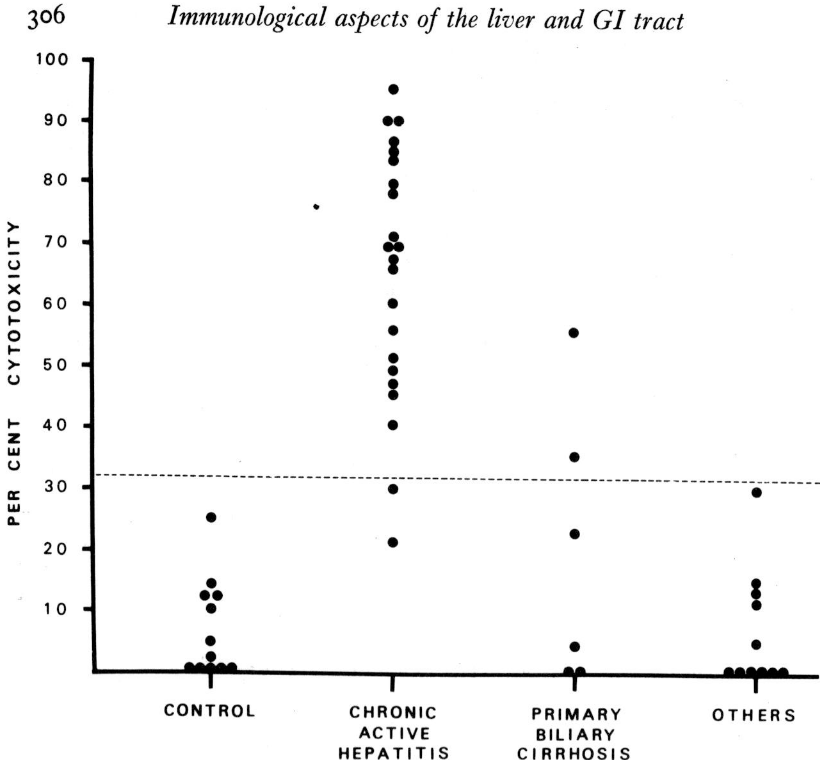

FIGURE 8.6 Percentage of hepatocytes killed after incubation for 48 hours with lymphocytes from patients with the various chronic liver diseases shown. The horizontal dotted line shows the upper limit of the normal range. (From Thomson, A. D. *et al.* (1974), reference 53)

to have been an important aetiological agent in those in the HBsAg-negative group who had an initial type B hepatitis. There are many ways in theory in which viruses can initiate an autoimmune reaction and any description of the interactions involved must be speculative. Recently, however, we have outlined one scheme which seems to fit the available facts[54] and has correctly predicted the results of some further experiments.

Interactions between T- and B-lymphocytes are, according to Allison, Denman and Barnes, of fundamental importance in the development of autoimmunity[55]. B-lymphocytes responsive to many of the self antigens are present in normal individuals but are only activated to produce antibodies when T-cells provide a 'helper effect'. Autoreactive T-cells are normally rendered unresponsive by small amounts of tissue antigens in the circulation, but T- and B-cell co-operation, with production of autoantibody, can occur if a new antigenic determinant is introduced, on or close to a self constituent, to which other T-cells can respond. The possibility that viral antigens on the surface of infected hepatocytes could provide such a new antigenic determinant and promote T- and B-cell co-operation formed the basis of our working hypothesis (Figure 8.7).

Both the HBsAg positive and some of the antigen negative cases are initiated by exposure to the hepatitis B virus. This enters some of the hepatocytes and towards the end of the incubation period, virus-associated antigens appear on the surface of infected cells. T-cells

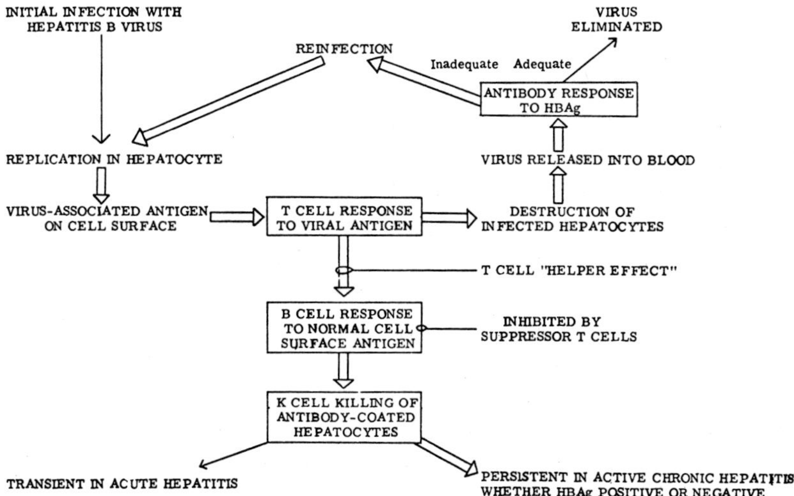

FIGURE 8.7 A working hypothesis to explain the induction and perpetuation of auto-immune liver injury in chronic active hepatitis. (From Eddleston, A. L. W. F. and Williams, R. (1974), reference 53)

recognizing these new determinants destroy the infected hepatocytes. Viral particles are released, some of which are capable of entering previously uninfected hepatocytes. This is normally prevented by the production of neutralizing antibody which interferes with the ability of the virus to penetrate liver cell membranes. However, those patients who go on to develop antigen-positive chronic active hepatitis either fail to produce enough antibody, or its affinity is too low and further penetration of the virus into uninfected hepatocytes is then possible. Initially the cycle of infection thus established will be phasic, but slight differences in the times required for viral replication in different hepatocytes will rapidly lead to a stable situation in which the rate of production of HBsAg will be constant and in any one area of the liver there will be infected cells at different stages of 'maturity'.

Another effect of T-cell stimulation is the activation of B-cells responsive to existing hepatocyte cell surface antigens including the liver-specific lipoprotein. Antibodies to this antigen are produced, and entering the liver bind to the surface of periportal hepatocytes. While fixation of complement is one possible mechanism leading to necrosis in this area, it is likely that K-cells would also be activated. These are morphologically identical to lymphocytes and, having receptors on their surface for the Fc portion of antibody molecules, are cytotoxic when bound to antibody-coated target cells[56]. The mononuclear cell infiltrate in the portal areas may largely represent K-cell aggregates.

The synthesis and release of the damaging autoantibody would normally be subject to control by suppressor T-cells[55] and in an uncomplicated acute hepatitis the autoimmune reaction initially generated is but transient. However, in HBsAg-positive chronic active hepatitis the autoantibody continues to be produced, in spite of normal suppressor T-cell function, because of the continuous activation of helper T-cells. On the other hand, in the HBsAg negative cases, suppressor T-cell function is defective and although the helper T-cell effect is only transient, the autoimmune response persists.

One of the predictions of this hypothesis is that the autoimmune liver damage is antibody-mediated, either directly or by the activation of K-cells. By removing either E or EAC rosetting cells from mixed peripheral blood lymphocytes of patients with chronic active hepatitis we have been able to obtain enriched T- and B-cell fractions which can be tested for cytotoxic activity on isolated hepatocytes. The results clearly indicate that the effector cells in this system have the capacity to form EAC rosettes (Figure 8.8) and this together with preliminary observations of the blocking effect of non-specific immune complexes strongly suggest that they are K-cells.

HL-A8 as a marker for defective suppressor T-cell function

Not only are histocompatibility antigens closely associated in animals with specific immune response genes[57], but they have also been identified as one of about 10 genetic factors which can promote a non-specific increase in antibody production[58]. The latter effect might be related to defective suppressor T-cell function as we have postulated in HBsAg-negative chronic active hepatitis. HL-A8 was detected in 62% of these cases[59] but in none of those with HBsAg positive disease in which, according to our hypothesis, suppressor T-cell function is normal. If HL-A8 were a marker of defective suppressor T-cell function, individuals possessing this antigen would have increased and prolonged antibody responses to autoantigens and foreign determinants, which

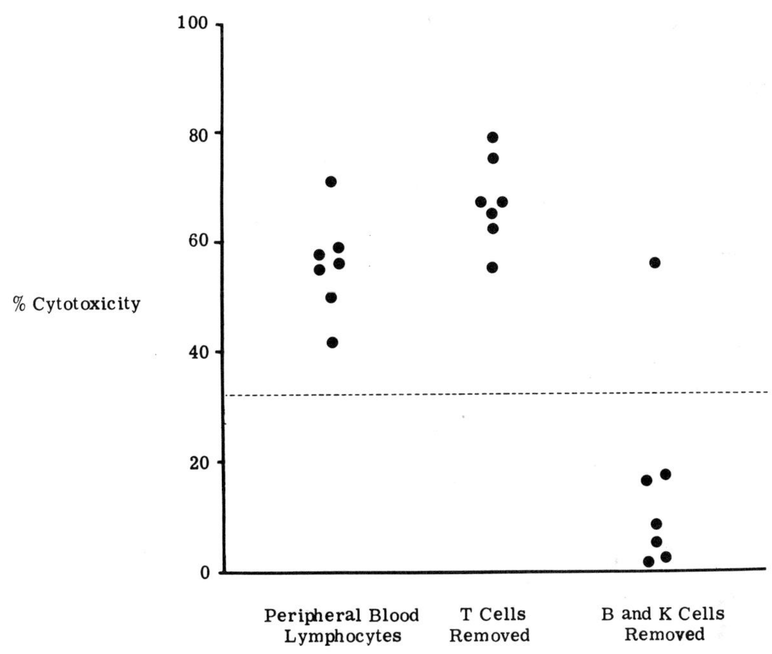

FIGURE 8.8 Effect of removal of T-cells or B-and K-cells on lymphocyte cytotoxicity to isolated hepatocytes. The peripheral blood lymphocytes were from seven patients with uncontrolled chronic active hepatitis. The T-cell-depleted preparations were obtained by removing lymphocytes forming E-rosettes and the B- and K-cell depleted fractions by removing cells forming EAC-rosettes. (From Cochrane, A. M. G. *et al.* In preparation)

would explain the high titre antibody to certain viral and bacterial antigens in many patients with HBsAg-negative chronic active hepatitis[60]. Furthermore, an increased frequency of HL-A8 has been reported in a wide variety of conditions associated with a positive Coombs test[61] as well as in thyrotoxicosis, idiopathic Addison's disease, juvenile diabetes mellitus, myasthenia gravis, gluten-sensitive enteropathy, dermatitis herpetiformis and childhood asthma[57]. In all these diseases a failure to suppress production of an antibody directed against either a self constituent or an extrinsic antigen could provide a rational explanation for the clinical and pathological changes.

Occurrence of multisystem involvement

Although antibody to the liver-specific lipoprotein may play a major role in the development of liver damage, there may well be other membrane antigens which are not liver-specific, and antibodies produced to these could cross-react with membrane components in other organs to produce the characteristic multisystem involvement. Direct evidence in support of this hypothesis comes from a recent study in which we showed first, sensitization to a kidney antigen, the Tamm-Horsfall glycoprotein, in patients with renal tubular acidosis associated with chronic active hepatitis, and, secondly, that antisera to this renal tubular antigen reacted with hepatocyte surface membranes in cryostat sections of normal human liver[62].

Drug-induced chronic active hepatitis

Adverse drug reactions resulting in abnormalities of hepatic structure and function are normally classified into those that are predictable and those that are idiosyncratic. Reactions in the latter category show no relationship to dose and cannot be produced in animals, and as they may be associated with skin rashes and eosinophilia in man, it is often assumed that hypersensitivity is involved. This impression is strengthened by the observation that in many cases there is a prompt relapse upon readministration of the drug. However, evidence of humoral or cell-mediated immunity to drugs in patients with 'drug hypersensitivity hepatitis' is scanty[63] and there has been little progress in our understanding of the mechanism responsible for these sometimes fatal reactions. Most present as an acute hepatitis but two drugs, oxyphenisatin and methyl dopa, have been implicated as aetiological agents in some cases of chronic active hepatitis.

Oxyphenisatin is a component of some laxative preparations and Reynolds, Peters and Yamada first described the development of chronic active hepatitis in patients who had been taking the drug for 6 months to 2 years[64]. The clinical presentation, results of laboratory tests and histological changes were identical to those seen in cases without a history of drug ingestion, but in all those who had been taking the laxative the disease regressed when oxyphenisatin was withdrawn. Rechallenge with the drug led to a prompt relapse of symptoms and biochemical evidence of further liver damage.

Although an acute hepatitis is a well recognized complication of treatment with methyl dopa[65], chronic active hepatitis is an uncommon reaction[66]. As with oxyphenisatin, the disease usually regresses when the drug is withdrawn, but in one reported case there was progression from acute to chronic liver damage after the drug had been stopped[67]. This case was also unusual in developing a positive Coombs test in the acute hepatitic phase.

Possible mechanisms

Information about autoimmune responses in drug-induced chronic active hepatitis is limited to the description of tissue antibodies and LE cells. However, the disease so closely resembles the usual pattern that it is tempting to suggest that the basic mechanisms in these cases are identical to those described earlier, the progressive liver damage being due to an autoimmune response directed at the hepatocyte surface lipoprotein. Thus, if the drug or one of its metabolites were incorporated in the liver cell membrane, the resulting change in surface structure could be similar to that induced by virus infection and might activate a T-cell response. By exerting a helper effect this would then initiate the autoimmune B-cell response which would persist as long as the drug continued to be administered. When it was withdrawn the action of suppressor T-cells would be unopposed and production of the auto-antibodies would cease. A defect in suppressor T-cell function could explain the progression to chronic liver disease after the drug had been stopped in the exceptional case of methyl dopa-induced chronic active hepatitis described earlier. The mechanism here would then be similar to that postulated in cases with acute type B hepatitis who successfully cleared the virus but went on to develop HBsAg-negative chronic active hepatitis.

Primary biliary cirrhosis

Although the frequent finding of antibodies in serum reacting with mitochondria (M-antibody) has directed attention to the possibility that autoimmune reactions may be important in pathogenesis, the aetiology of this condition remains obscure. Apart from one early report[69], there seems to be general agreement that the frequency of hepatitis B surface antigenaemia in these patients is little different from that in the normal population[70]. In our own series of 45 cases, the surface antigen was detected by radioimmunoassay in one[21], and only four of 17 patients showed cellular immunity to HBsAg (Figure 8.2). Thus it is unlikely, in these cases, that infection with the hepatitis B virus played a part in the aetiology.

Histologically, the earliest lesions consist of granulomata surrounding damaged interlobular bile ducts and it is conceivable that these are associated with an autoimmune reaction directed at bile duct epithelial cell antigens. Isolation of these antigens in order to test this hypothesis has proved difficult in man, mainly because of the technical problem of separating bile duct cells from hepatocytes. However if lining epithelial cells are normally shed into the lumen of bile ducts, then the relevant antigenic material might be obtained from bile. Indeed, in a preliminary study, we were able to show that eight of 10 patients with primary biliary cirrhosis had evidence of cellular immunity to a protein fraction from human bile. Antisera to this protein fraction raised in guinea pigs were shown by immunofluorescence to react with epithelial cells in septal and interlobular bile ducts in sections of human liver, indicating that the antigenic material in bile was derived from these cells. In a larger clinical study, 22 of 30 patients with primary biliary cirrhosis showed sensitization to the bile proteins and eight of 30 with chronic active hepatitis[71]. Negative results were obtained in all of 10 cases of extrahepatic biliary obstruction, and it is unlikely that the sensitization to bile duct epithelial cell antigens found in primary biliary cirrhosis was simply secondary to bile duct damage. However, much more evidence is needed before these reactions can be implicated in pathgensis.

ACKNOWLEDGEMENTS

I am grateful to all the research fellows who have contributed to the studies quoted and to Dr Roger Williams, the director of the Unit, for his encouragement. I am also indebted to Professor A. J. Zuckerman, Professor Deborah Doniach and Professor J. R. Batchelor for their most helpful collaboration, and to the Wellcome Trust for their continued support.

REFERENCES

1. World Health Organization Consultation on Viral Hepatitis (1970). Viral hepatitis and tests for the Australia (hepatitis-associated) antigen and antibody. *Bull. Wld. Hlth. Org.*, **42**, 957
2. Krugman, S., Giles, J. P. and Hammond, J. (1967). Infectious hepatitis—evidence for two distinctive clinical, epidemiological and immunological types of infection. *J. Amer. Med. Ass.*, **200**, 365
3. Mosley, J. W. (1965). The surveillance of transfusion-associated viral hepatitis. *J. Amer. Med. Ass.*, **193**, 1007
4. Blumberg, B. S. (1964). Polymorphisms of the serum proteins and the development of isoprecipitins in transfused patients. *Bull. N.Y. Acad. Med.*, **40**, 377
5. Blumberg, B. S., Gerstley, B. J. S., Hungerford, D. A., London, W. T. and Sutnick, A. I. (1967). A serum antigen (Australia antigen) in Down's syndrome, leukemia and hepatitis. *Ann. Intern. Med.*, **66**, 924
6. World Health Organization (1973). Viral hepatitis. *Report of a WHO Scientific Group. Tech. Rep. Ser. Wld. Hlth. Org. No. 512*
7. Almeida, J. D., Rubinstein, D. and Stott, E. J. (1971). New antigen–antibody system in Australia antigen-positive hepatitis. *Lancet*, **ii**, 1225
8. Feinstone, S. M., Kapikian, A. Z. and Purcell, R. H. (1973). Hepatitis A: detection by immune electron microscopy of a virus-like antigen associated with acute illness. *Science*, **182**, 1026
9. Almeida, J. D., Gay, F. W. and Wreghitt, T. G. (1974). Pitfalls in the study of hepatitis A. *Lancet*, **ii**, 738
10. Dienstag, J. L., Feinstone, S. M., Kapikian, A. Z. and Purcell, R. H. (1975). Immune electron microscopy and hepatitis A. *Lancet*, **i**, 102
11. Del Prete, S., Costantino, D., Doglia, M., Graziina, A., Ajdukiewicz, A., Dudley, F. J., Fox, R. A. and Sherlock, S. (1970). Detection of a new serum antigen in three epidemics of short incubation hepatitis. *Lancet*, **ii**, 579
12. Taylor, P. E., Almeida, J. D., Zuckerman, A. J. and Leach, J. M. (1972). Relationship of Milan antigen to abnormal serum lipoprotein. *Amer. J. Dis. Child*, **123**, 329
13. Nielsen, J. O., Dietrichson, O., Elling, P. and Christoffersen, P. (1971). Incidence and meaning of persistence of Australia antigen in patients with acute viral hepatitis: development of chronic hepatitis. *New Eng. J. Med.*, **285**, 1157
14. Gallagher, N. D. and Goulston, S. J. M. (1962). Persistent acute viral hepatitis. *Brit. Med. J.*, **i**, 906
15. Sidi, S., Michel, H. and Redeker, A. (1972). Unresolved (persistent) viral hepatitis. *Abstract 7th Meet. EASL, Arnhem*
16. Cooksley, W. G. E., Powell, L. W., Mistilis, S. P., Olsen, G., Mathews, J. D. and Mackay, I. R. (1972). Australia antigen in active chronic hepatitis in Australia: results in 130 patients from three centres. *Austr. N.Z. J. Med.*, **2**, 261

17. Bianchi, P., Bianchi Porro, C., Coltorti, M., Dardanoni, L., Del Vecchio Blanco, C., Fagiolo, U., Farini, R., Menozzi, L., Naccarato, R., Pagliaro, R., Spano, C. and Verme, G. (1972). Occurrence of Australia antigen in chronic hepatitis in Italy. *Gastroenterology*, **63**, 482
18. Gitnick, G. L., Gleich, G. J., Schoenfield, L. J., Baggenstoss, A. H., Sutnick, A. I., Blumberg, B. S., London, W. T. and Summerskill, W. H. J. (1969). Australia antigen in chronic active liver disease and cirrhosis. *Lancet*, **ii**, 285
19. Wright, R., McCollum, R. W. and Klatskin, G. (1969). Australia antigen in acute and chronic liver disease. *Lancet*, **ii**, 117
20. Sherlock, S., Fox, R. A., Niazi, S. P. and Scheuer, P. J. (1970). Chronic liver disease and primary liver-cell cancer with hepatitis-associated (Australia) antigen in serum. *Lancet*, **i**, 1243
21. Reed, W. D., Eddleston, A. L. W. F., Stern, R. B., Williams, R., Zuckerman, A. J., Bowes, A. and Earl, P. M. (1973). Detection of hepatitis-B antigen by radioimmunoassay in chronic liver disease and hepatocellular carcinoma in Great Britain. *Lancet*, **ii**, 690
22. Bulkley, B. H., Goldfinger, S. E., Heizer, W. D., Isselbacher, K. J. and Shulman, N. R. (1970). Distinctions in chronic active hepatitis based on circulating hepatitis-associated antigen. *Lancet*, **ii**, 1323
23. Lee, W. M., Reed, W. D., Mitchell, C. G., Galbraith, R. M., Eddleston, A. L. F. W., Zuckerman, A. J. and Williams, R. (1975). Cellular and humoral immunity to the heptitis-B surface antigen in active chronic hepatitis. *Brit. Med. J.*, **1**, 705
24. Reinicke, V., Dybkjaer, E., Poulsen, H., Banke, O., Lylloff, K. and Nordenfeld, E. (1972). A study of Australia-antigen-positive blood donors and their recipients, with special reference to liver histology. *New Eng. J. Med.*, **286**, 867
25. Woolf, I. L., Boyes, B. E., Jones, D. M., Whittaker, J. S., Tapp, E., MacSween, R. N. M., Renton, P. H., Stratton, F. and Dymock, I. W. (1974). Asymptomatic liver disease in hepatitis-B antigen carriers. *J. Clin. Path.*, **27**, 348
26. Hadziyannis, S., Vissoulis, C., Moussouros, A. and Afroudakis, A. (1972). Cytoplasmic localisation of Australia antigen in the liver. *Lancet*, **i**, 976
27. Gerstley, B. J. S., Custer, R. P., Blumberg, B. S., London, W. T., Sutnick, A. I. and Coyne, V. Z. (1972). Liver biopsies in patients with and without Australia antigen. *Arch. Path.*, **93**, 366
28. Grange, M. J., Erlinger, S., Teillet, F., Schlegal, N., Barge, J. and Degott, C. (1973). A possible relationship to treatment between hepatitis-associated antigen and chronic persistent hepatitis in Hodgkin's disease. *Gut*, **14**, 433
29. Le Bouvier, G. L. (1971). The heterogeneity of Australia antigen. *J. Infect. Dis.*, **123**, 671
30. Holland, P. V., Purcell, R. H., Smith, H. and Alter, H. J. (1972). Subtyping of hepatitis-associated antigen (HB Ag); simplified technique with counterelectrophoresis. *J. Immunol.*, **109**, 420

31. Iwarson, S., Magnius, L., Lindholm, A. and Lundin, P. (1973). Subtypes of hepatitis B antigen in blood donors and post-transfusion hepatitis: clinical and epidemiological aspects. *Brit. Med. J.*, **i**, 84
32. Kim, C. Y. and Tilles, J. G. (1971). Immunologic and electrophoretic heterogeneity of hepatitis-associated antigen. *J. Infect. Dis.*, **123**, 618
33. Van Kooten Kok-Doorschodt, H. J., Van den Akker, R. and Gispen, R. (1972). Determination and distribution of two types of hepatitis-associated antigen. *J. Infect. Dis.*, **126**, 117
34. Magnius, L. O., Berg. R., Fjorvatn, B., Espmark, J. A. and Svedmyr, A. (1972). Evidence for a change in the dominant subtypes of HBAg associated with clinical hepatitis. (In preparation, 1972; cited in Iwarson *et al.*[31])
35. Magnius, L. O., and Espmark, J. A. (1972). New specificities in Australia antigen positive sera distinct from the Le Bouvier determinants. *J. Immunol.*, **109**, 1017
36. Nielsen, J. O., Dietrichson, O. and Juhl, E. (1974). Incidence and meaning of the 'e' determinant among hepatitis-B antigen positive patients with acute and chronic liver diseases. *Lancet*, **ii**, 913
37. Magnius, L. O., (1975). Characterisation of a new antigen–antibody system associated with hepatitis B. *Clin. Exp. Immunol.*, **20**, 209
38. Hotchin, J. (1971). Virus, cell surface, and self: Lymphocytic choriomeningitis of mice. *Am. J. Clin. Path.*, **56**, 333
39. Nielsen, J. O., Reinecke, V., Dietrichson, O., Andersen, V., Thomsen, M. and Andersen, E. (1973). Immunological studies of Australia antigen carriers with and without liver diseases. *Clin. Exp. Immunol.*, **15**, 9
40. Yeung Laiwah, A. A. C. (1971). Lymphocyte transformation by Australia antigen. *Lancet*, **ii**, 470
41. Dudley, F. J., Giustino, V. and Sherlock, S. (1972). Cell-mediated immunity in patients positive for hepatitis-associated antigen. *Brit. Med. J.*, **iv**, 754
42. Lee, W. M., Reed, W. D., Mitchell, C. G., Woolf, I. L., Dymock, I. W., Eddleston, A. L. W. F., and Williams, R. (1975). Cell-mediated immunity to hepatitis B surface antigen in blood donors with persistent antigenaemia. *Gut*, **16**, 416
43. Walsh, J. H., Yalow, R. S. and Berson, S. A. (1970). Radioimmunoassay of Australia antigen. *Vox Sang.*, **19**, 217
44. Reed, W. D., Mitchell, C. G., Eddleston, A. L. W. F., Lee, W. M., Williams, R. and Zuckerman, A. J. (1974). Exposure and immunity to hepatitis-B virus in a liver unit. *Lancet*, **i**, 581
45. Mitchell, C. G., Smith, M. G. M., Golding, P. L., Eddleston, A. L. W. F. and Williams, R. (1972). Evaluation of the leucocyte migration test as a measure of delayed hypersensitivity in man. *Clin. Exp. Immunol.*, **11**, 535
46. Kempe, C. H. (1960). Studies on smallpox and complications of smallpox vaccination. *Pediatrics*, **26**, 176
47. Galbraith, R. M., Smith, M., Mackenzie, R. M., Tee, D. E., Doniach, D.

and Williams, R. (1974). High prevalance of seroimmunologic abnormalities in relatives of patients with active chronic hepatitis or primary biliary cirrhosis. *New Eng. J. Med.*, **290**, 63

48. Dawkins, R. L. and Joske, R. A. (1973). Immunoglobulin deposition in liver of patients with active chronic hepatitis and antibody against smooth muscle. *Brit. Med. J.*, **2**, 643
49. Smith, M. G. M., Golding, P. L., Eddleston, A. L. W. F., Mitchell, C. G., Kemp, A. and Williams, R. (1972). Cell-mediated immune responses in chronic liver diseases. *Brit. Med. J.*, **i**, 527
50. Hopf, U., Meyer zum Buschenfelde, K. H. and Freudenberg, J. (1974). Liver-specific antigen of different species. *Clin. Exp. Immunol.*, **16**, 117
51. Meyer zum Buschenfelde, K. H., Kossling, F. K. and Miescher, P. A. (1972). Experimental chronic active hepatitis in rabbits following immunization with human liver proteins. *Clin. Exp. Immunol.*, **11**, 99
52. Hopf, U. and Meyer zum Buschenfelde, K. H. (1974). Studies on the pathogenesis of the experimental active chronic hepatitis (ACH) in rabbits. *Digestion*, **10**, 306
53. Thomson, A. D., Cochrane, M. A. G., McFarlane, I. G., Eddleston, A. L. W. F. and Williams, R. (1974). Lymphocyte cytotoxicity to isolated hepatocytes in chronic active hepatitis. *Nature* (*Lond.*), **252**, 721
54. Eddleston, A. L. W. F., and Williams, R. (1974). Inadequate antibody response to HBAg or suppressor T-cell defect in development of active chronic hepatitis. *Lancet*, **ii**, 1543
55. Allison, A. C., Denman, A. M. and Barnes, R. D. (1971). Co-operating and controlling functions of thymus-derived lymphocytes in relation to autoimmunity. *Lancet*, **ii**, 135
56. MacLennan, I. C. M., Loewi, G. and Howard, A. (1969). A human serum immunoglobulin with specificity for certain homologous target cells, which induces target cell damage by normal human lymphocytes. *Immunology*, **17**, 897
57. McDevitt, H. O. and Bodmer, W. F. (1974). HL-A, immune-response genes, and disease. *Lancet*, **i**, 1269
58. Stiffel, C., Mouton, D., Bouthillier, Y., Henmann, A. M., Decreusefond, C., Mevel, J. C. and Biozzi, G. (1974). Polygenic regulation of general antibody synthesis in the mouse. In *Progress in Immunology*, *II*, Vol 2. L. Brent and E. J. Holborow (eds). p. 203. (Amsterdam: North Holland)
59. Galbraith, R. M., Eddleston, A. L. W. F., Smith, M. G. M., Williams, R., MacSween, R. N. M., Watkinson, G., Dick, Heather, Kennedy, L. A. and Batchelor, J. R. (1974). Histocompatibility antigens in active chronic hepatitis and primary biliary cirrhosis. *Brit. Med. J.*, **3**, 604
60. Triger, D. R., Kurtz, J. B., MacCallum, F. O., Wright, R. (1972). Raised antibody titres to measles and rubella viruses in chronic active hepatitis. *Lancet*, **i**, 665
61. Da Costa, J. A. G., White, A. G., Parker, A. C. and Grigor, G. B. (1974). Increased incidence of HL-A 1 and 8 in patients showing IgG or complement coating on their red cells. *J. Clin. Path.*, **27**, 353

62. Tsantoulas, D. C., McFarlane, I. G., Portmann, B., Eddleston, A. L. W. F. and Williams, R. (1974). Cell-mediated immunity to human Tamm–Horsfall glycoprotein in autoimmune liver disease with renal tubular acidosis. *Brit. Med. J.*, **4**, 491
63. Davis, M. and Williams, R. (1976). Drugs and the liver. In *Textbook of adverse drug reactions*, D. M. Davies (ed.). In press
64. Reynolds, T. B., Peters, R. L. and Yamada, S. (1971). Chronic active and lupoid hepatitis caused by a laxative, oxyphenisatin. *New Eng. J. Med.*, **285**, 813
65. Elkington, S. G., Schreiber, W. M. and Conn, H. O. (1969). Hepatic injury caused by L-alpha-methyldopa. *Circulation*, **40**, 589
66. Goldstein, G. B., Lam, K. C. and Mistilis, S. P. (1973). Drug-induced active chronic hepatitis. *Am. J. Dig. Dis.*, **18**, 177
67. Schweitzer, I. L. and Peters, R. L. (1974). Acute submassive hepatic necrosis due to methyldopa. A case demonstrating possible initiation of of chronic liver disease. *Gastroenterology*, **66**, 1203
68. Shikata, T., Uzawa, T., Yoshiwara, N., Akatsuka, T. and Yamazaki, S. (1974). Staining methods of Australia antigen in paraffin section–detection of cytoplasmic inclusion bodies. *Jap. J. Exp. Med.*, **44**, 25
69. Krohn, K., Finlayson, N. D. C., Jokelainen, P. T., Anderson, K. E. and Prince, A. M. (1970). Electron microscopical and immunological observations on the serum-hepatitis (SH) antigen in primary biliary cirrhosis. *Lancet*, **ii**, 379
70. Maddrey, W. C., Saito, S., Shulman, N. R. and Klatskin, G. (1972). Coincidental Australia antigenaemia in primary biliary cirrhosis. *Ann. Intern. Med.*, **76**, 705
71. Tsantoulas, D. C., McFarlane, I. G., Portmann, B., Eddleston, A. L. W. F. and Williams, R. (1974). Sensitisation to human bile proteins in primary biliary cirrhosis and active chronic hepatitis: demonstration of antigenic material in bile duct epithelial cells. *Digestion*, **10**, 305.

CHAPTER 9

Immune mechanisms in liver disease

FIORENZO PARONETTO

Many of the facts and ideas presented here will prove in the near future to be partially or entirely wrong. However (this review) will have served its purpose if one of its readers is interested enough to design and perform the experiments needed to show what is wrong and what is right.

JEAN BRACHET*

* Biochemical Cytology, Academic Press (1957).

Introduction

An increasing amount of evidence points to the importance of immunological mechanisms in the pathogenesis of certain liver diseases. The exact mechanism has not been pinpointed, in spite of the consensus of opinion favouring the importance of cell-mediated immunity (CMI). Such a large quantity of data in this field is being made known in such a short period of time that it remains fragmented and difficult to organize into a meaningful hypothesis. Although any hypothesis is subject to modification, with acquisition of new facts, it is imperative at this time to present an up-to-date summary and evaluation of the basic data that are available concerning the importance of each of the various mechanisms of immunologic reactions. Five major types of allergic reactions capable of producing tissue damage have been identified[1,2]. Evidence will be presented showing the participation of each of these immunological reactions in liver disease.

Type I reaction—Anaphylactic or immediate hypersensitivity

Type I reaction is characterized by the liberation of pharmacologically active mediators (e.g. histamine, serotonin, slow reactive substance of anaphylaxis) following the reaction of antigen with antibody-sensitized cells. Whether this immunological mechanism in liver disease is significant has not been thoroughly investigated. This is unfortunate because it has been ascertained that certain cases of drug hepatitis (e.g. those following administration of chlorpromazine or halothane) are characterized by blood and tissue eosinophilia. Additionally, the polyclonal hypergammaglobulinaemia so frequently observed in chronic liver diseases may be associated with an increase of IgE and a recent report seems to suggest an increase of IgE in chronic liver disease[3].

Type II reaction—Cytotoxic

Type II reaction is characterized by the reaction of antibodies with tissue cells in which the antigenic determinants are either unmodified or are modified by antigens or haptens. A variety of antibodies directed against tissue antigens have been described in patients with acute viral hepatitis or chronic hepatitis. These antibodies, however, are for the most part not liver-specific. They include smooth muscle antibodies; anti-mitochondrial or M-antibodies and antinuclear antibodies; antibodies to renal glomeruli and ductular cells; and antibodies to bile canaliculi[5], microsomes[6] and lymphocytes[7,8]. It has been suggested that these antibodies may damage liver cells by reacting or cross-reacting with liver antigens and may fix complement. There is, however, no evidence that these antibodies are capable of producing liver damage, since their presence does not correlate with the severity of the disease[9], and complement has not been convincingly demonstrated at the site of damage[4]. Furthermore, they do not possess cytotoxic activity against tissue cultures of liver cells[10]. Thus, the appearance and significance of these antibodies in certain patients with liver disease has been difficult to explain. Hypothetically, one may suggest that an alteration of T-lymphocytes, possibly suppressor T-lymphocytes or helper T-cells, may render B-lymphocytes capable of responding to a variety of auto-antigens[11]. These autoantibodies, however, may form circulating immune complexes that may be deposited in the kidneys. Thus, antinuclear antibodies have been detected in the kidneys of patients with chronic active hepatitis[12].

Type III reaction—Immune complex

Type III reaction is characterized by the deposition or formation of toxic antigen–antibody complexes. The hypergammaglobulinaemia frequently observed in patients with liver diseases is associated with a variety of antibodies against exogenous antigens such as bacterial intestinal antigens[13,14] or viral antigens (measles, rubella, and cytomegalovirus)[15,16]. Antibodies to hepatitis B core antigen (HB_cAg)[17] but not to hepatitis B surface antigen (HB_sAg)[18] have also been frequently described in patients with chronic hepatitis. It has been suggested that these antibodies may combine with the corresponding antigen localized in the liver and form cytotoxic immune complexes. Experiments have shown that the injection or formation of immune complexes in the liver may produce acute and chronic damage to that organ. An injection of preformed immune complexes produces large areas of hepatocellular necrosis[19]. In lymphocytic choriomeningitis, areas of hepatic necrosis are associated with the formation of immune complexes[20], and the repeated injection of various foreign sera induces a cirrhosis with localization of the antigen injected, of the corresponding antibody, and fixation of complement[19]. Also, in hepatic schistosomiasis, immune complexes may be formed around schistosoma ova[19].

The importance of immune complexes in the pathogenesis of liver diseases is not as clear in man. Serum complement levels decrease in various liver diseases[21]. Evaluation of these findings is complicated because the liver produces certain complement components, and a decrease of complement may reflect an altered liver synthetic activity. Low levels of complement (C_3 and C_4) correlate with low albumin levels, while Clq levels (a complement moiety not originating from the liver) are not altered in chronic liver damage[21]. More recent investigations using intravenous administration of radioiodinated C3 seem to suggest that the complement system might be activated in primary biliary cirrhosis[22].

Circulating immune complexes are detected in the serum by a variety of techniques, including the agar gel Clq precipitation test, radiolabelled Clq binding assay, or electron microscopy. With the first technique, immune complexes were rarely found in sera of patients with acute or chronic hepatitis[23], while the more sensitive radioimmunoassay has indicated the presence of immune complexes in patients with chronic hepatitis and HB_sAg[24]. Furthermore, immune complexes composed of HB_sAg and anti-HB_sAg (HB_sAb) have been detected in patients with HB-antigenaemia by electron microscopy, passive haemagglutination, and radioimmunoassay[25,26]. However, no correlation has been detected between serum immune complexes and severity of liver diseases[25,26]. Thus, immune complexes may be unrelated to liver damage. Rather, immune complexes may be responsible for the systemic manifestations observed in patients with liver diseases (e.g. rashes, arthritis, glomerulonephritis, angiitis). HB_sAg, IgG and complement (C_3) have been demonstrated in blood vessels[27,28] and renal glomeruli[28,29] of patients with HB_s-antigenaemia.

Although in the case of patients with renal disease immune complexes have been frequently observed in the kidney, it is difficult to detect complexes in the liver of patients with liver diseases. Since the mononuclear phagocytic system (MPS) of the liver is capable of removing and degrading large amounts of immune complexes, only a markedly decreased function of the phagocytic system of the liver may allow deposition of immune complexes in the liver parenchyma[30]. Decreased phagocytic activity of the hepatic MPS has been demonstrated in cirrhosis in man[31].

It is also possible that the MPS may be depressed in chronic hepatitis and impaired phagocytosis has been considered by some investigators to contribute to the development of cirrhosis[32] (see Chapter 7). Circulating antibody undisturbed by phagocytic cells may, however, reach the corresponding antigen and these result in the local formation of immune complexes. This would therefore occur independently of and without interference by the MPS.

The formation of toxic immune complexes in the liver has not been convincingly demonstrated. HBcAg can be demonstrated by electron microscopy, immunoelectron microscopy, and immunofluorescence in the nuclei of some patients with chronic hepatitis or in HB_sAg carriers receiving immunosuppressive therapy or undergoing haemodialysis treatment[33]. In these patients Ig can also be demonstrated in the nuclei. Since this Ig can be eluted at acid pH, it may be an antibody bound to an antigen[34]. Complement (C_3) was not demonstrated, or only rarely[28,34,35], suggesting either the formation of a noncomplement-fixing immune complex or that complement is unable to reach this antigen-antibody complex. Clq without Ig was demonstrated mainly in the nucleoli and considered an *in vitro* binding of Clq to nucleic acids[35]. Antibodies to hepatitis B virus may represent a protective mechanism interfering with the replication of the virus rather than participating in the formation of cytotoxic immune complexes. In chronic hepatitis HB_sAg has been demonstrated in the cytoplasm of hepatocytes[36], but complement and Ig were either not localized in these locations or were noted only rarely. The difficulty in demonstrating antigen-antibody/complement complexes consistently in areas of HB_sAg localization may reflect either failure to form complexes, the presence of noncomplement-fixing complexes, or a rapid catabolism of complement. Indeed, in the experimental Arthus reaction, complement disappears rapidly from the lesions[37].

In chronic hepatitis not associated with HB_sAg in the serum, Ig and complement were not localized in the liver. The only exception was the localization of IgG and complement in the early stages of primary biliary cirrhosis[19]. However, if immune complexes are involved in the early stage of the disease, progression over a period of many years to cirrhosis cannot be explained solely by the formation of immune complexes. In the latter stages of primary biliary cirrhosis there is no evidence of formation of immune complexes in the liver.

The formation or localization of immune complexes does not necessarily induce tissue damage *per se*. The hallmark of tissue damage by immune complexes is the accumulation of neutrophil polymorphs. The latter are rarely seen in acute or chronic liver damage. Thus, histological observations militate against an impotant role for immune complexes in acute or chronic liver damage. However, as in some forms of renal diseases, the formation of tissue damage induced by immune complexes may be independent of neutrophil accumulation[38]

It is difficult to discount the marked quantitative alteration of B-lymphocytes in liver diseases. In a variety of liver diseases both the absolute number and the percentage of B-cells is increased; thus, in acute viral hepatitis an increase of B cells is described, mainly of the lymphocytes bearing surface IgM, although in patients with fatty liver, alcoholic hepatitis and cirrhosis, B-lymphocytes are not altered numerically[8]; in chronic hepatitis B-lymphocytes are increased, especially those bearing surface IgA and IgM[8]; in primary biliary cirrhosis a striking increase of both the absolute numbers and the percentage of circulating B-lymphocytes bearing surface IgA, IgM and IgG has been reported[39]. In addition, null cells (cells without surface Ig, not identified by T-cell markers and most likely related to B-lymphocytes)[40] are increased in both chronic hepatitis and acute viral hepatitis[8]. The pathogenetic significance of these profound alterations is unclear at present. It is difficult to explain them as an inconsequential manifestation of an altered T-cell system. Recent evidence indicates that activated B-cells may act as suppressors of T-cell function[41].

Type IV reaction—Cell-mediated immunity or delayed hypersensitivity

Type IV reaction is mediated by mononuclear cells. Much has been said, written and hypothesized about the role of CMI in liver disease. The use of methods whose significance is still unclear may contribute to a cloudy assessment or, at times, even misinformation. The frequently claimed alteration of T-cells in liver disease has been derived by the study of parameters improperly considered as specific functions of T-cells e.g. phytohaemagglutinin (PHA) stimulation and leucocyte migration inhibition tests. The data gathered to date using various parameters thought to be correlates of T-lymphocyte function will be described.

Table 9.1 MODIFICATION OF CORRELATES OF CMI IN LIVER DISEASES

	Acute viral hepatitis	*Resolving acute viral hepatitis*	*Chronic active hepatitis*	*Primary biliary cirrhosis*
T-cells, absolute number	↓ (8)	N (8)	↓ (8, 43)	N (39)*
B-cells, absolute number	↑ (8)		↑ (8)	↑ (39)
LT by PHA	↓ (99, 100, 104)	N (54)	V (43, 47, 48, 50, 53, 54)	↓ (46, 50, 51)
LT by HB_sAg	V (47, 54)	+ (54, 62–64)	O or + (occasionally) (47,54)	
MIF or LIF test by HB_sAg	+ (54, 78–84)	O (78–82)	O or + (54, 78, 79, 84)	
LIF test by liver Ag	O or +(rarely) (70, 72, 73, 83, 84)		+ (67, 69–72, 84)	+ (67–70)
Lymphocytotoxicity to liver cells	+ (87)	O (87)	+ (87, 89–91)	+ (87,91)

Numbers in parentheses refer to reference numbers.
V = controversial
↑ = increased incidence
↓ = decreased incidence
N = normal reactivity
O = no reactivity
+ = test positive
* = increase in active rosette-forming cells
LT = lymphocyte transformation test
MIF = macrophage migration inhibition test
LIF = leukocyte migration inhibition test

T-lymphocytes

Available information indicates that the absolute numbers of T-lymphocytes decrease in both HB_sAg-positive and HB_sAg-negative acute viral hepatitis[8] as in other viral diseases[42]. The lymphocytes return to normal values when the hepatitis resolves. In chronic carriers of HB_sAg without liver damage, the number of T-lymphocytes is not different from controls; but in chronic hepatitis T-lymphocytes show a statistically significant decrease[8,43] that is independent of the presence in the serum of HB_sAg or antibodies. A depression of T-lymphocytes has also been reported in alcoholic hepatitis even in the absence of cirrhosis[44]. In primary biliary cirrhosis, however, the total number of T-lymphocytes is not altered[39], suggesting that a decrease of T-lymphocytes is not *per se* an epiphenomenon in chronic liver damage. These findings will be better interpreted when the actual distribution of T- and B-lymphocytes in the liver becomes known.

Skin testing

A decrease of reactivity to ubiquitous antigens or to specific sensitization with dinitrochlorobenzene has been reported in patients with alcoholic liver disease[45] and in patients with primary biliary cirrhosis[45] and chronic active hepatitis[47,48]. No alteration in reactivity was observed in patients with acute viral hepatitis[47].

Lymphocyte stimulation by mitogens

A markedly increased spontaneous activation of lymphocytes has been observed in patients with acute viral hepatitis and chronic active hepatitis[47,49]. When lymphocytes are stimulated by mitogens the results have been contradictory, probably because of a lack of evaluation of the dose- and time-response curves. Thus, depression of lymphocyte response to mitogens may revert to stimulation when a dose response to mitogen is performed. Although a depression of lymphocyte stimulation by PHA has been reported in primary biliary cirrhosis and acute viral hepatitis[46,50,51,100,101,104] no alterations were observed in chronic HB_sAg carriers without liver diseases[52,53]. In chronic hepatitis the results are controversial: stimulation[43,47], decrease[48,50], and no alteration[53,54] have all been reported.

An altered reactivity to PHA has been considered an alteration of T-lymphocytes. More recent investigations using highly purified human preparations of T- and B-lymphocytes indicate that both B- and T-lymphocytes are capable of reacting to PHA and other mitogens[55]. Therefore, an altered reactivity to PHA cannot at the present state of our knowledge be considered exclusively a reflection of an alteration of T-lymphocytes.

Lymphocyte stimulation by antigens

Stimulation of lymphocytes by liver extracts has been observed only in some patients with chronic hepatitis. The difficulty in obtaining uniform results may be related to the production of a disturbingly high background level by spontaneous stimulation of lymphocytes and to the presence in liver extracts of an inhibitor of lymphocyte stimulation[56]. In alcoholic hepatitis lymphocytes have been stimulated by alcoholic hyalin[57], and in some cases of drug hepatitis lymphocytes may be stimulated by the drug involved (antibiotics, anti-inflammatory drugs, hypoglycaemic agents, anaesthetics)[58–61]. HB_sAg stimulates lymphocytes of patients recovering from HB_sAg-positive acute viral hepatitis[54,62–64]. Lymphocyte reactivity seems to exhibit subtype specificity[65]. These data suggest that CMI is necessary to clear hepatitis B virus. Little is known, however, of the activity of lymphocytes in the presence of HB_cAg, which may be the virus itself. Furthermore, the test of lymphocyte transformation is not necessarily a correlate of T-lymphocyte activity, since both T- and B-lymphocytes may be specifically stimulated by antigens[66].

Inhibition of leucocyte migration by antigen

This test has also been considered a correlate of T-cell function, and has been utilized in the study of reactivity to liver antigen and HB_sAg. Inhibition of migration in the presence of liver extract or liver-specific proteins has been described in patients with chronic active hepatitis, primary biliary cirrhosis and in alcoholic patients[67,73]. Other substances that inhibit migration of leukocytes are mitochondrial[74] and biliary proteins[68] in patients with primary biliary cirrhosis, and alcoholic haylin in patients with alcoholic hepatitis[75]. The specificity of these reactions has not yet been completely ascertained. Extracts of kidney[70] and parotid gland[67] have been used as controls by some investigators, and a positive reactivity has been considered a reflection of renal tubular acidosis and the sicca complex. These are considered a frequent complication of chronic liver diseases (see Chapter 8). On the other hand, the reactivity to mitochondria in patients with primary biliary cirrhosis is not typical of the disease, since it was also observed in patients with thyroiditis and diabetes[76,77].

Somewhat controversial results have been obtained using HB_sAg in patients with liver disease. Patients with acute viral hepatitis show inhibition of migration,[54,78–84] which disappears when the patient recovers[78–82], a finding, however, not confirmed by some investigators[63,85]. In both HB_sAg-positive and HB_sAg-negative chronic active hepatitis the HB_sAg failed to inhibit migration of leukocytes in all or some patients[54,78,79,84]. The variability of these results may reflect either technical difficulties or the use of unpurified or partially purified antigens. To date, the reactivity of HB_cAg has not been investigated.

From a pathogenetic point of view, these data are difficult to interpret because increased reactivity may reflect either a beneficial attempt to liberate the liver of a noxious agent or an autoaggressive damaging activity. Conversely, a lack of reactivity may be harmful if it reflects tolerance to an injurious agent. Since the hepatitis B virus has two different antigenic systems represented by HB_sAg and HB_cAg, one may also envisage a different, perhaps even a contrasting, reactivity to the two antigenic systems. More recent studies indicate that the phenomenon of inhibition of migration in the presence of antigens is not exclusive to T-lymphocytes, since both T- and B-lymphocytes are capable of producing inhibitory factors when stimulated by antigens[86].

Cytotoxicity of lymphocytes

Since the previous method may reflect a non-harmful sensitization, it has been considered important to ascertain whether lymphocytes are endowed with cytotoxic activity against the patient's liver cells. The purified lymphocytes of patients with chronic active hepatitis and acute viral hepatitis, but not those of control patients, are cytotoxic against the patient's liver cells grown in tissue culture[87] (Figure 9.1). More recently, cytotoxicity of lymphocytes was detected against a variety of heterologous liver cells, both normal and abnormal, but not against human fibroblasts. This suggests a specific reactivity against normal liver antigens[88]. Patients with chronic hepatitis display the most dramatic activity, but the reactivity is not seen in some patients treated with immunosuppressive agents. The cytotoxic activity seems to be decreased by blocking factors present in the serum of patients. Cytotoxicity of lymphocytes can be detected in patients with chronic hepatitis using both isolated autologous liver cells[89,90] and xenogeneic hepatocytes (rabbit)[91]. Cytotoxic activity of lymphocytes is blocked by incubation of lymphocytes with liver-specific proteins (lipoprotein)[91]. The type of

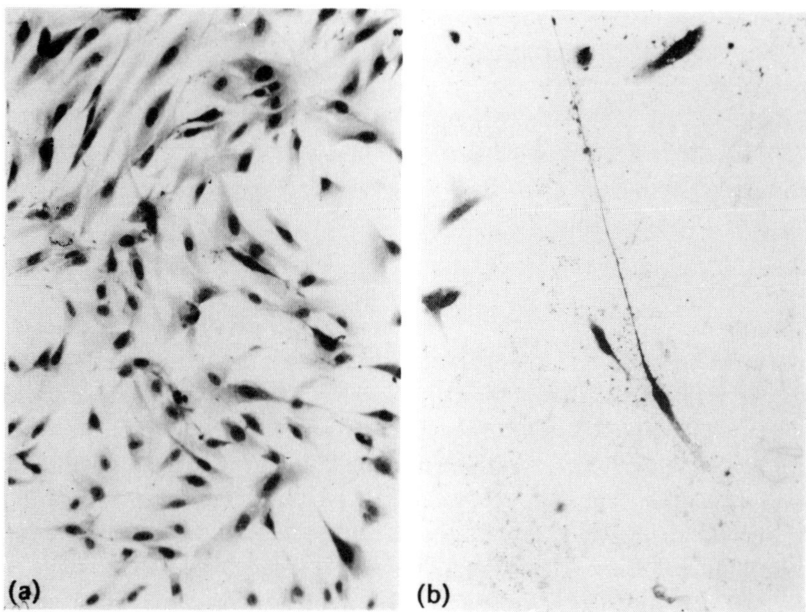

FIGURE 9.1 Liver cells from a patient (V.E.) with chronic active hepatitis: (a) treated with culture medium only, (b) treated for 3 days with patient's lymphocytes. Note the cellular debris and the few surviving hepatocytes that are shrunken or markedly altered

lymphocytes involved in the cytotoxic reaction is not known at present.

These investigations of *in vitro* cytotoxic activity of lymphocytes suggest an *in vivo* activity directed against antigens normally present in the liver and not formed *de novo* by viral or other toxic agents, although these agents seem to be necessary in the triggering of the sensitization.

Type V reaction—Antibody dependent cytotoxicity of lymphocytes

Type V immunologic reaction is the antibody dependent cytotoxicity of lymphocytes. It has been proven that certain antibodies bound to target cells induce an immunologically specific cytotoxicity in normal unsensitized lymphocytes or may potentiate the cytotoxicity of immune lymphocytes[2]. This phenomenon may play a role in certain human diseases (e.g. thyroiditis)[92] and in the reactivity to certain tumours (bladder and choriocarcinoma)[93,94]. While this pathogenetic mechanism is suggested in the liver lesions observed in rabbits immunized with liver antigens[95], various experiments performed *in vitro* indicate that antibodies (smooth muscle antibodies, M-antibodies and HB_sAb) do not render normal or patients' lymphocytes cytotoxic against autochthonous or heterologous liver cells[96].

Blocking factors

Serum from patients with liver diseases (primary biliary cirrhosis, alcoholic hepatitis and cirrhosis)[97–105] may contain factors which block the stimulation of lymphocytes. Blocking factors for the cytotoxic activity of lymphocytes have also been observed in some patients with chronic hepatitis[87,89,90,106]. More recently, it has been demonstrated that liver cells may contain a high-molecular-weight protein capable of inhibiting both the transformation of lymphocytes and the production of migration inhibitory factors[56]. Thus, it is conceivable that either a specific liver protein liberated in the serum by liver damage, or antibodies, or immune complexes, or some other factors may interfere with the sensitization and cytotoxic activity of lymphocytes.

Genetic factors

The recent developments in immunogenetics suggest a link between antigenic response and certain HL-A antigens. This avenue of investigation has now been actively pursued in patients with liver disease, especially those with HB_sAg. It is not known whether HL-A antigens share antigenic determinants with hepatitis B virus or represent receptors capable of binding hepatitis B virus, or are linked to immune response genes. The latter may control the host response to the virus.

HB_sAg-negative chronic active hepatitis patients in Australia, in the United States, and in England have a statistically significant increase of the phenotype HL-A I-8[107–109]. In contrast preliminary observations indicate that patients with HB_sAg-positive chronic active hepatitis lack the antigen HL-A8[110], and children with HB_sAg chronic hepatitis frequently exhibit the W5 antigen in locus 4[110]. Patients with chronic persistent hepatitis but not those with chronic active hepatitis had an increase of W18[7].

A genetic background has not so far been detected in patients with primary biliary cirrhosis. The distribution of HL-A antigens in primary biliary cirrhosis is not different from that found in control groups[109].

Clearly further investigation is needed to establish firmly the genetic background of patients with chronic hepatitis.

Immunological mechanisms in acute hepatitis (viral and drug-induced)

In acute viral hepatitis induced by hepatitis B virus the available evidence indicates that liver damage is mediated not by a direct tissue damaging activity of the virus but by an immunological reaction against the virus. The humoral response against both HB_sAg and HB_cAg appears early in the disease but it seems to be preceded by a cellular response to HB_sAg[81]. Most investigators have reported a positive assay for macrophage migration inhibition factor (MIF) or leucocyte migration inhibition factor (LIF). The number of T-lymphocytes is decreased; sensitization to liver antigens also seems to occur but is ephemeral. The most likely hypothesis is that hepatitis B virus induces synthesis of viral antigens on the surface of some liver cells. This is supported by the fact that the HB_sAg appears to occur on the surface of hepatocytes in the preicteric state[111]. B-cells or T-cells become sensitized to viral antigens and produce cytolysis of liver cells containing the antigens. Destruction of virus-containing cells is focal and quick, and the patient recovers. At this stage, HB_sAg or HB_cAg is no longer detected in the liver[36] because the affected cells are destroyed by lymphocytes cytotoxic for liver cells. The presence of leucocyte migration inhibition factor seems to correlate with the ability of the patient to clear the virus. Antibodies are formed and they may be involved in blocking replication or spread of hepatitis B virus; however a direct cytotoxic activity of antibodies is not excluded.

Several important points are at present still not clarified: (1) is hepatitis B virus cytotropic for T- or B-cells, and does the decrease in T-cells represent a selective killing or inhibition of T-cells or a sequestration of these cells in the liver? (2) Does lymphocyte activation (MIF and LIF production, cytotoxicity) involve T- and B-cells? (3) Why is lymphocyte production of MIF and LIF by HB_sAg not associated with stimulation and blast transformation? (4) Are humoral antibodies protective or cytotoxic either by fixing complement or by eliciting antibody dependent lymphocyte cytotoxicity? (5) Is sensitization directed only against HB_sAg or also against HB_cAg? (6) Are macrophages and Kupffer cells important in this viral disease? (7) Is fulminant hepatitis caused by lack of antibody formation, cellular reactivity, or massive deposition of immune complexes in the liver—or by other known immunological factors? It is possible that the answers to these questions will also elucidate the pathogenesis of acute hepatitis induced by hepatitis A virus or by some drugs that induce a picture indistinguishable from acute viral hepatitis (halothane hepatitis, marsilid hepatitis, colcemid hepatitis).

Immunological mechanisms in chronic hepatitis

Chronic active hepatitis is a disease characterized, as the name implies by (a) chronicity of more than 6 months, (b) activity, especially prolonged elevation of serum transaminases, high levels of IgG and frequent serological abnormalities (see Chapter 8), and (c) hepatitis that is characterized morphologically by the presence of periportal hepatitis with accumulation of mononuclear cells in the portal tract with extension to the lobular periphery where hepatocytes are destroyed (piecemeal necrosis).

It is most likely that chronic active hepatitis is a disease of multiple aetiologies. At least three major types have been identified:

(a) HBAg-associated chronic active hepatitis, characterized by the presence in the serum of HB_sAg[4] or HB_cAb[18] and in the liver by a few hepatocytes with groundglass appearance and cytoplasmic HB_sAg[36]. Other hepatocytes may display HB_cAg in the nuclei[36]. The various types of hepatitis B virus may be demonstrated by immunofluorescence, electron microscopy, immunoelectron microscopy[33] and also by histological[112] and immunologic stains[113] in paraffin-embedded tissues. The incidence of this type differs in various parts of the world;

(b) autoimmune chronic active hepatitis seen mainly in young females with marked serological abnormalities (high titres of smooth muscle antibody, antinuclear antibody and positive LE tests) and without evidence of hepatitis B virus infection,

(c) drug-associated chronic active hepatitis described in some patients after prolonged administration of certain drugs (oxyphenisatin, alpha methyl dopa)[114].

In addition it is important to differentiate the immunological abnormalities in chronic active hepatitis from those seen in other chronic hepatitis, e.g. chronic persistent hepatitis (chronic portal hepatitis) and protracted acute hepatitis (lobular hepatitis)[115]. Unfortunately the frequent changes in classification of chronic liver diseases have contributed to confusion and disparity in the criteria used for the diagnosis. Therefore, it may be difficult at times to compare data from different laboratories.

The reason why acute viral hepatitis progresses to a chronic stage in only a few patients is unknown. Genetic factors which govern the immune response are probably important, and future studies will hopefully clarify the importance of HL-A 1-8 in chronic hepatitis. It is possible that those patients with acute viral hepatitis who have inherited a particular immune response gene (Ir) respond to a viral infection with an abnormal series of immunologic processes that may lead to the chronicity of the disease. Unfortunately, the HL-A system is only closely related to and does not necessarily mirror the alteration of the Ir locus.

T-cells are numerically decreased with a corresponding increase of B-cells in chronic active hepatitis[8,43]. It is not known at present whether there is a general decrease or an increase of cellular immunity; both hypo- and hyper-reactivity to PHA has been described[43,47,48,50,53,54]. The data on CMI to HB_sAg are also controversial. Leucocyte migration inhibition factor production in the presence of HB_sAg in patients with HB_s antigenaemia was described only in a few patients or is completely absent[67,69–72]. A recent report from England suggests, however, that both HB_sAg-positive and HB_sAg-negative chronic hepatitis patients exhibit cellular and humoral immunity to HB_sAg[84]. Sensitization to liver antigens is frequently observed in chronic active hepatitis[67,69–72,84]. Specific cytotoxic activity of lymphocytes against liver cells is present in these patients[87,89–91], and this reactivity is directed not only to autologous but also to normal homologous liver antigens. Thus, hyporeactivity to HB_sAg seems to be associated with hyperreactivity against some liver antigens. Reactivity against the latter antigens might be responsible for hepatocellular damage. In chronic hepatitis also, a variety of important questions remain unanswered: (1) Does the decrease of T-cells represent a decrease of suppressor cells or a sequestration of T-cells in the liver and is the increase of B-cells responsible for CMI? (2) Are the hepatic cells protected from a massive cytolytic activity of lymphocytes because the hepatitis B virus antigen is not represented on the surface of the hepatocytes? (3) Can the reactivity to various antigenic determinants of hepatitis B virus have different perhaps opposite *in vivo* effects? (4) What is the relationship between various lymphocytic factors in chronic hepatitis—LIF, MIF, and lymphocyte transformation? (5) Are new antigens formed in the liver, and are these responsible for the sensitization? (6) Are HB_c antibodies, frequently detected in patients with chronic hepatitis, protective or cytotoxic or eliciting tissue-damaging immune complexes? (7) Does a difference in the immunological reactivity lead to a picture of chronic persistent hepatitis rather than chronic active hepatitis? (8) Does HB_sAg-negative chronic hepatitis exhibit a similar pathogenetic mechanism to HB_sAg-positive chronic hepatitis but have a different aetiological factor?

Immunological mechanisms in primary biliary cirrhosis

Primary biliary cirrhosis is a disease of unknown aetiology, with a relative benign course over a number of years. Middle-aged women are affected predominantly. Histologically the disease is characterized by chronic non-suppurative cholangitis with progressive destruction, inflammation and scarring of the septal and interlobular bile ducts. This process eventually leads to cirrhosis. In the early lesions the epithelial cells of the bile ducts are damaged and surrounded by lymphocytes, histiocytes and plasma cells[116]. Occasionally lymphoid aggregates and granulomata may be seen. At this stage Ig and complement may be localized in the bile ducts[19]. Besides the histological and immunopathological findings, the association of primary biliary cirrhosis with other autoimmune diseases (e.g. Sjögren syndrome)[117,118] the presence of M-antibody and other antibodies (see Chapter 8), and the increased serum levels of rheumatoid factors and Ig especially IgM[19] support an immune pathogenesis for the disease.

Early in the disease an alteration of CMI seems to occur with an increase of active rosette forming cells (a subpopulation of lymphocytes that seems to demonstrate lymphocytes actively involved in CMI), a marked increase of B-cells[39], and a decrease of lymphocyte stimulation by PHA related both to impairment of lymphocyte responsiveness[46,51] as well as the occurrence of serum inhibitory factors[97,98].

The recently demonstrated increase of leucocyte migration inhibition factor in the presence of liver and bile antigens[67,70] and cytotoxicity of lymphocytes against liver cells[87,90] indicate a specific, probably harmful, immune reactivity against liver antigens. In this disease it is of paramount importance to characterize the lymphocytes and antigens involved in the reaction, especially the nature (helper cells, killer cells) of the increase of active E-rosettes.

Conclusions

Available information indicates that genetic factors may govern the altered CMI in some liver diseases. Chronicity of liver disease may be associated with a cytotoxic activity of lymphocytes directed against normal liver antigens, suggesting the appearance of cells with auto-aggressive activity. The relative importance of T- and B-cells is not known. The study of the function and the localization in the liver of subpopulations of T- and B- cells may prove of importance. After many years of studies the roles of immune complexes, antibodies and blocking factors in liver diseases are still not clarified, and the possibility of an antibody dependent lymphocytic cytotoxicity must be entertained.

REFERENCES

1. Coombs, R. R. A. and Gell, P. G. H. (1962). The classification of allergic reactions underlying disease. In *Clinical Aspects of Immunology*, P. G. H. Gell and R. R. A. Coombs (eds.) p. 317 (Philadelphia: F. A. Davis Company)
2. Perlmann P, and Holm, G. (1969). Cytotoxic effects of lymphoid cells *in vitro*. *Adv. Immunol.*, **11**, 117
3. Van Epps, D. E., Strickland, R. G. and Williams, R. C. Jr. (1975). Elevated IgE levels in liver disease. *Clin. Res.*, **23**, 106A

4. Paronetto, F. (1973). Immunologic aspects of liver disease. *Postgrad. Med.*, **53**, 156
5. Linder, E., Miettinen, A., Kurki, P. and Alftan, O. (1974). Liver-specific bile canalicular antibodies. *Lancet*, **ii**, 1275
6. Smith, M. G. M., Williams, R., Walker, G., Rizzetto, M. and Doniach, D. (1974). Hepatic disorders associated with liver/kidney microsomal antibodies. *Br. Med. J.*, **2**, 80
7. Bertrams, J., Reis, H. E., Kuwert, E. and Selmair, H. (1974). Hepatitis associated antigen (HAA), HL-A antigens and autolymphocytotoxins (CoCoCy) in chronic aggressive and chronic persistent hepatitis. *Z. Immun. Forsch.*, **146**, 300
8. DeHoratius, R. J., Strickland, R. G. and Williams, R. C. Jr. (1974). T- and B-lymphocytes in acute and chronic hepatitis. *Clin. Immunol. Immunopath.*, **2**, 353
9. Doniach, D. (1970). The concept of an 'autoallergic' hepatitis. *Proc. Royal Soc. Med.*, **63**, 527
10. Paronetto, F., Gerber, M. and Vernace, S. J. (1973). Immunologic studies in patients with chronic active hepatitis and primary biliary cirrhosis. I. Cytotoxic activity and binding of sera to human liver cells grown in tissue culture. *Proc. Soc. Exp. Biol. Med.*, **143**, 756
11. Allison, A. C., Denman, A. M. and Barnes, R. D. (1971). Co-operating and controlling functions of thymus-derived lymphocytes in relation to autoimmunity. *Lancet*, **ii**, 135
12. Sevc, K. C., Blair, J. D. and Kaplan, M. H. (1967). Immunopathologic studies of systemic lupus erythematosus (SLE). I. Tissue-bound immunoglobulins in relation to serum antinuclear immunoglobulins in systemic lupus and in chronic liver disease with LE cell factor. *J. Clin. Invest.*, **46**, 558
13. Bjørneboe, M., Prytz, H. and Ørskov, F. (1972). Antibodies to intestinal microbes in serum of patients with cirrhosis of the liver. *Lancet*, **i**, 58
14. Triger, D. R., Alp, M. H. and Wright, R. (1972). Bacterial and dietary antibodies in liver disease. *Lancet*, **i**, 60
15. Triger, D. R., Kurtz, J. B., MacCallum, F. O. and Wright, R. (1972). Raised antibody titres to measles and rubella viruses in chronic active hepatitis. *Lancet*, **i**, 665
16. Triger, D. R., Kurtz, J. B. and Wright, R. (1974). Viral antibodies and autoantibodies in chronic liver disease. *Gut*, **15**, 94
17. Shulman, N. R. (1970). Hepatitis-associated antigen. *Am. J. Med.*, **49**, 669
18. Brzosko, W. J., Madalinski, K., Krawczynski, K. and Nowoslawski, A. (1973). Duality of hepatitis B antigen and its antibody. I. Immunofluorescence studies. *J. Infect. Dis.*, **127**, 424
19. Paronetto, F. (1969). Hetero-iso and autoimmune phenomena in the liver. In *Textbook of Immunopathology*, P. A. Miescher and H. J. Müller-Eberhard (eds.) p. 562 (New York: Grune and Stratton, Inc.)

20. Oldstone, M. B. A. and Dixon, F. J. (1970). Pathogenesis of chronic disease associated with persistent lymphocytic choriomeningitis viral infection. II. Relationship of the antilymphocytic choriomeningitis immune response to tissue injury in chronic lymphocytic choriomeningitis disease. *J. Exp. Med.*, **131**, 1
21. Finlayson, N. D. C., Krohn, K., Fauconnet, M. H. and Anderson, K. E. (1972). Significance of serum complement levels in chronic liver disease. *Gastroenterology*, **63**, 653
22. Potter, B. J., Elias, E. and Jones, E. A. (1974). Hypercatabolism of the third component of complement in primary biliary cirrhosis. *Digestion*, **10**, 305
23. Agnello, V., Koffler, D., Eisenberg, J. W., Winchester, R. J. and Kunkel, H. G. (1971). Clq precipitins in the sera of patients with systemic lupus erythematosus and other hypocomplementemic states: characterization of high and low molecular weight types. *J .Exp. Med.*, **134**, 228s
24. Nydegger, U. E., Lambert, P. H., Gerber, H. and Miescher, P. A. (1974). Circulating immune complexes in the serum in systemic lupus erythematosus and in carriers of hepatitis B antigen. Quantitation by binding to radiolabelled Clq. *J. Clin. Invest.*, **54**, 297
25. Prince, A. M. and Trepo, C. (1971). Role of immune complexes involving SH antigen in pathogenesis of chronic active hepatitis and polyarteritis nodosa. *Lancet*, **i**, 1309
26. Trepo, C. G., Zuckerman, A. J., Bird, R. C. and Prince, A. M. (1974). The role of circulating hepatitis B antigen/antibody immune complexes in the pathogenesis of vascular and hepatic manifestations in polyarteritis nodosa. *J. Clin. Path.*, **27**, 863
27. Gocke, D. J., Hsu, K., Morgan, C., Bombardieri, S., Lockshin, M. and Christian, C. L. (1971). Vasculitis in association with Australia antigen. *J. Exp. Med.*, **134**, 330s
28. Nowoslawski, A., Krawczynski, K., Brzosko, W. J. and Madalinski, K. (1972). Tissue localization of Australia antigen immune complexes in acute and chronic hepatitis and liver cirrhosis. *Am. J. Path.*, **68**, 31
29. Brzosko, W. J., Krawczynski, K., Nazarewicz, T., Morzycka, M. and Nowoslawski, A. (1974). Glomerulonephritis associated with hepatitis B surface antigen immune complexes in children. *Lancet*, **ii**, 477
30. Paronetto, F. and Popper, H. (1965). Aggravation of hepatic lesions in mice by *in vivo* localization of immune complexes (Auer hepatitis). *Am. J. Path.* **47**, 549
31. Biozzi, G. and Stiffel, C. (1965). The physiopathology of the reticuloendothelial cells of the liver and spleen. In *Progress in liver diseases*, H. Popper and F. Schaffner (eds.) **2**, p. 166 (New York: Grune and Stratton)
32. Bjørneboe, M. and Prytz, H. (1975). Kupffer cells and cirrhosis. *Lancet*, **i**, 45
33. Gerber, M. A. and Paronetto, F. (1974). Hepatitis B antigen in human tissues. In *The Liver and its diseases*, F. Schaffner, S. Sherlock and

C. M. Leevy (eds.) p. 54 (New York: International Medical Book Corporation)

34. Gerber, M. A., Brodin, A., Steinberg, D., Vernace, S., Chen-Ping, Y. and Paronetto, F. (1972). Periarteritis nodosa, Australia antigen and lymphatic leukemia. *N. Eng. J. Med.*, **286**, 14
35. Edgington, T. S. and Ritt, D. J. (1971). Intrahepatic expression of serum hepatitis virus-associated antigens. *J. Exp. Med.*, **134**, 871
36. Gudat, F., Bianchi, L., Sonnabend, W., Thiel, G., Aenishaenslin, W. and Stalder, G. A. (1975). Pattern of core and surface expression in liver tissue reflects state of specific immune response in hepatitis B. *Lab. Invest.*, **32**, 1
37. Cochrane, C. G., Wiegle, W. O. and Dixon, F. J. (1959). The role of polymorphonuclear leukocytes in the initiation and cessation of Arthus vasculitis. *J. Exp. Med.*, **110**, 481
38. Henson, P. M. (1971). Release of biologically active constituents from blood cells and its role in antibody-mediated tissue injury. In *Progress in Immunology*, B. Amos (ed.) p. 155 (New York: Academic Press)
39. Colombo, M., Vernace, S. J. and Paronetto, F. (1974). T- and B-lymphocytes in primary biliary cirrhosis. *Gastroenterology*, **67**, 783
40. Chess, L., Levine, H., MacDermott, R. P. and Schlossman, S. F. (1975). The maturation of human null cells into B-cells. *Fed. Proc.*, **34**, 1031
41. Katz, S. I., Parker, D. and Turk, J. L. (1974). B-cell suppression of delayed hypersensitivity reactions. *Nature* (*Lond.*), **251**, 550
42. Wybran, J. and Fudenberg, H. H. (1973). Thymus-derived rosette-forming cells in various human disease states: Cancer, lymphoma, bacterial and viral infections, and other diseases. *J. Clin. Invest.*, **52**, 1026
43. Tolentino, P., Pasino, M., Braito, A., Astaldi, A. Jr. and Giacchino, R. (1974). Impaired T-lymphocyte function in chronic hepatitis? *Digestion*, **10**, 331
44. Bernstein, I. M., Webster, K. H., Williams, R. C. Jr. and Strickland, R. G. (1974). Reduction in circulating T-lymphocytes in alcoholic liver disease. *Lancet*, **ii**, 488
45. Berenyi, M. E., Straus, B. and Cruz, D. (1974). *In vitro* and *in vivo* studies of cellular immunity in alcoholic cirrhosis. *Am. J. Digest. Dis.*, **19**, 199
46. Fox, R. A., Scheuer, P. J., James, D. G., Sharma, O. and Sherlock, S. (1969). Impaired delayed hypersensitivity in primary biliary cirrhosis. *Lancet*, **i**, 959
47. Sodomann, C.-P., Havemann, K. and Martini, G. A. (1974). Cellular immune reactions in the course of virus hepatitis. *Digestion*, **10**, 328
48. Toh, B. H., Roberts-Thomson, I. C., Mathews, J. D., Whittingham, S. and Mackay, I. R. (1973). Depression of cell-mediated immunity in old age and the immunopathic diseases, lupus erythematosus, chronic hepatitis and rheumatoid arthritis. *Clin. Exp. Immunol.*, **14**, 193
49. Maerker-Alzer, G., Schumacher, K. and Gross, R. (1974). Detection of

lymphocytes with increased DNA-synthesis in the peripheral blood of patients with active chronic hepatitis. *Klin. Wschr.*, **52**, 190

50. Pettigrew, N. M., Russell, R. I., Goudie, R. B. and Chaudhuri, A. K. R. (1972). Evidence for a role of hepatitis virus B in chronic alcoholic liver disease. *Lancet*, **ii**, 724
51. MacSween, R. N. M., Galbraith, I., Thomas, M. A., Watkinson, G. and Ludlam, G. B. (1973). Phytohaemagglutinin (PHA) induced lymphocyte transformation and *Toxoplasma gondii* antibody studies in primary biliary cirrhosis. *Clin. Exp. Immunol.*, **15**, 35
52. Sutnick, A. I., Bugbee, S. J., London, W. T., Loeb, K. A., Peyretti, F., Litwin, S. and Blumberg, B. S. (1973). Lymphocyte function in normal people with persistent Australia antigen. *J. Lab. Clin. Med.*, **82**, 79
53. Nielsen, J. O., Reinicke, V., Dietrichson, O., Andersen, V., Thomsen, M. and Andersen, E. (1973). Immunological studies of Australia antigen carriers with and without liver diseases. *Clin. Exp. Immunol.*, **15**, 9
54. Warnatz, H. (1974). Immune reactions to hepatitis B antigen in acute and chronic hepatitis. *Acta Hepato-Gastroenterol.*, **21**, 237
55. Chess, L., MacDermott, R. P. and Schlossman, S. F. (1974). Immunologic functions of isolated human lymphocyte subpopulations. 1. Quantitative isolation of human T- and B-cells and response to mitogens. *J. Immunol.*, **113**, 1113
56. Schumacher, K., Maerker-Alzer, G., and Wehmer, U. (1974). A lymphocyte-inhibiting factor isolated from normal human liver. *Nature (Lond)*., **251**, 655
57. Sorrell, M. F. and Leevy, C. M. (1972). Lymphocyte transformation and alcoholic liver injury. *Gastroenterology*, **63**, 1020
58. Opolon, P., Cartron, J., Chicot, D. and Caroli, J. (1969). Application of the lymphoblast transformation test to the diagnosis of drug-induced hepatitis. *Presse Med.*, **77**, 2041
59. Holland, P. and Mauer, A. M. (1964). Drug-induced *in vitro* stimulation of peripheral lymphocytes. *Lancet*, **i**, 1368
60. Sarkany, I. (1967). Lymphocyte transformation in drug hypersensitivity. *Lancet*, **i**, 743
61. Paronetto, F. and Popper, H. (1970). Lymphocyte stimulation induced by halothane in patients with hepatitis following exposure to halothane. *New Eng. J. Med.*, **283**, 277
62. De Gast, G. C., Houwen, B. and Nieweg, H. O. (1973). Specific lymphocyte stimulation by purified, heat-inactivated hepatitis-B antigen. *Br. Med. J.*, **4**, 707
63. Yeung Laiwah, A. A. C., Chaudhuri, A. K. R. and Anderson, J. R. (1973). Lymphocyte transformation and leucocyte migration-inhibition by Australia antigen. *Clin. Exp. Immunol.*, **15**, 27
64. Pettigrew, N. M., Russell, R. I., Goudie, R. B. and Chaudhuri, A. K. R. (1972). Evidence for a role of hepatitis virus B in chronic alcoholic liver disease. *Lancet*, **ii**, 724

65. De Gast, G. C., Houwen, B., Que, G. S. and Nieweg, H. O. (1974). Lymphocyte stimulation by subtypes of HB_sAg. *Digestion*, **10**, 327
66. Bloom, B. R. (1971). *In vitro* approaches to the mechanism of cell-mediated immune reactions. *Adv. Immunol.*, **13**, 101
67. Bacon, P. A., Berry, H. and Bown, R. (1972). Cell-mediated immune reactivity in liver disease. *Gut.* **13**, 427
68. Eddleston, A. L. W. F., McFarlane, I. G., Mitchell, C. G., Reed, W. D. and Williams, R. (1973). Cell-mediated immune response in primary biliary cirrhosis to a protein fraction from human bile. *Br. Med. J.*, **4**, 274
69. Miller, J., Mitchell, C. G., Eddleston, A. L. W. F., Smith, M. G. M., Reed W. D. and Williams, R. (1972). Cell-mediated immunity to a human liver-specific antigen in patients with active chronic hepatitis and primary biliary cirrhosis. *Lancet.* **ii**, 296
70. Smith, M. G. M., Golding, P. L., Eddleston, A. L. W. F., Mitchell, C. G., Kemp, A. and Williams, R. (1972). Cell-mediated immune responses in chronic liver diseases. *Br. Med. J.*, **1**, 527
71. Meyer zum Büschenfelde, K. H., Knolle, J. and Berger, J. (1974). Celluläre immunreaktionen gegenüber homologen leberspezifischen antigenen (HLP) bie chronischen Leberentzundungen. *Klin. Wschr.*, **52**, 246
72. Vergani, C., Oldoni, T. and Dioguardi, N. (1974). Leucocyte migration inhibition in liver disease. *J. Clin. Path.*, **27**, 772
73. Mihas, A. A., Bull, D. M. and Davidson, C. S. (1974). Cellular immune reactivity to liver tissue in alcoholic hepatitis. *Gastroenterology*, **67**, 816
74. Hardt, F., Nerup, J. and Bendixen, G. (1960). Antihepatic cellular hypersensitivity in hepatic cirrhosis. *Lancet*, **i**, 730
75. Zetterman, R. K., Chen, T. and Leevy, C. M. (1974). Role of altered lymphocyte function in alcoholic liver disease. *Gastroenterology*, **67**, 837
76. Richens, E. R., Irvine, W. J., Williams, M. J., Hartog, M. and Ancill, R. J. (1974). Cellular hypersensitivity to mitochondrial antigens in diabetes mellitus and its relationship to the presence of circulating auto-antibodies. *Clin. Exp. Immunol.*, **17**, 71
77. Wartenberg, J., Doniach, D., Brostoff, J. and Roitt, I. M. (1973). Leucocyte migration inhibition with mitochondria in human auto-immune thyroid disorders. *Clin. Exp. Immunol.*, **14**, 203
78. De Moura, M. C., Vernace, S. J. and Paronetto, F. (1975). Cell-mediated immune reactivity to hepatitis B surface antigen in liver diseases. *Gastroenterology*, **69**, 310
79. Dudley, F. J., Giustino, V. and Sherlock, C. (1972). Cell-mediated immunity in patients positive for hepatitis-associated antigen. *Br. Med. J.*, **4**, 754
80. Gerber, M. J., Phuangsab, A., Vittal, S. B. V., Dourdourekas, D., Steigmann, F. and Clowdus, B. F. (1974). Cell-mediated immune response to hepatitis B antigen in patients with liver disease. *Am. J. Dig. Dis.*, **19**, 637

81. Ibrahim, A. B., Vyas, G. N. and Perkins, H. A. (1975). Immune response to hepatitis B surface antigen. *Infect. Immun.*, **11**, 137
82. Irwin, G. R. Jr., Hierholzer, W. J. Jr., Cimis, R. and McCollum, R. W. (1974). Delayed hypersensitivity in hepatitis B: Clinical correlates of *in vitro* production of migration inhibition factor. *J. Infect. Dis.*, **130**, 580
83. Knolle, J., Meyer zum Büschenfelde, K. H., Bolte, J. P. and Berger, J. (1973). Celluläre Immunreaktionen gegenüber dem Hepatitisassoziierten antigen (HAA) und homologen leberspezifischen Protein (HLP) bei akuten HAA-positiven Hepatitiden. *Klin. Wschr.*, **51**, 1172
84. Lee, W. M., Reed, W. D., Mitchell, C. G., Galbraith, R. M., Eddleston, A. L. W. F., Zuckerman, A. J. and Williams, R. (1975). Cellular and humoral immunity to Hepatitis-B surface antigen in active chronic hepatitis. *Br. Med. J.*, **1**, 705
85. Frei, P. C., Erard, P. and Zinkernagel, R. (1973). Cell-mediated immunity to hepatitis-associated antigen (HAA) demonstrated by leucocyte migration test during and after acute B hepatitis. *Biomedicine*, **19**, 379
86. Rocklin, R. E., MacDermott, R. P., Chess L., Schlossman, S. F. and David, J. R. (1974). Studies on mediator production by highly purified human T- and B-lymphocytes. *J. Exp. Med.*, **140**, 1303
87. Paronetto, F. and Vernace, S. J. (1975). Immunological studies in patients with chronic active hepatitis. Cytotoxic activity of lymphocytes to autochthonous liver cells grown in tissue culture. *Clin. Exp. Immunol.*, **19**, 99
88. Paronetto, F., Vernace, S. J. and Colombo, M. (1975). Further studies on the cytotoxic activity of lymphocytes against liver cells in patients with chronic hepatitis (CH). *Gastroenterology* **68**, 965
89. Geubel, A. P., Keller, R. H. Summerskill, W. H. J., Stobo, J. D., Tomasi, T. B. and Shorter, R. G. (1975). Cytotoxicity of autologous and normal lymphocytes against isolated liver cells from patients with chronic active liver disease (CALD). *Gastroenterology*, **68**. 1084
90. Wands, J. R. and Isselbacher, K. J. (1975). Lymphocyte cytotoxicity to autologous liver cells in chronic active hepatitis. *Proc. Nat. Acad. Sci.* (*USA*), **72**, 1301
91. Thomson, A. D., Cochrane, M. A. G., McFarlane, I. G., Eddleston, A. L. W. F. and Williams, R. (1974). Lymphocyte cytotoxicity to isolated hepatocytes in chronic active hepatitis. *Nature* (*Lond.*), **252**, 721
92. Calder, E. A., Penhale, W. J., McLenan, D., Barnes, E. W. and Irvine, W. J. (1973). Lymphocyte-dependent antibody-mediated cytotoxicity in Hashimoto thyroiditis. *Clin. Exp. Immunol.*, **14**, 153
93. Hakala, T. R., Lange, P. H., Castro, A. E., Elliott, A. Y. and Fraley, E. E. (1974). Antibody induction of lymphocyte-mediated cytotoxicity against human transitional-cell carcinomas of the urinary tract. *New Eng. J. Med.*, **291**, 637
94. Wunderlich, J. R., Rosenberg, E. B. and Connolly, J. M. (1971). Human lymphocyte-dependent cytotoxic antibody and mechanisms of target cell

destruction *in vitro*. *In Progess in Immunology*, B. Amos (ed.) p. 473 (New York: Academic Press)

95. Hopf, U. and Meyer zum Büschenfelde, K. H. (1974). Studies on the pathogenesis of experimental chronic active hepatitis in rabbits. **II.** Demonstration of immunoglobulin on isolated hepatocytes. *Br. J. Exp. Path.*, **55**, 509
96. Paronetto, F. Unpublished observations
97. Fox, R. A., Dudley, F. J., Samuels, M., Milligan, J. and Sherlock, S. (1973). Lymphocyte transformation in response to phytohaemagglutinin in primary biliary cirrhosis: The search for a plasma inhibitory factor. *Gut*, **14**, 89
98. MacSween, R. N. M. and Thomas, M. A. (1973). Lymphocyte transformation by phytohaemagglutinin (PHA) and purified protein derivative (PPD) in primary biliary cirrhosis. *Clin. Exp. Immunol.*, **15**, 523
99. Hsu, C. C. S. and Leevy, C. M. (1971). Inhibition of PHA-stimulated lymphocyte transformation by plasma from patients with advanced alcoholic cirrhosis. *Clin. Exp. Immunol.*, **8**, 749
100. Winter, G. C. B., McCarthy, C. F., Read, A. E. and Yoffey, J. M. (1967). Development of macrophages in phytohaemagglutinin cultures of blood from patients with idiopathic steatorrhoea and with cirrhosis. *Br. J. Exp. Path.*, **48**, 66
101. Mella, B. and Lang, D. J. (1967). Leukocyte mitosis: Suppression *in vitro* associated with acute infectious hepatitis. *Science*, **155**, 80
102. Mella, B. A. and Taswell, H. F. (1970). Suppression of leukocyte mitosis by sera of hepatitis-implicated donors. *Am. J. Clin. Path.*, **53**, 141
103. Willems, F. T., Melnick, J. L. and Rawls, W. E. (1969). Viral inhibition of the phytohaemagglutinin response of human lymphocytes and application to viral hepatitis. *Proc. Soc. Exp. Biol.*, **130**, 652
104. Newble, D. I. Holmes, K. T., Wangel, A. G. and Forbes, I. J. (1975). Immune reactions in acute viral hepatitis. *Clin. Exp. Immunol.*, **20**, 17
105. Newberry, W. M., Shorey, J. W., Sandford, J. P. and Combes, B. (1973). Depression of lymphocyte reactivity to phytohaemagglutinin by serum from patients with liver disease. *Cell. Immunol.*, **6**, 87
106. Wands, J. R., Perrotto, J. L., Alpert, E. and Isselbacher, K. J. (1975). Cell-mediated immunity in acute and chronic hepatitis. *J. Clin. Invest.*, **55**, 921
107. Mackay, I. R. and Morris, P. J. (1972). Association of autoimmune active chronic hepatitis with HL-AI, 8. *Lancet*, **ii**, 793
108. Page, A., Sharp, H. and Yunis, E. (1975). HL-A and MLC typing studies in patients with active chronic hepatitis. *Fed. Proc.*, **34**, 1017
109. Galbraith, R. M. Eddleston, A. L. W. F., Smith, M. G. M., Williams, R., MacSween, R. N. M., Watkinson, G., Dick, H., Kennedy, L. A. and Batchelor, J. R. (1974). Histocompatibility antigens in active chronic hepatitis and primary biliary cirrhosis. *Br. Med. J.*, **3**, 604
110. Barbanti, M., Reali, G. and Tolentino, P. (1974). Sistema maggiore

dell'istocompatibilita e malattie. Studio delle epatiti croniche HBAg-positive. *Bull. Ist. Sieroterapico Milanese*, **53**, 4

111. Barker, L. F., Chisari, F. V., McGrath, P. P., Dalgard, D. W., Kirschstein, R. L., Almeida, J. D., Edgington, T. S., Sharp, D. G., and Peterson, M. R. (1973). Transmission of Type B viral hepatitis to chimpanzees. *J. Infect. Dis.*, **127**, 648
112. Shikata, T., Uzawa, T., Yoshiwara, N., Akatsuka, T. and Yamazaki, S. (1974). Staining methods of Australia antigen in paraffin section. Detection of cytoplasmic inclusion bodies. *Jap. J. Exp. Med.*, **44**, 25
113. Huang, S. (1975). Immunohistochemical demonstration of hepatitis B core and surface antigens in paraffin sections. *Lab. Invest.*, **33**, 88
114. Guidelines for diagnosis of therapeutic drug-induced liver injury in liver biopsies (1974). *Lancet*, **i**, 854.
115. Popper, H. and Schaffner, F. (1971). The vocabulary of chronic hepatitis. *New Eng. J. Med.*, **284**, 1154
116. Rubin, E., Schaffner, F. and Popper, H. (1973). Primary biliary cirrhosis: chronic nonsuppurative destructive cholangitis. *Am. J. Pathol.*, **46**, 387
117. Alarcón-Segovia, D., Díaz-Jouanen, E. and Fishbein, E. (1973). Features of Sjögren's syndrome in primary biliary cirrohosis. *Ann. Int. Med.*, **79**, 31
118. Golding, P. L., Bown, R. and Stuart-Mason, A. (1971). Studies on multisystem involvement in active chronic hepatitis and primary biliary cirrhosis. In *Immunology of the liver*, M. Smith and R. William (eds.) p. 194 (Philadelphia: F. A. Davis Company)

CHAPTER 10

Autoimmune diseases of the liver

R. N. M. MacSween and P. A. Berg

In this chapter we propose to deal with certain forms of chronic liver disease in which autoimmune aetiological mechanisms have been invoked and in particular those forms in which serum autoantibodies are commonly demonstrated. These include various forms of chronic active hepatitis, and the more homogeneous disease entity primary biliary cirrhosis. We will describe the morphological and clinical features, the clinicopathological and immunological associations in these diseases, and briefly discuss their medical management.

Chronic active hepatitis

INTRODUCTION

Chronic active hepatitis presents an extremely variable clinical picture of poorly defined aetiology, with a spectrum of disease pattern in which acute and chronic inflammatory processes co-exist. In the early stages it may resemble an episode of acute viral hepatitis; it pursues a pattern of relapse and remission, the duration of each phase being unpredictable. In some instances the disease may revert to an inactive form, in others there may be a rapid progression to hepatic cirrhosis, while in further instances the cirrhosis evolves more slowly. In these latter stages the disease pattern is that of an established cirrhosis. Many patients may not present until this late stage, having been previously symptom free and with no history of any earlier acute episode.

This relatively serious progressive chronic hepatitis with hypergammaglobulinaemia was described in 1950 by Waldenstroem[1], and a year later by Bearn and his colleagues[2]. Bearn *et al.* described 12 patients, 11 of whom were women less than 35 years, in whom the liver showed a histological picture of a severe periportal plasma cell infiltration with parenchymal necrosis, and in whom there were extremely high serum globulin levels. Saint *et al.* in 1953[3], observed an 'infectious hepatitis' in 39 patients, with a poor prognosis, and because of the progressive inflammatory process in the liver, applied the term 'active chronic hepatitis'. The link with viral hepatitis was also further noted by Joske and King, describing a severe form of progressive 'post-viral' hepatitis[4]. The demonstration of LE cells in these patients[4,5] and the occurrence of accompanying rheumatoid arthritis like phenomena aroused suspicion of an association with systemic lupus erythematosus (SLE) and the term lupoid was applied[5-7]. Such an association has not, however, been confirmed and today one can recognize that the clinical patterns are virtually exclusive: (a) in SLE minimal, if any, changes occur in the hepatic parenchyma, (b) renal involvement, often an early symptom of SLE, is a rare complication in chronic active hepatitis, and (c) the spectrum and specificity of antinuclear antibodies (ANA) in SLE are substantially different from those in chronic active hepatitis.

Various other terms have been applied to this form of liver disease, including plasma cell hepatitis, active juvenile cirrhosis, hypergammaglobulinaemic hepatitis, chronic aggressive hepatitis and chronic hepatitis of women at the menopause[8,9]. The term chronic active hepatitis is now, however, generally recommended for this disease process. The diagnosis is often established only after examination of a liver biopsy, and we propose therefore to first outline the morphological characteristics of the disease.

Morphological features

A study group of the European Association for the Study of the Liver in a recommended classification of chronic hepatitis[10] subdivided it into a chronic persistent benign form and a chronic active form which might show mild or severe degrees of activity and in which the prognosis was poor. In chronic persistent hepatitis there is a chronic inflammatory cell infiltrate in the portal tracts, which may be enlarged and show a degree of portal fibrosis. However, this inflammatory cell infiltrate remains confined to the portal tracts, the limiting plate is intact, and there is no septal disruption of the normal lobular architecture. There may be small foci of parenchymal liver cell necrosis, but such changes are minimal.

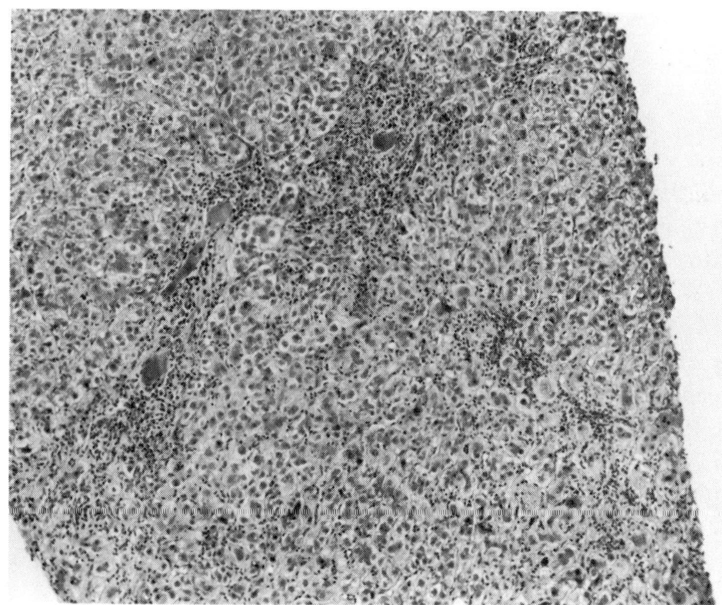

FIGURE 10.1 Needle biopsy of liver from a patient with chronic active hepatitis. Note the diffuse chronic inflammatory cell infiltrate involving both portal areas and lobules. Haematoxylin and eosin × 85

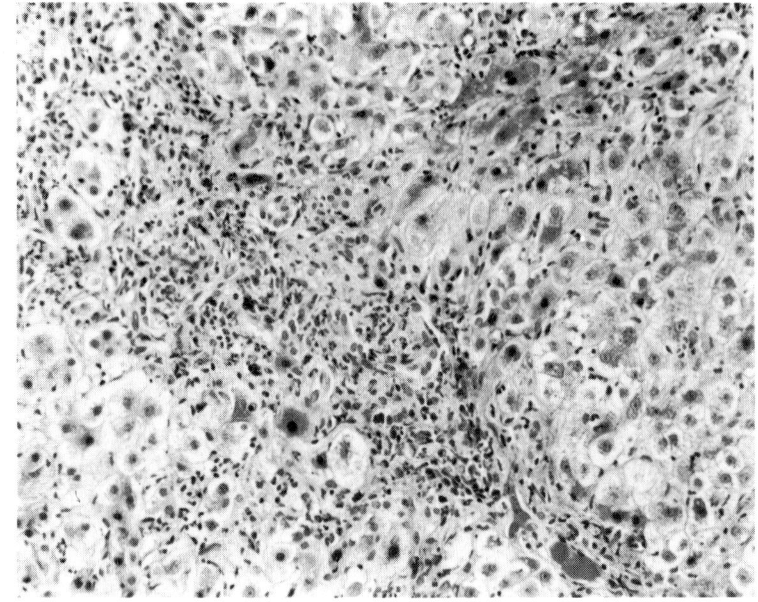

FIGURE 10.2 Same material as in Figure 10.1. There is an intense chronic inflammatory cell infiltrate of the portal area, with extensive erosion of the limiting plate and periportal piecemeal necrosis. Foci of liver cell necrosis are present within the neighbouring lobules, and acidophilic degeneration of individual hepatocytes is also evident. Haematoxylin and eosin × 223

In chronic active hepatitis there is an intense chronic inflammatory process, mainly lymphocytes but with variable numbers of plasma cells[11,12], involving both the portal tracts and the lobules (Figure 10.1). The inflammatory infiltrate in the portal area is intense; it spills over into the neighbouring parenchyma so that the limiting plate is eroded and difficult to define. The peripheral hepatocytes show degenerative changes, and individual and groups of hepatocytes become swollen and surrounded by the chronic inflammatory cells (Figure 10.2). These changes constitute piecemeal necrosis. In places regenerating cells at the periphery of the lobules give rise to pseudo-rosette formation (Figure 10.3). The entire process has been referred to as periportal hepatitis[13].

In addition to these features there is also lobular involvement—lobular hepatitis—which tends to be diffuse in contrast to acute viral hepatitis where the changes are more marked centrilobularly. In the early stages, however, the morphological differential diagnosis may be difficult. There are accompanying degenerative changes in hepatocytes

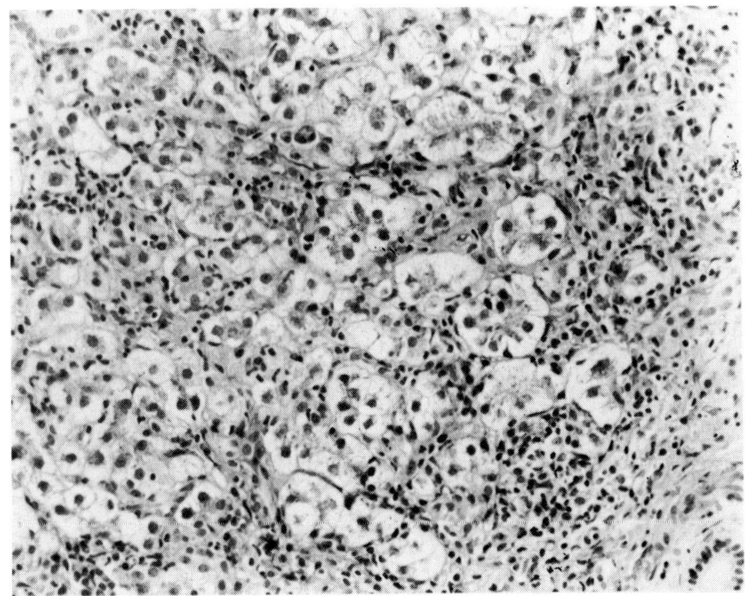

Figure 10.3 Same material as in Figures 10.1 and 10.2. Active regeneration with pseudo-rosette or gland-like formations at margins of lobules. There is also swelling and degenerative changes of many hepatocytes. Haematoxylin and eosin × 223

with focal liver cell necrosis, ballooning degeneration, and the formation of acidophil bodies. There is a generalized reactive hyperplasia of Kupffer cells.

The degree of inflammatory reaction may vary from area to area, and in addition varies with clinical relapse and remission. In severe acute exacerbations and with progression to a more chronic stage the lobular structure becomes disturbed by connective tissue septa which link up portal tracts or central veins and portal tracts; this has been referred to as 'bridging necrosis', and in some instances the septa may be passive, due to parenchymal cell loss and collapse, rather than active and due to progressive fibrosis. There is usually continuing subacute necrosis of hepatocytes[14], and in severe cases the diffuse multilobular involvement has been referred to as multilobular necrosis[15]. Further descriptive terms which have been used include subacute hepatitis, and chronic necrotizing hepatitis[16–18], but all are regarded as being the histological correlates of chronic active hepatitis[19–21].

With progressive subdivision of the parenchyma and the appearance of regenerating nodules the pattern becomes that of an established macronodular cirrhosis. Cholestasis of variable degree is usually present. In some cases there is proliferation of intra and inter-lobular bile ducts, and in some there may be destructive processes involving these and resembling the lesions seen in primary biliary cirrhosis[21]. Recently Baggenstoss *et al.*[15] have drawn attention to the possible prognostic value of some of these morphological features. In a study in which 20–26 patients were present in each sub-group they noted that with multilobular necrosis, bridging necrosis or chronic active hepatitis without these changes, cirrhosis developed in 40%, 27% and 8% respectively. These observations, however, remain to be confirmed.

In chronic active hepatitis associated with hepatitis B antigenaemia hepatocytes with a ground-glass cytoplasm may be noted. While these *per se* are not specific indicators of such infection immunofluorescent techniques[22] or orcein stain[23] can be used to confirm the presence of the antigen within these hepatocytes.

Viral and immunological markers

On the basis of viral and autoantibody markers chronic active hepatitis may be classified as follows:

1. Hepatitis B (HB) positive. In this group serum autoantibodies may sometimes occur, but in our experience are usually present only in low titres.
2. HB negative/autoantibody negative.
3. HB negative/autoantibody positive.

A further smaller group would include those drug-induced forms in which, e.g. methyl-dopa and oxyphenisatin have been implicated.

It is with the third group that this account is principally concerned, in that this represents that form of chronic active hepatitis which seems to be indeed autoimmune. However, it has to be emphasized that clinically and morphologically there may be little to distinguish between the various groups and the possibility cannot be excluded that a final common pathway, irrespective of the initial 'triggering agent' may lead to the establishment of the chronicity of the disease process (see Chapter 8). In particular the role of hepatitis A virus, and other hepatitis associated virus, remains to be clarified and this will follow as methods for identifying such viruses are developed.

* * *

Incidence of HB virus and serum autoantibodies: Three different autoantibodies occur in chronic active hepatitis: antinuclear antibody (ANA), smooth muscle antibody (SMA) and anti-mitochondrial antibody (M-antibody)[24]. The frequency and distribution of hepatitis B surface antigen (HBsAg), hepatitis B anti-surface antigen antibody (HBsAb), and of these autoantibodies in a series of 425 patients with chronic liver disease are presented in Tables 10.1 and 10.2.* Only limited conclusions, however, can be drawn from this data partly because of the selectivity of the case material and partly because biopsies were not performed in all patients. In analysing 215 needle biopsy-confirmed cases of chronic active hepatitis, 42% were HB associated (i.e. HBsAg or HBsAb positive), 26% were autoimmune (i.e. SMA/ANA or M-antibody positive) and the remaining 32% had neither viral nor immunological markers (Table 10.3).

Table 10.1 INCIDENCE OF HB VIRUS ASSOCIATION IN 425 PATIENTS WITH CHRONIC LIVER DISEASE

Diagnosis	*No. of patients*	*Sera positive for HBsAg**	*HBsAb†*	*%HBsAg/HBsAb positive*
Chronic active hepatitis (All biopsy proven)	215	66	26	42
Established cirrhosis (Biopsies in 161)	210	48	43	42

* Radioimmunoassay
† Passive haemagglutination

Heterogeneity of M-antibody: The M-antibodies in chronic active hepatitis seem to have different specificities as compared with the M-antibody found in sera from patients with primary biliary cirrhosis. As shown in Figure 10.4 they also react with a second antigen which has been found to be specific for the pseudo-lupus erythematosus (PLE) syndrome, which is now known to be drug induced[25–29]. Highly purified 'PLE antigen' fractions contain small globular particles 2·8–3·5 nm in size, much smaller than the primary biliary cirrhosis antigen which consists of 10-13 nm particles. Although there is no doubt that this

* Collaborative studies by one of us (P.A.B.) with Dr H. Lindner (DRK-Krankenhaus, Hamburg) and Dr H. Bannaski (Klinik Kempfenhausen).

Table 10.2 DISTRIBUTION OF SERUM AUTOANTIBODIES IN 425 PATIENTS (SAME SERIES AS TABLE 10.1) WITH CHRONIC LIVER DISEASE

	HB positive	*HB negative*	
No. of patients	178 (42%)	247 (58%)	
Male/female ratio	61/117	170/77	
Autoantibodies*	Titre $<1/20$	Titre $<1/20$	Titre $>1/30$
ANA/SMA	41	26	57
M-antibody	—	—	62†

* Figures given are for only those sera which did contain autoantibodies at the titres stated

† M-antibody positive—24 with chronic active hepatitis and 38 with primary biliary cirrhosis

Table 10.3 HB VIRUS AND SERUM AUTOANTIBODIES IN 215 PATIENTS WITH NEEDLE BIOPSY PROVEN CHRONIC ACTIVE HEPATITIS

Group	*No. of patients*	*Male/female ratio*
HB associated (HBsAg/HBsAb)	90 (42%)	31/59
Autoimmune (Ab titres $>1/20$)	57* (26%)	54/3
HB negative/autoantibody negative	68 (32%)	32/36

* Autoantibody distribution: ANA 8; ANA/SMA 33; M-antibody 6; M-antibody/ANA/SMA 10

antigen is specific for the pseudo-lupus syndrome interpretations of the results obtained with M-positive chronic active hepatitis sera are much more difficult to interpret since no completely purified antigen fractions were used in the complement fixation tests. Thus reactions with other cytoplasmic constituents, e.g. microsomes, were not firmly excluded. At this stage we prefer therefore to speak of a reaction with the PLE-associated antigen, since the fraction used in the tests contained approximately 60% of the total antigen showing PLE-activity.

One hundred and fifteen sera, giving a positive mitochondrial staining pattern on immunofluorescence, have been examined by complement fixation testing against these two antigens, and the results are summarized in Table 10.4. All patients whose sera reacted exclusively with the 'PBC antigen' manifested the classical clinical, biochemical and

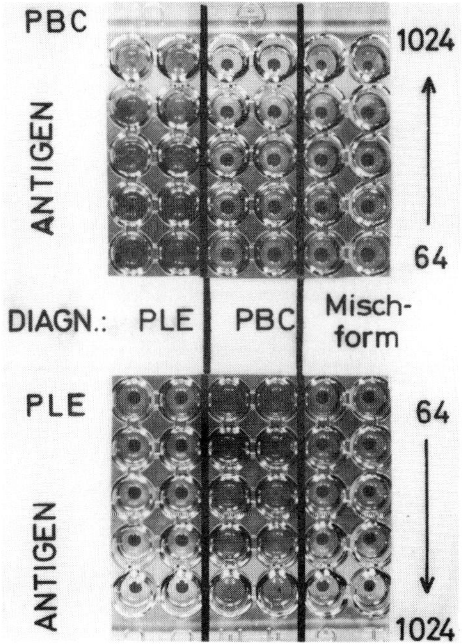

FIGURE 10.4 Complement fixation tests using two antigen fractions: primary biliary cirrhosis antigen ('PBC antigen') and pseudo-lupus erythematosus syndrome antigen ('PLE antigen')*. The sera tested all contained M-antibody on immunofluorescent screening. However, the two antigen fractions discriminate between the PLE and PBC sera. The serum from an M-antibody positive chronic active hepatitis (Misch-form) binds complement with both antigen fractions.

(* PBC antigen-free surcose gradient fraction containing approximately 60% PLE antigen and other cytoplasmic constituents)

pathological features of primary biliary disease, thus confirming the reliability of this antigen–antibody reaction as a marker of this disease. The patients whose sera reacted with both antigens showed a mixed clinical picture of chronic active hepatitis and primary biliary cirrhosis, and histologically were frequently diagnosed as chronic active hepatitis or as cryptogenic cirrhosis, and less frequently as primary biliary cirrhosis.

Thus on the basis of autoantibody testing it is now possible to distinguish three different groups of autoimmune hepatitis:

1. ANA- and SMA-positive chronic active hepatitis.
2. M-antibody (heterogeneous) positive chronic active hepatitis.
3. M-antibody (homogeneous) positive primary biliary cirrhosis.

For want of a better term, and bearing in mind what we have already said, we will refer to group 1 as the lupoid variety. This term does imply the possible immuno-pathogenesis of the disease and distinguishes it from the M-antibody positive form.

Table 10.4 HETEROGENEITY OF M-ANTIBODY: COMPLEMENT FIXATION (CF) TESTS USING 115 CHRONIC LIVER DISEASE SERA GIVING A TYPICAL M-ANTIBODY IMMUNOFLUORESCENT STAINING PATTERN

Antigen	*No. of sera giving positive CF*	*Male/female ratio of patients*
'PBC' and 'PLE'*	54	43/11
'PBC'	40	39/1
'PLE'	1	1/0

* PBC antigen-free sucrose gradient fraction containing approximately 60% PLE antigen and other cytoplasmic constituents

Twenty sera were negative or gave weakly positive CF tests with both antigens

ANA/SMA POSITIVE CHRONIC ACTIVE HEPATITIS—LUPOID HEPATITIS

Early stage with acute onset: This form of chronic active hepatitis occurs predominantly in young girls, and may manifest itself as early as 10–15 years of age[2,6,19,31]. The clinical presentation may resemble that of acute viral hepatitis, with an influenza-like illness, moderate pyrexia, nausea, polyarthralgia, pale stools and dark urine[11,12]. There may be a history of pruritus, and of right hypochondrial pain. Endocrine changes such as dysmenorrhea or amenorrhea may antedate these symptoms by many months. On clinical examination there is moderate jaundice, there is usually tender hepatomegaly, and the spleen is palpable in most instances.

Biochemically the bilirubin is seldom higher than 5–8 mg%[31], but the serum alanine and aspartate transaminase levels are raised to 300–500 I.U. units per litre. The alkaline phosphatase level may be temporarily slightly raised. The prothrombin time, haptoglobin, and cholesterol levels are unremarkable, and the haematological findings are not usually abnormal. In contrast to acute viral hepatitis the serum immunoglobulin levels are elevated from the start and may vary between 2–3 times the normal. This increase is mainly in the IgG class, but IgA and IgM may show slight simultaneous increases[32,33]. The ESR is almost always greater than 30 mm (Westergren) in the first hour, whereas in acute viral hepatitis it is seldom over 10 mm[34].

Serological findings

Antinuclear and smooth muscle antibodies, readily demonstrable by immunofluorescent techniques are present in high titre[7,24], and in earlier publications as already mentioned, attention was drawn to the frequent association with LE cells. The antinuclear antibodies produce a homogeneous or speckled staining pattern on immunofluorescence and are directed against nucleo-protein antigens[35]. Davies and Read recently found anti-DNA antibodies in 17 of 36 patients with chronic active hepatitis, and of these 36, 26 also had antinuclear antibodies[36]. In no instance have we been able to demonstrate M-antibody in these patients, with early chronic active hepatitis, and in our experience high titres of M-antibody and ANA are virtually mutually exclusive. MacKay, however, found M-antibody in 5% of his cases of lupoid hepatitis[32]. In contrast to our findings in HBsAg positive viral hepatitis[37], antibodies against vascular endothelium are not found in these patients.

Clinical course

The clinical course in a typical case of lupoid hepatitis is illustrated in Figure 10.5. The patient (M.B.) born in 1955 was first noted to have jaundiced sclera in school and was referred to hospital in July 1972. There were no other cases of hepatitis at the school. At that time the serum bilirubin was 4·7 mg% and the alanine and aspartate transaminases were moderately raised at 170 I.U./litre. There was no past history of note apart from measles and mumps in childhood. The menarche occurred in 1970. In January 1972 she developed amenorrhea and this was treated in April 1972 with estradiol.

On admission to hospital the bilirubin was increased to 5 mg%, the transaminase levels were in excess of 300 I.U./litre, and tests for HB_SAg were negative. The serum immunoglobulins were increased $\times 2\frac{1}{2}$ above normal. Following the institution of corticosteroid (prednisolone) therapy a fall in transaminase levels occurred, followed by a subsequent increase on their withdrawal. D-penicillamine therapy was then commenced, but she developed a severe agranulocytosis and this had led to her admission to the Med. Klinik at Tübingen in January 1973, where she has been treated since. At this time the serum immunoglobulins

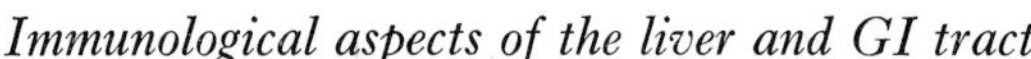

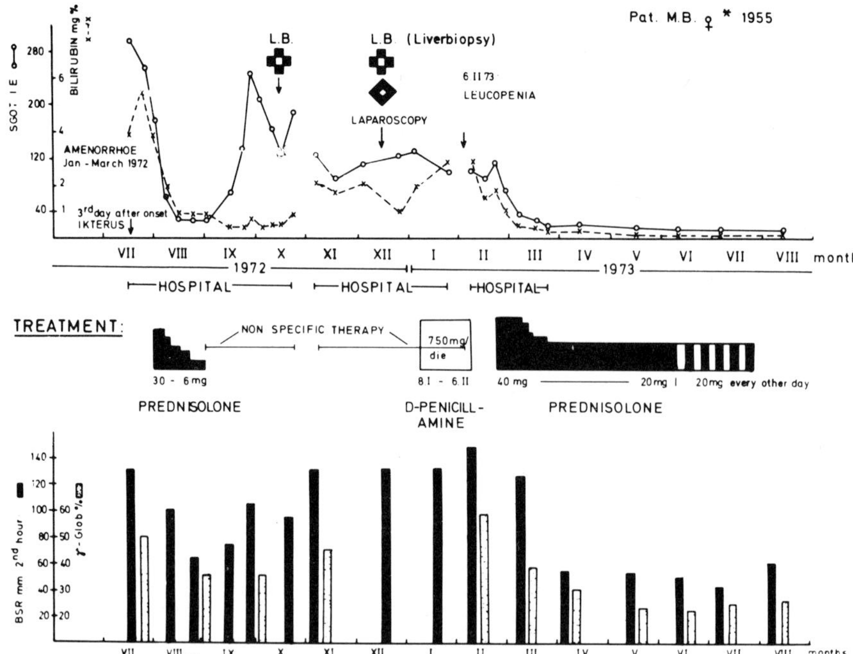

FIGURE 10.5 Early stage and progress of lupoid hepatitis in a 17-year-old female patient. In the upper block the sequential changes in serum alanine transaminase (SGOT—I.U./litre) and bilirubin (mg%) are shown; in the lower block the BSR erythrocyte sedimentation rate (BSR—mm 2nd hour) and immunoglobulin levels (normal range 15–20%) are shown

were × 3 above normal, and ANA was demonstrated in a titre of 1/2000. Steroid therapy was re-instituted in March 1973, and the serum transaminase and serum bilirubin showed a progressive return to normal, and the immunoglobulins also became normal some 13 months later. When last tested (May 1975) ANA was demonstrable to a titre of 1/20. SMA has remained weakly positive throughout. Liver biopsy in October 1972 and in December 1972 showed classical features of chronic active hepatitis. The most recent biopsy in 1974 showed portal tract fibrosis, regenerative hepatocytes, and Kupffer cell hyperplasia. More recent laparoscopic examination showed an early hepatic cirrhosis.

We have observed similar findings in a further five patients, of age range 10-16 years, who have been under our care since 1971. All had ANA in varying titres but present persistently; SMA was also sometimes found, but HBsAg and HBsAb have been consistently absent. Multi-system involvement, previously noted not infrequently in lupoid hepatitis[31,38], has not been a feature in these cases. Disturbances in lung diffusion, thyroid dysfunction, and inflammatory bowel disease have been actively excluded. In one of these patients we have noted raised serum amylase and diastase levels over a 2-year period, and so a chronic (? autoimmune) pancreatitis must be considered.

The occurrence of symptoms such as arthralgia, purpura, pleuritis and nephritis suggested immune complex phenomena. A reduction of C_4 in all forms of chronic liver disease (particularly in association with hypergammaglobulinaemia), and decreased levels of C_3 have also been reported in chronic active hepatitis[39–42]. These findings, however, do not necessarily indicate the occurrence of immune complexes, and could result from a reduced hepatic synthetic rate or from an increased catabolism of these factors as part of the hepatitis *per se*. A number of other immunological phenomena have been described in lupoid hepatitis, but these do not have any essential diagnostic significance. Rheumatoid factor, and gastric and thyroid microsomal antibodies, are frequently observed[24], but are generally only temporarily present. A false positive Wassermann reaction may occur, and in contrast to HBsAg associated chronic active hepatitis, these patients also have high titres of rubella and measles antibodies[43]. There have been few reports on the frequency of cryoglobulins. Where they have been demonstrated they appear to be predominantly of a mixed type, and in three cryoprecipitates examined antibody activity against smooth muscle and IgG (rheumatoid factor) could be demonstrated[44]. Jori and Buonanno[45] examined 11 patients with cryoglobulinaemia and in all instances the liver showed histological evidence of either chronic persistent or chronic active hepatitis.

Late stage with insidious onset: Lupoid hepatitis more commonly pursues a subclinical course and presents only in the later stages[19]. The patients present with general malaise, lethargy, and loss of appetite. There are no features to suggest an acute hepatitis, and the diagnosis is suspected only when the serum transaminases are found to be elevated. On occasion they present with mild jaundice. Hepatosplenomegaly is almost invariable, the liver being of a firm consistency. There may be spider naevi and occasionally ascites. If the patients present because of an acute exacerbation the liver function tests show a pattern similar to that found in early lupoid hepatitis, with transaminases in excess of 300 I.U./litre and elevation of immunoglobulins, particularly IgG. The bilirubin is only moderately raised, but in relapse can increase to 10–15 mg%. The alkaline phosphatase is normal or only marginally increased. Estimations of hepatic synthetic activity vary depending on the degree of disease activity, and the prothrombin time fibrinogen factors V and VII, and serum albumin fluctuate accordingly. The bromsulphthalein retention test is almost always abnormal.

Morphologically the liver shows typical features of chronic active hepatitis and in some there may already be an established macronodular cirrhosis. In acute exacerbations an extensive lobular hepatitis may be superadded. Bile duct lesions may also be seen and the differentiation from primary biliary cirrhosis may then be more difficult[12,15,19]. Klatskin and Kantor[46] reported on 22 patients, all M-antibody positive, who had atypical progressive primary biliary cirrhosis, and in 19 of whom the histological pattern showed an established cirrhosis which they described as postnecrotic. They concluded that the syndrome of postnecrotic cirrhosis with evidence of cholestasis represented a late manifestation of primary biliary cirrhosis. However, the differential diagnosis in such cases can be difficult. Presumed overlap between primary biliary cirrhosis and chronic active hepatitis are described both on the basis of the morphology and of the clinical course[9,21,47–49], and the serological findings in both of M-antibody and ANA would further support this[50]. However, we believe the M-antibody positive chronic active hepatitis exhibits a particular type of progress which can also be distinguished from the ANA positive chronic active or lupoid hepatitis.

M-ANTIBODY (HETEROGENEOUS) POSITIVE CHRONIC ACTIVE HEPATITIS

This type affects mainly middle-aged women around or after the menopause[9,51]. The initial symptoms may simulate acute viral hepatitis with tiredness, loss of energy, occasionally pruritus, fever and rigors. The liver and spleen are palpably enlarged. The bilirubin can be transiently raised to 10–15 mg%, and the alkaline phosphatase is almost invariably increased although perhaps less than that seen in classical primary biliary cirrhosis. In contrast to lupoid hepatitis both the IgG and IgM can simultaneously be elevated. Multisystem involvement seems to appear more frequently than in primary biliary cirrhosis or lupoid hepatitis and in a retrospective analysis we found a number of patients who in addition had rheumatoid arthritis, scleroderma, Sjøgren's syndrome, myocarditis, and pulmonary interstitial fibrosis. Serologically the M-antibody is of the heterogeneous type previously described, its titre fluctuating during the course of the illness. ANA and SMA may be transiently positive but usually in low titre.

The clinical courses of two such patients' cases are illustrated in Figures 10.6 and 10.7. The female patient (E.J.) died in 1970 as a result of bleeding from esophageal varices; liver biopsy had been refused and no autopsy was performed. The insidious course, with symptoms resembling cholangitis, the acute exacerbations, multisystem involvement, the early detected simultaneous elevation of IgG and IgM and the raised alkaline phosphatase are observations which resemble those found in primary biliary cirrhosis. The course of the disease with a lack of any progressive increase in transaminase and bilirubin levels militate against such a diagnosis and favour either chronic active hepatitis or the mixed form showing in addition features of biliary involvement.

Similarly with patient L.M. (Figures 10.7 and 10.8) primary biliary cirrhosis was considered as the initial diagnosis because of the elevated

Clinical	1955	1956	1960	1963	1965	1968	1969	1970
	Cholangitis	Menopause (Age 54 yr)	Tiredness Pyrexia Weight loss	Pyrexia Rigors Hepato-splenomegaly Sicca syndrome Polyarthritis (hands) Pancytopenia	No pruritus Pulmonary diffusion abnormality		Radiologically diagnosed: Esophageal varices Pulmonary interstitial fibrosis Corticosteroids 30–7·5 mg/day	
***Laboratory indices**								
			ESR	80/115	90/132	65/108	62/94	35/70
			SGOT	33	31	24	35	26
			Bilirubin	1·5	1·7	1·8	2·4	3·4
			Alkaline phos-phatase	116	116	66	93	60
			Immuno-globulins	32 IgM ↑ IgG ↑	42	35	48 IgM ↑ ↑ IG ↑	34
			Autoantibodies				ANA and SMA Positive M-antibody (heterogen-ous) —strongly positive	

FIGURE 10.6 Clinical and laboratory data in a patient E.J. (d.o.b. 2.7.03) with M-antibody (heterogeneous) chronic active hepatitis

* ESR—mm 1st hour/2nd hour; SGOT (serum aspartate transaminase—I.U./litre); bilirubin—mgm%; alkaline phosphatase—I.U./ml; immunoglobulins—relative % (normal 15–20%)

Clinical					
Tiredness Epigastric fullness	Hepatomegaly Diabetes mellitus	Radiology —cholelithiasis —peribronchitis Metalcaptase commenced	Hepato-splenomegaly Good general health	Dyspnea ST depression on ECG Azathioprine commenced	Progressive weight loss —5 kg
1966	1967	1971	1972	1973	1974
**Laboratory indices*					
ESR	32/58	63/95	60/100	56/95	25/55
SGOT	13	67	11	31	18
Bilirubin	0·2	1·0	0·5	0·8	0·5
Alkaline phosphatase	—	Raised	Normal	Normal	Normal
Immuno-globulins	23	40 IgG 20·0 IgM 3·25	25 IgG 15·6 IgM 2·97	28 IgG 21·6 IgM 4·6	32 IgG 26·0 IgM 4·36
Autoantibodies				ANA and SMA strongly positive; M-antibody (heterogenous) positive	

FIGURE 10.7 Clinical and laboratory data in a patient L.M. (d.o.b. 2.8.10; Wenckebach State Hospital, Berlin, courtesy of Prof W. D. Germer), with M-antibody (heterogeneous) chronic active hepatitis

* Indices as in Figure 10.6; absolute levels for IgG and IgM—mg/ml

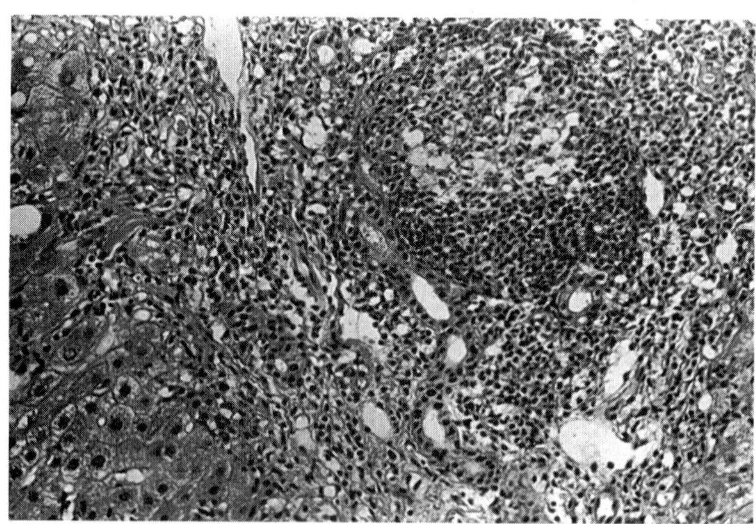

FIGURE 10.8 Liver biopsy from patient L.M. (Figure 10.7) in 1972 (courtesy of Prof C. J. Lüders, Berlin). There is a pronounced chronic inflammatory cell infiltrate of the widened portal area, with spill over into the parenchyma, and with early ductular proliferation. In addition (lower L. quadrant), there is granulomatous destruction of normal bile duct elements. Haematoxylin and eosin × 112

serum alkaline phosphatase and IgM. Subsequently, however, the characteristic increase in bilirubin seen in the latter stages of primary biliary cirrhosis was not manifest, and the alkaline phosphatase became normal. Histologically, a liver biopsy in 1967 showed a fatty liver with some periportal chronic inflammation. In 1971 liver biopsy showed features in keeping with chronic active hepatitis; a further biopsy in 1972 showed more pronounced chronic inflammation of the portal areas with cirrhosis and in addition features suggesting primary biliary cirrhosis (Figure 10.8). To date, however, we have not seen transition into a classical primary biliary cirrhosis in any of these patients. In the late stages the morphological pattern is that of a macronodular cirrhosis.

Klatskin and Kantor[46] in a series of 77 patients with chronic active hepatitis found eight with M-antibody in titres of 1/10 to 1/4000. In six of these patients, all over 40 years, the alkaline phosphatase was raised. Histologically some changes similar to those in primary biliary cirrhosis were seen, but the interlobular bile ducts were intact. In patients with cryptogenic cirrhosis these authors found only two cases with M-antibody in titres of 1/100 to 1/160, and in one of these the M-antibody was transient. Histologically the livers showed a 'post-necrotic' (macronodular) cirrhotic pattern.

The interpretation of these findings is primarily of interest in relation to the symptoms and signs of the pseudo-lupus syndrome. These resemble serum sickness with recurring bouts of fever, arthralgia, myositis, pleuritis and pericarditis, and the syndrome is now considered to be drug induced.[25-29]. There is today no doubt that therapeutic agents can produce a clinical picture resembling chronic active hepatitis and primary biliary cirrhosis[57], and with the typical serum autoantibody profiles[53]. Martini and Dölle[54] drew attention in 1960 to the frequency of laxative abuse by women developing cryptogenic cirrhosis perimenopausally. Autoantibodies develop in halothane-induced hepatitis and, although initially considered to be antimitochondrial, more recent evidence suggests that they are directed against a microsomal antigen[30,53].

One could speculate that in the chronic active hepatitis associated with heterogeneous M-antibody, a hypersensitivity reaction to some exogenous or therapeutic agent might play a supplementary role in the clinical picture. Conceivably, such a hypersensitivity reaction superimposed on a basic organ-specific autoimmune hepatitis of a cell-mediated immune nature could, with the development of circulating immune complexes, lead to symptomatic multisystem manifestations.

Medical management

At present the medical management of chronic active hepatitis is the same irrespective of the possible aetiology and/or serological findings. The mainstay of therapy is the corticosteroids, and carefully controlled trials in England, Denmark and the USA indicate that they alone or combined with the immunosuppressant azathioprine (immuran) increase the survival rate in both younger and older patients even with advanced chronic active hepatitis[55–59]. Corticosteroids (prednisolone) may be used alone, or else may be combined with azathioprine. Azathioprine alone seems to be less effective and should therefore not be used in this way[56]. The initial steroid dosage should be of the order of 30–40 mg/day, and the maintenance dose will have to be individually 'titrated' against the clinical and biochemical findings, but is generally of the order of 7·5–20 mg/day. Alternate day therapy with prednisolone appears to be less effective than daily administration. The combination with azathioprine has the advantage that the steroid dose may be reduced thus decreasing the risk of steroid-induced side effects. After an initial dose of 100 mg a maintenance dose of 50–75 mg/day of azathioprine is adequate, and is combined with maintenance doses of 5–10 mg/day of prednisolone.

The duration of therapy is dependent on the patients' clinical progress. Too rapid or too early a reduction in medication can result in clinical relapse which may be more difficult to control than the initial attack. Long-term therapy must therefore be aimed at, and consequently the side effects of osteoporosis, bleeding from ulcers, diabetes mellitus, and recurrent infections have to be accepted as not infrequent complications.

It is not always easy to determine at what point in time to initiate chemotherapy. Spontaneous remissions probably occur more frequently than are appreciated and are obscured by the immediate initiation of chemotherapy. The early form of lupoid hepatitis is best treated consistently and *ab initio*. In an older age group with only moderate elevations of IgG, low titres of serum autoantibodies and lack of extrahepatic manifestations, one should have regard for the complications of long-term immunosuppressive therapy and follow the spontaneous course of the disease for a period. Repeated and regular liver biopsies should in all cases be carried out to assess the adequacy of medical management.

Primary biliary cirrhosis

Introduction

Although the first case was described by Addison and Gull in 1851[60], the term primary biliary cirrhosis was first applied to the disease by Dauphinee and Sinclair in 1949[61]. The disease has been variously known as hypertrophic hepatic cirrhosis, chronic intrahepatic obliterating cholangitis, cholangiolitic or pericholangiolitic biliary cirrhosis xanthomatous biliary cirrhosis, and chronic non-suppurative destructive cholangitis[62–70]. Ahrens and his colleagues[71] clearly separated biliary cirrhosis into primary and secondary types distinguishing between them respectively on the basis of the small radicle and major duct biliary obstruction present. In 1965 Walker *et al.*[72] using an immunofluorescent technique first described an autoantibody (the M-antibody) in the serum of patients with primary biliary cirrhosis, an antibody directed against cell mitochondria and which was neither organ nor species specific. The M-antibody is found in the serum of over 90% of patients, and this highly selective association has resulted in the more frequent recognition of the disease and it has therefore come to be more clearly defined. It presents as a much more homogeneous disease entity than chronic active hepatitis, and the diagnosis is frequently suggested on the clinical history and biochemical findings.

Clinical course

Sex and age

The disease predominantly affects women in middle age. In our experience of some 137* patients the female to male ratio was 20:1[73], but in other large series approximately 10% of the patients are male. Any explanation of the aetiology of the disease must take cognisance of this marked sex difference. The mean age at presentation in our series

* Collaborative studies by one of us (R.N.M.Mc.S.) with Dr Geoffrey Watkinson and Dr Sheila Ross, Western Infirmary, Glasgow.

was 55 years, and although the range was from 30 to 76 years, the very large majority presented in the 5th or 6th decade.

Mode of presentation

The disease is of insidious onset, and characteristically the patient presents with either a history of intractable pruritus, worse at night, or with mild jaundice frequently accompanied by intense pruritus. The pruritus may result in referral to dermatologists, or the obstructive pattern of the liver function tests may result in surgical intervention but with no evident extrahepatic obstruction demonstrable. Pruritus may antedate the onset of jaundice for as long as 10 years, and in some patients this may be true despite continuing biochemical and histological evidence of progressive hepatocellular damage. Other less frequent modes of presentation include the incidental discovery of hepatomegaly, raised serum alkaline phosphatase or the presence of M-antibody, the occurrence of vague upper abdominal pain often localised to the right hypochondrium, and only very infrequently is presentation delayed till the onset of portal hypertension and its complications.

Liver function tests

The pattern of routine liver function tests in a series of 36 patients and the sequential pattern of tests in one patient are shown in Figures 10.9 and 10.10 respectively. Many patients show only a mild degree of bilirubinaemia in the earlier stages; a progressive slow rise takes place over the last few years, but only infrequently are levels in excess of 20 mg/100 ml attained. The most characteristic abnormality is the marked elevation of the serum alkaline phosphatase level, this from the earliest stage of presentation, but with a tendency for a fall to occur in the later stages of the disease. The serum transaminases show moderate elevations of the order of 100 I.U./litre, with the glutamic aspartate transaminase (SGOT) usually slightly higher than the alanine transaminase (SGPT). The serum cholesterol is elevated in more than 50% of patients and may occasionally attain very high levels (in excess of 1500 mg/100 ml). This has recently been shown to be due to reduced cholesterol metabolism secondary to a reduced conversion to bile salts, which are retained in biliary cirrhosis[74].

Clinical signs

Skin pigmentation, resembling an intense sun tan, most marked on the

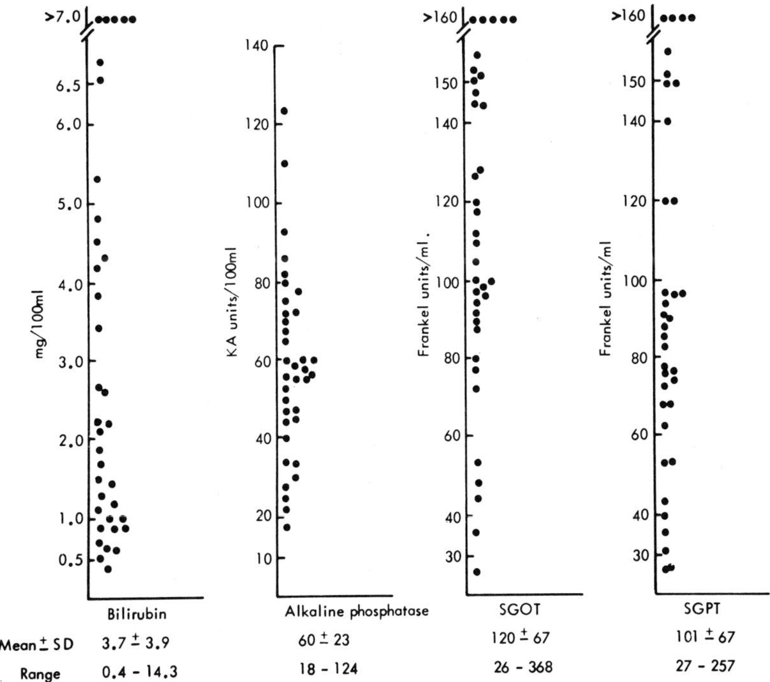

FIGURE 10.9 Results of liver function tests in 36 patients with primary biliary cirrhosis. Bilirubin—mg/100 ml; alkaline phosphatase—King Armstrong Units/100 ml; serum aspartate (SGOT) and alanine transaminases (SGPT)—Frankel Units/ml. (Normal values < 40 units/ml).

exposed parts, but also present on the trunk and in skin folds, is a characteristic feature in half the patients, and this pigmentation may develop simultaneously with the pruritus or may occasionally antedate the pruritus. Xanthomata/xanthelasma occur in a third of patients, usually in the later stages, and are associated with serum cholesterol levels in excess of 600 mg/100 ml. A very few patients develop xanthomatous neuropathy[74].

The degree of hepatomegaly varies, in approximately a third being slight, in a third of moderate degree and in a third massive with the liver edge being palpable in the right iliac fossa. We have been impressed in some patients with progressive hepatic enlargement over a period of years.

Splenomegaly, usually only of a moderate degree, occurs in a little more than half of patients and may be associated with haematological evidence of hypersplenism in 20%. Clinical and radiological evidence of portal hypertension is uncommon in the early stages of the disease[75],

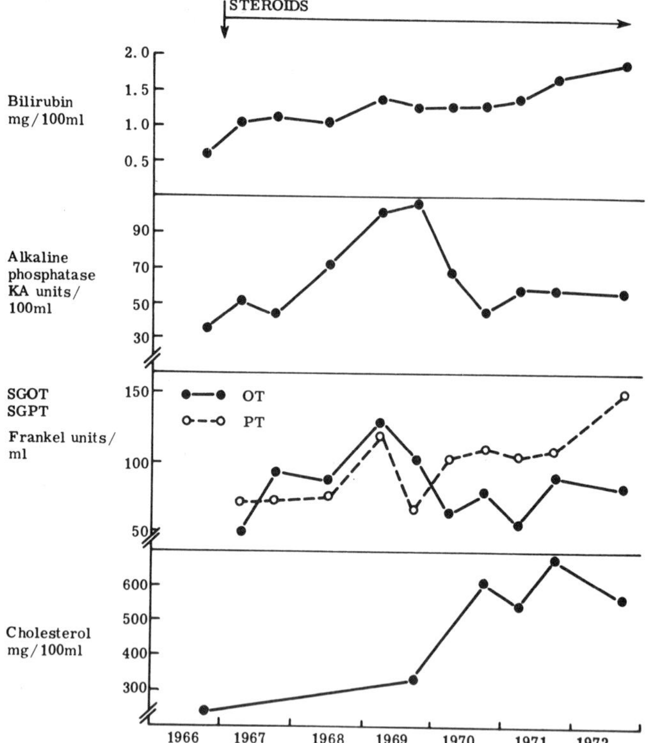

FIGURE 10.10 Pattern of sequential liver function tests in a female patient (53 years at presentation) with primary biliary cirrhosis. Liver biopsy in 1970 showed Stage 3 changes

but later this may be found in up to 50% of cases[76], and fatal bleeding from esophageal varices may occur in 25%. Ascites and hepatic encephalopathy occur uncommonly and only in the later stages of primary biliary cirrhosis.

Prognosis and cause of death

The mean duration of the liver disease in a series of 52 fatal cases in our own series was 5 years, with a range from 6 months to 15 years. Survival periods of 11–18 years have been recorded by others[71,77–79]. Progressive hepatocellular failure was the primary cause of death in 70% of these 52 patients, and, as previously mentioned, gastrointestinal bleeding occurred in 13 of the 52 (25%). A primary hepatocellular carcinoma supervened in three of the 52 patients (6%). Death in the remaining patients was due to incidental unrelated causes, and in particular, despite the hyperlipidaemia, cardiovascular disease was not a prominent feature. This has been the experience of others[78,79], and is contrary to Schaffner's assertion that 10% of patients had significant cardiovascular disease[80].

Morphological features

Although the disease is called primary biliary cirrhosis *ab initio*, the term is rather a misnomer in that a true cirrhosis with linkage of fibrous septa, disruption of normal architecture and the development of regenerating nodules occurs later in the pathological process. The pathological changes have been described in a number of recent studies[14,70,81–83], and are divided into four stages as follows.

Stage 1

Specific bile duct injury (Figures 10.11 and 10.12). This is characterized by the destruction of the small interlobular or septal bile ducts and the process has been accurately described as that of a non-suppurative destructive cholangitis[70]. The epithelium of affected bile ducts becomes irregular and swollen with vacuolation of the cell cytoplasm and heaping up of the cells producing irregular distortion of the luminal margin. Occasional lymphocytes and plasma cells may be seen invading through and within the basement membrane of the affected ducts[81,82]. Surrounding these ducts there is a dense mixed inflammatory cell infiltrate predominantly of lymphocytes and plasma cells, but with conspicuous numbers of macrophages often containing PAS positive granules, and a few neutrophil polymorphs. This chronic inflammatory cell infiltrate also involves the rest of the involved portal tracts, and may sometimes form focal aggregates in which lymphoid follicles occur. However, the limiting plate usually remains intact, and the abutting hepatocytes are conspicuously normal. Some mild Kupffer cell hyperplasia is, however, usually evident. Cholestasis is not seen, sometimes even in the presence of clinical jaundice. Granuloma formation is seen in approximately a third of cases, sometimes with multinucleate giant cells, and direct granulomatous destruction of bile duct elements may be a feature. In less than 5% of cases aggregates of foamy macrophages—xanthoma cells—may be present in portal tracts or at the periphery of lobules. These changes initially affect only a proportion of the portal tracts and in

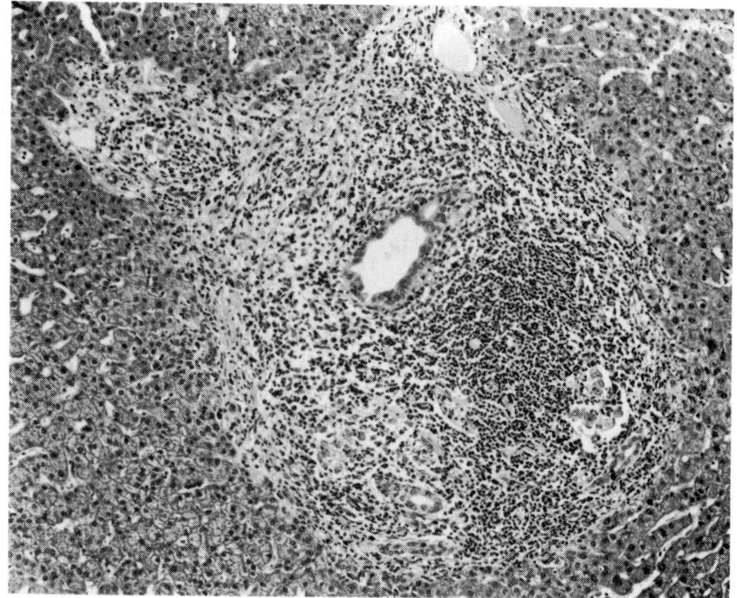

FIGURE 10.11 Stage 1 of primary biliary cirrhosis with an intense partly focal chronic inflammatory cell infiltrate of a portal area; the bile duct present appears abnormal, and granulomatous destruction of further biliary radicles is evident in the lower right quadrant. Haematoxylin and eosin × 90

biopsy at this stage normal portal tracts with intact spared bile ducts are found.

Stage 2

Ductular proliferation (Figure 10.13). With progressive destruction of the normal bile ducts, compensatory ductular proliferation develops. The portal tracts become enlarged, and virtually all of them are involved at this stage. The mixed chronic inflammatory cell infiltrate begins to spill over into the surrounding parenchyma. There is an accompanying proliferation of fibrous tissue, and with extension of these from the portal tracts the lobules become involved in the inflammatory process with focal piecemeal necrosis of the peripheral hepatocytes. Cholestasis may be present at this stage and is characteristically peripheral in the lobule. Deposits of Mallory's hyaline may also appear in peripheral hepatocytes and are seen in 25% of cases[84].

Stage 3

Scarring. In this stage fibrous scarring develops and extension of

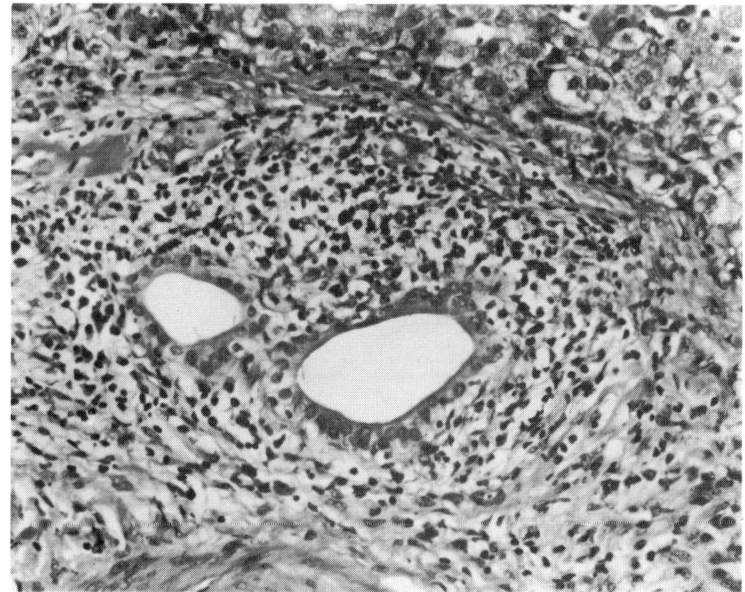

FIGURE 10.12 Irregular swelling and vacuolation of bile duct epithelium with lymphocytic invasion of the basement membrane in Stage 1 of primary biliary cirrhosis. Haematoxylin and eosin × 223

fibrous septae from the portal tracts occurs tending to surround individual lobules in a monolobular pattern. Bile duct elements are by now conspicuously scant, the ductular proliferation tends to become less marked, and the chronic inflammatory cell infiltrate less intense with the residual infiltration often forming focal aggregates. Peripheral cholestasis becomes more evident, and there is continuing inflammatory damage and piecemeal necrosis of hepatocytes.

Stage 4

Established cirrhosis (Figure 10.14). With linking up of fibrous septa a true biliary cirrhosis of a monolobular pattern becomes established, and is accompanied by the development of regenerating nodules producing gross distortion of the normal hepatic architecture. A further reduction in the intensity of the chronic inflammatory cell infiltrate occurs. There is now usually an intense degree of cholestasis at the periphery of the nodules. At this stage the features are those of an end-stage micronodular cirrhotic liver in which pointers to the true diagnosis of a primary biliary disease process are provided by the lack of bile duct elements, the

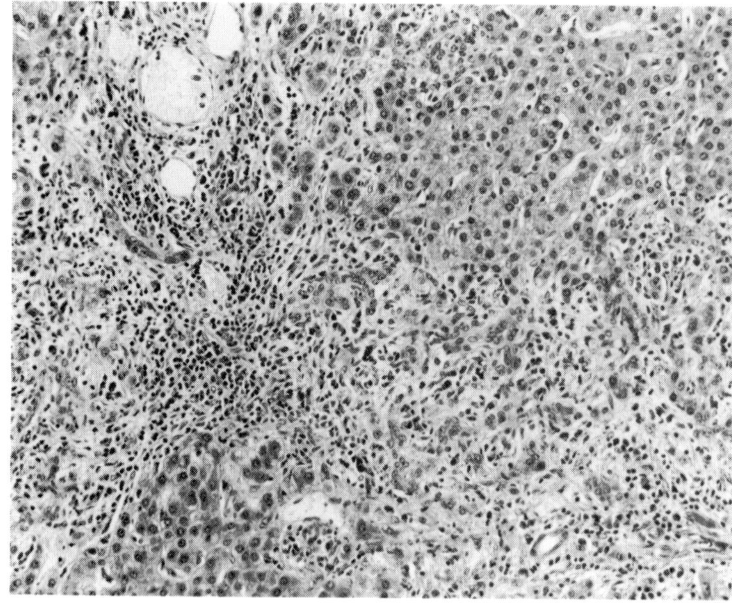

FIGURE 10.13 Stage 2 of primary biliary cirrhosis with irregular enlargement of portal area, prominent ductular proliferation and extension of chronic inflammatory cell infiltrate into neighbouring lobules. Haematoxylin and eosin × 136

presence of focal chronic inflammatory cell aggregates and the peripheral distribution of the cholestasis.

Immunological abnormalities

While some of the pathological features just described are the morphological expressions of an immune reaction, it has only been since the description of the M-antibody[72], that primary biliary cirrhosis has come to be regarded as a possible autoimmune or immune mediated disease. It is appropriate therefore to examine those clinico-immunological associations that have been described.

Serum autoantibodies

In our series of 137 patients the M-antibody was present in 97%[73], and it is now generally accepted that this marker occurs usually in more than 90% of cases[24,46,75,82,85,86]. In the present series no attempt was made to examine for M-antibody (heterogeneous) by complement fixation testing (v.s.). The antibody in all cases was demonstrated by a

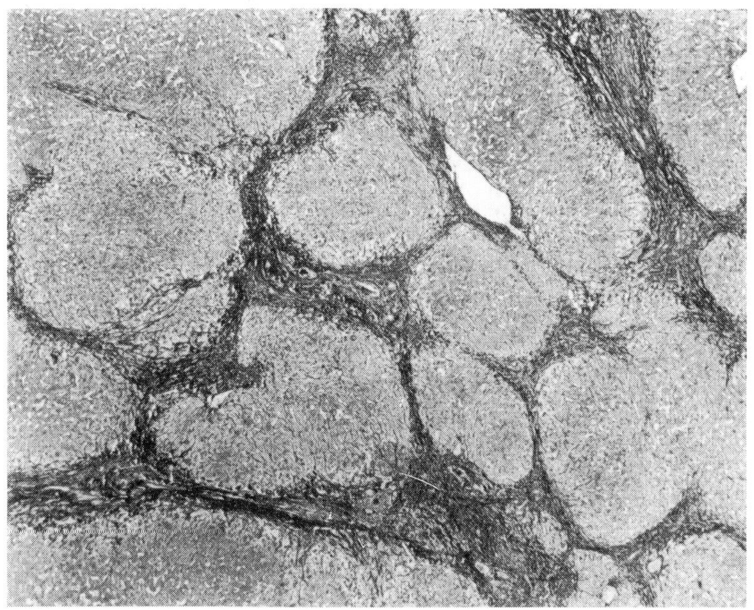

FIGURE 10.14 End stage primary biliary cirrhosis with an established microdular cirrhotic pattern. Gordon and Sweet's reticulin × 137

simple indirect immunofluorescent technique using rat kidney as substrate[82]. Any cell type rich in mitochondria can, however, be used in the test. Affected patients without antibody appear to be no different from those which are seropositive. The antibody is present in high titre, and in over 80% of our patients the titre was 1/128 or greater. It is directed against a lipoprotein antigen constituent of the inner membrane of mitochondria[87,88], and although predominantly present in the IgG class, it may also occur in the IgA and IgM globulin fractions[85]. Neither the presence nor the titre of M-antibody has been shown to correlate with any other clinical or serological parameter in primary biliary cirrhosis. The titre does not vary with severity or progression of the disease, nor has it been of value as a prognostic or therapeutic index, persisting in one patient in whom orthotopic transplantation was performed[85].

However, the presence of the M-antibody is of considerable differential diagnostic value. Except in a very small number of cases with both conditions, we have yet to find the antibody in the serum of proven cases of extrahepatic obstruction, the main differential diagnosis in patients suspected of having primary biliary cirrhosis. With one exception[89], as yet unconfirmed, the general experience has been that M-antibody occurs in less than 2% of patients with simple extrahepatic obstruction and then in only low titre[46,90]. Reference has already been made to the occurrence of M-antibody with different antigentic specificities in some patients with chronic active hepatitis and the PLE syndrome. Transient low titre M-antibody has been noted in a very small percentage of patients with drug induced liver damage[91]. The mechanisms of its induction are not understood nor is there any evidence as yet of its having any pathogenetic or deleterious cytopathological role in any of these disease processes.

The prevalence of other autoantibodies[35,92–95] in our series is summarized in Table 10.5. Smooth muscle antibody (18% positive) was no more frequent than in controls, although other workers have reported this antibody in 30–50% of primary biliary cirrhosis patients but usually in low titre[24,85,96]. The extact significance, if any, of the bile canalicular antibody is not yet clear. The antibody occurred concurrently with smooth muscle antibody in 13 of the 39 patients in whom it was found. This antibody may also occur in a significant number of patients with acute hepatitis[93], and while it was considered as a possible organ specific antibody, recent reports of its occurrence in a number of non-hepatic diseases and the different immunofluorescent staining patterns produced require further investigation[97].

Our observation that rheumatoid factor was present in 64% of patients with primary biliary cirrhosis is comparable to the 68% preva-

Table 10.5 SERUM AUTOANTIBODIES IN PRIMARY BILIARY CIRRHOSIS (PBC) PATIENTS AND IN AGE- AND SEX-MATCHED CONTROLS

	PBC % *positive*	*Controls* % *positive*
* Smooth muscle antibody (111)	18	13·5
* Bile canalicular antibody (111)	35·1	20·7
* Antinuclear antibody (112)	11·6	14·3
† Thyroglobulin antibody (113)	2·6	2·6
‡ Rheumatoid factor (114)	64·0	15·8

* Tested by immunofluorescent techniques[92,93,135]
† Tested by a tanned red cell agglutination technique[94]
‡ Tested by a slide agglutination technique[95] (Rheumaton, Warner Laboratories Ltd.)

lence reported by Paronetto *et al.*[98], and like them we found the antibody to be present in low titre—72% with a titre of 1/64 or less (R_3 latex kit—Warner Laboratories Ltd.)[95]. The significance of rheumatoid factor in the sera of primary biliary cirrhosis patients and in the sera of patients with a variety of chronic diseases is not known.

Immunoglobulins and complement

Increases in all three major classes of immunoglobulin have been described[96,99–101]. The IgM level is most consistently elevated, the IgG level usually and the IgA level less frequently. Increased IgM levels were found by us in 82% of a series of 73 patients, and with a mean elevation of 174% as compared with controls[101]. These serum immunoglobulin pattern changes, however, are not diagnostic and in particular are of limited value in differentiating between primary biliary disease and extrahepatic obstruction. The antigenic specificities of the immunoglobulins are not known, and the mechanisms of development remain uncertain (see Chapter 7).

Normal levels of the third component of complement (C_3) have been reported[101,102]. Potter and his colleagues, however, reported increased levels of C_3, and of total haemolytic complement activity (CH_{50}) and decreased levels of C_4 in well compensated primary biliary cirrhosis. Both the C_3 and CH_{50} levels however, were decreased in primary biliary cirrhosis patients who had developed ascites[42]. These findings were different from those in patients with chronic active hepatitis and cryptogenic cirrhosis, and suggested definable differences between the three diseases in terms of the pattern of changes in serum complement. In more recent studies these same workers have demonstrated hypercatabolism of C_3 in primary biliary cirrhosis patients, with an increase in the fractional catabolic rate accompanied by an increased synthetic rate, results which they interpreted as indicating that the complement system was activated[103].

Cell-mediated immune responses

Examination of cell-mediated immune responses have been carried out primarily as an attempt to define possible pathogenetic mechanisms in primary biliary cirrhosis (see Chapters 8 and 9). The results obtained both by *in vivo* skin testing and *in vitro* testing of lymphocyte responses to mitogenic agents, suggest that patients with the disease are anergic[104,105]. There is debate as to whether this anergic state antedates the development of primary biliary cirrhosis or whether it is a secondary manifestation. In our own studies using phytohaemagglutinin stimulation of peripheral blood lymphocytes, impaired responsiveness was demonstrable in asymptomatic patients in whom the liver biopsy showed Stage 1 histological changes[105]. It is still not clear whether the *in vivo* and *in vitro* results indicate an intrinsic defect in or quantitative reduction of T lymphocytes, or whether the results are due to the readily demonstrable serum inhibitory factors which are found in these patients[106]. Paronetto and his colleagues[107] have shown a marked increase in the numbers of a circulating subpopulation of lymphocytes actively involved in cell mediated immune mechanisms accompanied by a marked increase of B lymphocytes (see Chapter 9).

Clinical associations

Clinical overlap between the various autoimmune diseases is well recognized, in particular in the organ specific group involving thyroid, stomach and adrenal. Primary biliary cirrhosis has been shown to be associated with rheumatoid arthritis, the sicca complex (keratoconjunctivitis sicca and xerostomia) and Sjøgren's syndrome, with systemic sclerosis and other components of the CRST syndrome (calcinosis cutis, Raynaud's phenomenon, sclerodactyly and telangiectasia). In addition reference has already been made to the apparent overlap which can occur with chronic active hepatitis.

In our series rheumatoid arthritis was reported in 10 of 137 patients (7%) comparable to the 6% described by Sherlock and Scheuer[108]. We found keratoconjunctivitis sicca in 12 of 31 patients (39%), considerably less than the 72% incidence reported by Golding and his colleagues[109], and ten-fold higher than Sherlock's experience[108]. Those patients with the sicca complex showed no other differences when compared with the series as a whole. In a series of patients with the sicca complex or Sjøgren's syndrome, the M-antibody was found in 10 of 134 patients nine of whom showed clinical and/or biochemical evidence of liver disease and in three of whom liver biopsy showed features of primary biliary cirrhosis[110]. The association between primary biliary cirrhosis and the sicca complex appears real. It is of interest that in both diseases there is hypergammaglobulinaemia, an increased incidence of non-organ specific autoantibodies and evidence of impaired cell mediated immunity. Furthermore, as Schaffner[111] has pointed out, there are histological similarities between the lesions in the salivary and lachrymal glands and those in the liver.

Reynolds and his colleagues[112,113] first drew attention to the association of the CRST syndrome and primary biliary cirrhosis, describing its occurrence in six of 41 cirrhotic patients. A further 14 examples of this association have since been reported[46,114,115], and in our series of 137 patients features of the CRST syndrome were present in six. Thus the co-existence of the CRST syndrome in primary biliary cirrhosis is approximately 6%. Klatskin and Kantor[46] noted that the incidence of primary biliary cirrhosis in their series of 29 patients with various facets of the CRST syndrome was 38%. The occurrence of liver disease in systemic sclerosis appears to be low, Bartholomew *et al.* finding cirrhosis in only seven of 72 cases[116]. Levrat *et al.*[117] have recently described a patient with primary biliary cirrhosis, systemic sclerosis and Sjøgren's syndrome, and Schaffner has seen two similar cases[111]. The occurrence of these rare disease complexes is of considerable interest, and it is tempting to speculate that similar mechanisms modified by certain host factors are responsible for their pathogenesis.

Clinical and/or serological evidence of thyroid disease was found in seven (5%) of our series of patients, which is comparable to the 6% incidence of thyroiditis reported by Sherlock and Scheuer[108]. Doniach and Walker[85] found thyroid specific antibodies in 15% of 100 patients with primary biliary cirrhosis. An association of interstitial pulmonary fibrosis and chronic liver disease has been noted[118], and this was a complication in two (1·5%) of our patients.

Medical management

No specific treatment for primary biliary cirrhosis has been discovered. In general, corticosteroids and more recently azathioprine have been used. No trials of corticosteroid therapy have been carried out, and in fact Sherlock[75] categorically states that they are contraindicated because of hastening of the osteoporosis which complicates the late stage of the disease. Azathioprine is currently being used in an international 'double blind' trial (sponsored by the International Association for the Study of the Liver). Ross *et al.* however in a controlled trial involving 22 patients have reported negative results with this drug[119].

The intense pruritus can be well controlled by the oral use of cholestyramine, a bile acid sequestering resin. The secondary metabolic bone disease is ameliorated by the administration of vitamin D[120] and intravenous calcium infusion in addition have been reported as of benefit in the relief of bone pain[121]. In the few cases in which xanthomatous neuropathy develops, treatment by plasmapheresis has been found beneficial[74].

Conclusions

In view of the close embryological and anatomical relationships between hepatocytes and biliary epithelium, it has been inferred by some workers that overlap between the disease processes involving these structures is not surprising. The unifying postulate[50], that as a result of a continuing autoimmune process affecting hepatocytes or bile ducts, progression ensues to chronic active hepatitis or primary biliary cirrhosis, or to cryptogenic cirrhosis depending on the varying degree of involvement of these cell types, is probably too simple. The fact that the two diseases can exist as separate distinct entities is not consistent with such a concept. Further evidence against this view is also provided by the association of HBAg with some forms of chronic active hepatitis[33,51,122–127], and of the histocompatibility antigen HLA-8 with HBAg negative chronic active hepatitis; neither of these associations has been shown for primary biliary cirrhosis[127,128]. The differing specificities of the M-antibodies as reported in this chapter provides further evidence for there being two separate disease entities.

Although the recognition and definition of chronic active hepatitis as an autoimmune disorder was initially based on a relatively insensitive test with limited specificity, this concept has gained widespread general acceptance. The various subdivisions which we have outlined on the basis of virological and autoantibody markers are not sharply defined, and in fact they may show some of the same immune phenomena so that some authors have rejected the validity of a separate pathogenesis for the autoimmune form[38,129–135]. Meantime as a result of greater refinements in immunological investigation, such as the demonstration of cell mediated immunity against liver specific antigens, it has become possible to think in terms of autoaggressive mechanisms which bear a close relationship to the course of chronic active hepatitis whether it be HBAg associated or otherwise[135–137]. Similar techniques need to be applied in primary biliary cirrhosis and the definition of the host immune defect must become the central problem in attempts to explain the progressive chronicity in these forms of hepatitis[138].

The characterization of antigens specific for different forms of chronic liver disease (i.e. the attempt to define the various antibody specificites more precisely) seems to us a reasonable approach which will provide immunological tests better able to differentiate between them. In addition they may help explain their interrelationships with each other and with other disease entities (Figure 10.15). The association of the

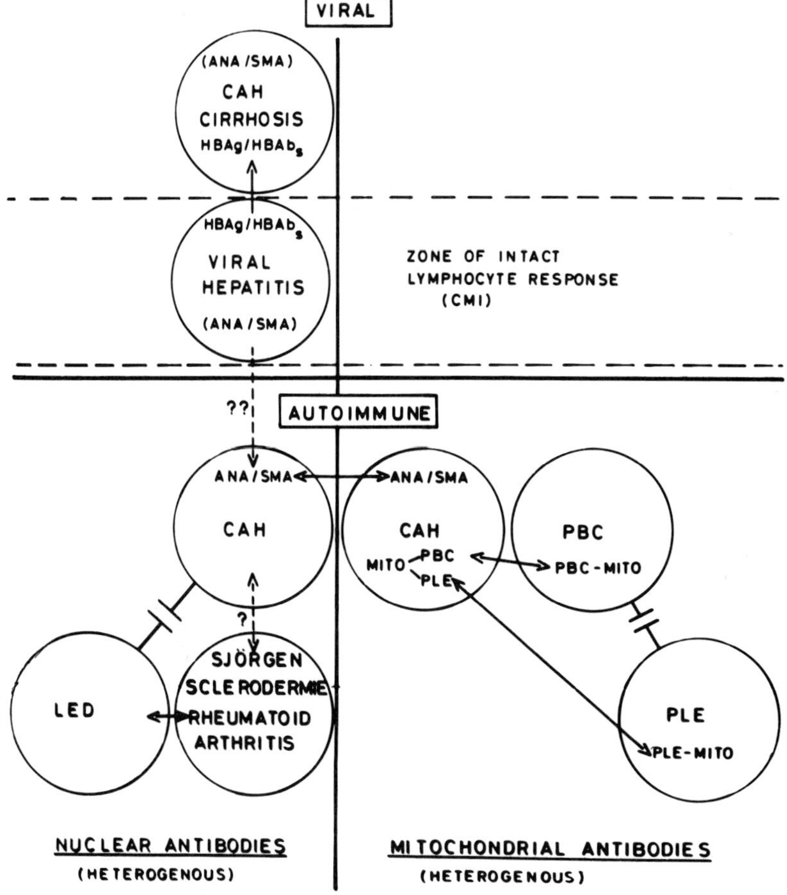

FIGURE 10.15 The different types of autoimmune liver diseases and their relationship to viral B hepatitis and other collagen diseases. LED—lupus erythematosus; CAH—chronic active hepatitis; PBC—primary biliary cirrhosis; PLE*—pseudo-lupus erythematosus. ANA—antinuclear antibodies; SMA—smooth muscle antibodies; Mito—anti-mitochondrial antibodies; CMI—cell mediated immunity.

(* PBC antigen-free sucrose gradient fraction containing approximately 60% PLE antigen and other cytoplasmic constituents)

PLE antigen with a drug induced hypersensitivity disease[25], raises hope of developing other test systems able to distinguish between virus-induced and drug-induced chronic hepatitis. The reports of the isolation of specific antigens from the pool of nuclear antigens[139,140], and the further characterization of the antigen system of smooth muscle, together with the possible associations of these antigens with defined disease processes, are advances which may help further our understanding of some forms of chronic liver disease.

REFERENCES

1. Waldenstroem, J. (1950). Leberblutproteine und Nahrungsgenesis—Stoffwechsel. Report of session: Bad Kissingen, special volume 15, p. 8
2. Bearn, A. G., Kunkel, H. G. and Slater, R. J. (1956). The problem of chronic liver disease in young women. *Am. J. Med.*, **21**, 3
3. Saint, E. G., King, W. E., Joske, R. A. and Finckh, E. S. (1953). The course of infectious hepatitis with special reference to prognosis and the chronic stage. *Aust. Ann. Med.*, **2**, 113
4. Joske, R. A. and King, W. E. (1955). The 'L.E. cell' phenomenon in active chronic viral hepatitis. *Lancet*, **ii**, 477
5. Mackay, I. R., Taft, L. I. and Cowling, D. C. (1956). Lupoid hepatitis. *Lancet*, **ii**, 1323
6. Mackay, I. R. and Wood, I. J. (1962). Lupoid hepatitis: a comparison of 22 cases with other types of chronic liver disease. *Quart. J. Med.*, **31**, 485
7. Mackay, I. R. and Whittingham, S. (1967). Autoimmune chronic hepatitis. *Postgraduate Med.*, **41**, 72
8. Mistilis, S. P. and Blackburn, C. R. B. (1970). Active chronic hepatitis. *Am. J. Med.*, **48**, 484
9. Sherlock, S. (1970). The immunology of liver disease. *Am. J. Med.*, **49**, 693
10. de Groote, J., Desmet, V. J., Gedigk, P., Korb, G., Popper, H., Poulsen, H., Scheuer, P., Schmid, M., Thaler, H., Uehlinger, E. and Wepler, W. (1968). A classification of chronic hepatitis. *Lancet*, **ii**, 626
11. Schmid, M. (1971). Einteilung und Klinik der chronischen Hepatitis. *Leber, Magen, Darm*, **1**, 56
12. Thaler, H. (1973). Systematische, morphologische und klinische Probleme der chronischen Hepatitis. *Internist Berlin*, **14**, 604
13. Popper, H. and Schaffner, F. (1971). The vocabulary of chronic hepatitis. *New Engl. J. Med.*, **284**, 1154
14. Scheuer, P. J. (1973). In *Liver Biopsy Interpretation*, 2nd ed., p. 33 (London: Bailliere Tindall)
15. Baggenstoss, A. H., Summerskill, W. H. J. and Ammon, H. V. (1974). The morphology of chronic hepatitis. In *The Liver and its Diseases.*

F. Schaffner, S. Sherlock and C. M. Leevy (eds.) p. 199 (New York: Intercontinental Medical Book Corporation)

16. Tisdale, W. A. (1963). Subacute hepatitis. *New Engl. J. Med.*, **268**, 85
17. Boyer, J. L. and Klatskin, G. (1970). Pattern of necrosis in acute viral hepatitis. Prognostic value of bridging (subacute hepatic necrosis). *New Engl. J. Med.*, **283**, 1063
18. Selmair, H., Vido, I., Wildhirt, E. and Ostmans, H. (1970). Die chronisch nekrotisierende Hepatitis. *Dtsch. Med. Wschr.* **95**, 1397
19. Schmid, M. (1966). *Die chronische Hepatitis: Vergleichende klinische und biologische Untersuchungen.* (Berlin–Heidelberg–New York: Springer)
20. Wepler, W. (1974). Die sogenannte chronische nekrotisierende Hepatitis. In *Chronische Hepatitis—Zirrhosen*, p. 14 (Stuttgart: Georg Thieme Verlag)
21. Wildhirt, E. (1974). Die chronische-nekrotisierende Hepatitis. In *Chronische Hepatitis—Zirrhosen*, p. 70 (Stuttgart: Georg Thieme Verlag)
22. Hadziyannis, S. J., Vissoulis, C., Moussouros, A. and Afroudakis, A. (1972). Cytoplasmic localisation of Australian antigen in the liver. *Lancet*, **i**, 976.
23. Shikata, T., Uzawa, T., Yoshiwara, N., Akatsuka, T. and Yamazaki, S. (1974). Staining methods of Australia antigen in paraffin section—detection of cytoplasmic inclusion bodies. *Jap. J. Exp. Med.*, **44**, 25
24. Doniach, D., Roitt, I. M., Walker, J. G. and Sherlock, S. (1969). Tissue antibodies in primary biliary cirrhosis, active chronic (lupoid) hepatitis, cryptogenic cirrhosis and other liver diseases and their clinical implications. *Clin. Exp. Immunol.*, **1**, 237
25. Berg, P. A., Binder, T., Linduer, H., Bannaski, H., Maas, D., Henning, H. and Brügel, H. (1975). Heterogenität mitochondrialer Autoantikörper. Zur serologischen Diagnose der primär-biliären Zirrhose und des Pseudo-Lupus erythematodes mit Hilfe von zwei verschiedenen Antigenfraktionen. *Dtsch. Med. Wschr.*, **100**, 1123
26. Berg, P. A., Traunecker, U. and Märker, A. (1973). Mitochondrial antibodies in non-hepatic diseases. *Germ. Med. Monthly*, **3**, 58
27. Maas, D. and Schubothe, H. (1973). Ein Lupus-erythematodes-ähnliches Syndrom mit antimitochondrialen Antikörpern. *Dtsch. Med. Wschr.*, **98**, 131
28. Grob, P. J., Müller-Schoop, J. W., Häcki, M. A. and Joller-Jemelka, H. (1975). Drug induced pseudolupus. *Lancet*, **ii**, 144
29. Maas, D., Schubothe, H., Seenekamp, J., Genth, E., Maerker-Alzer, G., Droese, M., Hartl, P. W. and Schumacher, K. (1975). Zur Frage einer Induzierbarkeit des Pseudo-LE-Syndroms durch Arzneimittel. Vorläufige Ergenbnisse von Erhebungen bei 58 Fällen. *Dtsch. Med. Wschr.*, **100**, 1555
30. Rizzetto, M., Swana, G. and Doniach, D. (1973). Microsomal antibodies in active chronic hepatitis and other disorders. *Clin. Exp. Immunol.*, **15**, 331

31. Maclachlan, M. J., Rodnan, G. P., Cooper, W. M. and Fennell, R. H. (1965). Chronic active (lupoid) hepatitis. A clinical, serological and pathological study of 20 patients. *Ann. Intern. Med.*, **62**, 425
32. Mackay, I. R. (1972). Chronic hepatitis. *Canad. Med. Ass. J.*, **106**, 519
33. Schumacher, K. (1975). Immunpathologie der chronischen Hepatitis. *Gastroenterologie und Stoffwechsel.* (Stuttgart: Georg Thieme Verlag)
34. Berg, P. A. and Brandt, H. (1974). Die chronische-aggressive (lupoide) Hepatitis: Diagnose, Differentialdiagnose und Therapie. *Therapiewoche*, **24**, 6, 521
35. Beck, J. S. (1961). Variations in the morphological patterns of 'autoimmune' nuclear fluorescence. *Lancet*, **i**, 1203
36. Davis, P. and Read, A. E. (1975). Antibodies to double-stranded (native) DNA in active chronic hepatitis. *Gut*, **16**, 413
37. Berg, P. A. (1974). Immune response in acute viral hepatitis. *Clin. Gastroenterol.*, **3**, 255
38. Golding, P. L., Smith, M. and Williams, R. (1973). Multisystem involvement in chronic liver disease. Studies on the incidence and pathogenesis. *Am. J. Med.*, **55**, 772
39. Grob, P. J., Jemelka, H. J. and Müller, J. W. (1971). B_1A and SH antigen in chronic hepatitis. *Gastroenterology*, **61**, 91
40. Kourilsky, O., Leroy, C. and Peltier, A. P. (1973). Complement and liver cell function in 53 patients with liver disease. *Amer. J. Med.*, **55**, 783
41. Thompson, R. A., Carter, R., Stokes, R. P., Geddes, A. M. and Goodall, J. A. D. (1973). Serum immunoglobulins, complement component levels and autoantibodies in liver disease. *Clin. Exp. Immunol.*, **14**, 335
42. Potter, B. J., Trueman, A. M. and Jones, E. A. (1973). Serum complement in chronic liver disease. *Gut*, **14**, 451
43. Triger, D. R., Kurtz, J. B. and Wright, R. (1974). Viral antibodies and autoantibodies in chronic liver disease. *Gut*, **15**, 94
44. Roux, M. E. B., Florin-Christensen, A., Arana, R. M. and Doniach, D. (1974). Paraproteins with antibody activity in acute viral heptatitis and chronic autoimmune liver diseases. *Gut*, **15**, 396
45. Jori, G. P. and Buonanno, G. (1972). Chronic hepatitis and cirrhosis of the liver in cryoglobulinaemia. *Gut*, **13**, 610
46. Klatskin, G. and Kantor, F. S. (1972). Mitochondrial antibody in primary biliary cirrhosis and other diseases. *Ann. Intern. Med.*, **77**, 533
47. Ruckstuhl, P., Cueni, B. and Schmid, M. (1971). Chronisch aggressive Hepatitis in Kombination mit chronisch destruierender nicht eitriger Cholangiitis (sog. primär-biliäre Zirrhose). *Schweiz. Med. Wschr.*, **101**, 741
48. Christoffersen, P., Poulsen, H. and Scheuer, P. J. (1972). Abnormal bile duct epithelium in chronic aggressive hepatitis and primary biliary cirrhosis. *Hum. Pathol.*, **3**, 227
49. Lüders, C. J., Kruck, P., Henning, H. and Look, D. (1974). Histologische und klinische Untersuchungen zur Differentialdiagnose der

aggressiven chronischen Hepatitis und der primären biliären Leberzirrhose. *Z. Gastroenterologie*, **12**, 467

50. Doniach, D. and Walker, J. G. (1969). A unified concept of autoimmune hepatitis. *Lancet*, **i**, 813
51. Doniach, D. (1972). Autoimmunity in liver diseases. In *Progress in Clinical Immunology*. R. S. Schwartz (ed.). p. 45. Vol. 1 (New York: Grune and Stratton)
52. Klatskin, G. (1974). Drug-induced hepatic injury. In *The Liver and its diseases*. F. Schaffner, S. Sherlock and C. M. Leevy (eds.) p. 163 (New York: Intercontinental Medical Book Corporation)
53. Doniach, D. (1974). Autoimmunity in liver diseases in relation to genes, drugs and viruses. In *Progress in Immunology*. L. Brent and J. Holborow (eds.). Vol. 4, p. 231 (North Holland Publishing Company)
54. Martini, G. A. and Dölle, W. (1960). Idiopathische Leberzirrhose bei Frauen in der Menopause. *Klin. Wschr.*, **38**, 13
55. Cook, G. C., Mulligan, R. and Sherlock, S. (1971). Controlled prospective trial of corticosteroid therapy in active chronic hepatitis. *Quart. J. Med.*, **40**, 159
56. Soloway, R. D., Summerskill, W. H. J., Baggenstoss, A. H., Geall, M. G., Gitnick, G. L., Elveback, L. R. and Schoenfield, L. J. (1972). Clinical biochemical and histological remission of severe chronic active liver disease: a controlled study of treatments and early prognosis. *Gastroenterology*, **63**, 820
57. Murray-Lyon, I. M., Stern, R. B. and Williams, R. (1973). Controlled trial of prednisone and azathioprine in active chronic hepatitis. *Lancet*, **1**, 735
58. Copenhagen Study Group (1974). Sex, ascites and alcoholism in survival of patients with cirrhosis. Effect of Prednisone. *New Engl. J. Med.*, **291**, 271
59. Summerskill, W. H. J., Ammon, H. V. and Baggenstoss, A. H.(1974). Treatment of chronic hepatitis. In *The Liver and its diseases*. F. Schaffner, S. Sherlock and C. M. Leevy (eds.) p. 216 (New York: Intercontinental Medical Book Corporation)
60. Addison, T. and Gull, W. (1851). On a certain affection of the skin vitiligoidea—δ-plana, β-Tuberosa. *Guy's Hosp. Rep.*, **7**, 265
61. Dauphinee, J. A. and Sinclair, J. C. (1949). Primary biliary cirrhosis. *Canad. Med. Ass. J.*, **61**, 1
62. Hanot, V. (1976). *Etude sur une forme de cirrhose hypertrophique du foie (cirrhose hypertrophique avec ictère chronique)* (Paris: Baillière)
63. Klemperer, P. (1937). Chronic intrahepatic obliterating cholangitis. *J. Mt. Sinai Hosp.*, **4**, 279
64. Karsner, H. T. (1943). Morphology and pathogenesis of hepatic cirrhosis. *Am. J. Clin. Pathol.* **13**, 569
65. Rossie, R. (1930). *Henke u Lubarsch, Handbuch de Speziellen Pathologischen Anatomie und Histologie*, Vol. V, pt. I, Berlin
66. Watson, C. J. and Hoffbauer, F. W. (1946). Problem of prolonged

hepatitis with particular reference to cholangiolitic type and to development of cholangiolitic cirrhosis of the liver. *Ann Intern. Med.*, **25**, 195

67. Thannhauser, S. J. (1950). *Lipidoses, Diseases of the Cellular Lipid Metabolism*, 2nd ed. (New York: Grune and Stratton)
68. Thannhauser, S. J. and Magendantz, H. (1938). The different clinical groups of xanthomatous diseases: a clinical physiological study of 22 cases. *Ann. Intern. Med.*, **11**, 1662
69. MacMahon, H. E. and Thannhauser, S. J. (1949). Xanthomatous biliary cirrhosis (clinical syndrome). *Ann Intern. Med.*, **30**, 121
70. Rubin, E., Schaffner, F. and Popper, H. (1965). Primary biliary cirrhosis. *Am. J. Pathol.*, **46**, 387
71. Ahrens, E. H. Jr., Payne, M. A., Kunkel, H. G., Eisenmenger, W. J. and Blondheim S. H. (1950). Primary biliary cirrhosis. *Medicine (Baltimore)*, **29**, 299
72. Walker, J. G., Doniach, D., Roitt, I. M. and Sherlock, S. (1965). Serological tests in diagnosis of primary biliary cirrhosis. *Lancet*, **i**, 827
73. MacSween, R. N. M., Ross, Sheila K, Williamson, J. and Watkinson, G. (1975). Primary biliary cirrohsis, Clinical and immunological associations. (In preparation)
74. Turnberg, L. A., Mahoney, M. P., Gleeson, M. H., Freeman, C. P. and Gowenlock, A. H. (1972). Plasmaphoresis and plasma exchange in the treatment of hyperlipaemia and xanthomatous neuropathy in patients with primary biliary cirrhosis. *Gut*, **13**, 976
75. Sherlock, S. (1974). The presentation and diagnosis of 100 patients with primary biliary cirrhosis. In *The Liver and its Diseases*, F. Schaffner, S. Sherlock and C. M. Leevy (eds.) p. 227. (New York: Intercontinental Medical Book Corporation)
76. Kew, M. C., Varma, R. R., Santos, H. D., Scheuer, P. J. and Sherlock, S. (1971). Portal hypertension in primary biliary cirrhosis. *Gut*, **12**, 496
77. Foulk, W. T., Baggenstoss, A. H. and Butt, H. R. (1964). Primary biliary cirrhosis: re-evaluation by clinical and histologic study of 49 cases. *Gastroenterology*, **47**, 354
78. Hoffbauer, F. W. (1960). Primary biliary cirrhosis. Observations on the natural course of the disease in 25 women. *Am. J. Dig. Dis.*, **5**, 348
79. Sherlock, S. (1959). Primary biliary cirrhosis (chronic intrahepatic obstructive jaundice). *Gastroenterology*, **37**, 574
80. Schaffner, F. (1969). Serum cholesterol in primary biliary cirrhosis. *Gastroenterology*, **56**, 1111
81. Williams, G. E. (1965). Pericholangiolitic biliary cirrhosis. *J. Pathol. Bact.*, **89**, 23
82. Goudie, R. B., MacSween, R. N. M. and Goldberg, D. M. (1966). Serological and histological diagnosis of primary biliary cirrhosis. *J. Clin. Pathol.*, **19**, 527
83. Scheuer, P. J. (1967). Primary biliary cirrhosis. *Proc. Roy. Soc. Med.*, **60**, 1257

84. MacSween, R. N. M. (1973). Mallory's ('alcoholic') hyaline in primary biliary cirrhosis. *J. Clin. Path.*, **26**, 340
85. Doniach, D. and Walker, J. G. (1972). Immunopathology of liver disease. In *Progress in Liver Diseases*. H. Popper and F. Schaffner (eds.) vol. IV, p. 381 (New York and London: Grune and Stratton).
86. Kantor, F. S. and Klatskin, G. (1967). Serological diagnosis of primary biliary cirrhosis: a potential clue to pathogenesis. *Trans. Ass. Am. Physicians*, **80**, 267
87. Berg, P. A., Muscatello, U., Horne, R. W., Roitt, I. M. and Doniach, D. (1969). Mitochondrial antibodies in primary biliary cirrhosis. II. The complement fixing antigen as a component of mitochondrial inner membranes. *Br. J. Exp. Pathol.* **50**, 200
88. Ben-Yoseph, Y., Shapira, E. and Doniach, D. (1974). Further purification of the mitochondrial inner membrane autoantigen reacting with primary biliary cirrhosis sera. *Immunology*, **26**, 311
89. Lam, K. C., Mistilis, S. P. and Perrott, N. (1973). Positive tissue antibody tests in patients with prolonged extrahepatic biliary obstruction. *New Engl. J. Med.*, **286**, 1400
90. Doniach, D., Walker, J. G., Roitt, I. M. and Berg, P. A. (1970). 'Autoallergic' hepatitis. *New Engl. J. Med.*, **282**, 86
91. Doniach, D. and Walker, G. (1974). Progress report. Mitochondrial antibodies (AMA). *Gut*, **15**, 664
92. Johnson, G. D., Holborow, E. J. and Glynn, L. E. (1965). Antibody to smooth muscle in patients with liver disease. *Lancet*, **ii**, 878
93. MacSween, R. N. M., Armstrong, E. M., Gray, K. G. and Mason, M. (1973). Bile canalicular antibody in primary biliary cirrhosis and in other liver diseases. *Lancet*, **i**, 1419
94. Fulthorpe, A. J., Roitt, I. M., Doniach, D. and Couchman, K. (1961). A stable sheep cell preparation for detecting thyroglobulin autoantibodies and its clinical application. *J. Clin. Pathol.*, **14**, 654
95. MacSween, R. N. M., Hughes, Hazel, Breen, Catriona, Kitchen, P. Cathcart, Brenda and Buchanan, W. W. (1974). A comparative study of some commercially available tests for rheumatoid factor. *J. Clin. Pathol.*, **27**, 368
96. Hadziyannis, S., Scheuer, P. J., Feizi, T., Naccarato, R., Doniach, D. and Sherlock, S. (1970). Immunological and histological studies in primary biliary cirrhosis. *J. Clin. Pathol.*, **23**, 95
97. Diederichsen, H. (1975). Bile canalicular antibodies in non-hepatic diseases. *Lancet*, **i**, 1142
98. Paronetto, F., Schaffner, F. and Popper, H. (1964). Immunocytochemical and serologic observations in primary biliary cirrhosis. *New Engl. J. Med.*, **271**, 1122
99. Feizi, T. (1968). Immunoglobulins in chronic liver disease. *Gut*, **9**, 193
100. Hobbs, J. R. (1967). Serum proteins in liver disease. *Proc. Roy. Soc. Med.*, **60**, 1250
101. MacSween, R. N. M., Horne, C. H. W., Moffat, A. J. and Hughes,

H. M. (1972). Serum protein levels in primary biliary cirrhosis. *J. Clin. Pathol.*, **25**, 789

102. Fox, R. A., Dudley, F. J. and Sherlock, S. (1971). The serum concentration of the third component of complement βlc/βla in liver disease. *Gut*, **12**, 574

103. Potter, B. J., Elias, E. and Jones, E. A. (1974). Hypercatabolism of the third component of complement in primary biliary cirrhosis. *Digestion*, **10**, 303 (Abstract).

104. Fox, R. A., James, D. G., Scheuer, P. J., Sharma, O. and Sherlock, S. (1969). Impaired delayed hypersensitivity in primary biliary cirrhosis. *Lancet*, **i**, 959

105. MacSween, R. N. M., Galbraith, I., Thomas, M. A., Watkinson, G. and Ludlam, G. B. (1973). Phytohaemagglutinin (PHA) induced lymphocyte transformation and *Toxoplasma gondii* antibody studies in primary biliary cirrhosis. *Clin. Exp. Immunol.*, **15**, 35

106. MacSween R. N. M. and Thomas, M. A. (1973). Lymphocyte transformation by phytohaemagglutinin (PHA) and purified protein derivative (PPD) in primary biliary cirrhosis. Evidence of serum inhibitory factors. *Clin. Exp. Immunol.*, **15**, 523

107. Colombo, M., Vernace, S. J. and Paronetto, F. (1974). T and B lymphocytes in primary biliary cirrhosis. *Gastroenterology*, **67**, 783. (Abstract)

108. Sherlock, S. and Scheuer, P. J. (1973). The presentation and diagnosis of 100 patients with primary biliary cirrhosis. *New Engl. J. Med.*, **289**, 674

109. Golding, P. L., Bown, R., Mason, A. M. S. and Taylor, E. (1970). 'Sicca Complex' in liver disease. *Brit. Med., J.*, **4**, 340

110. Whaley, K., Webb. J., McAvoy, B. A., Hughes, G. R. V., Lee, P., MacSween, R. N. M. and Buchanan, W. W. (1973). Sjøgren's syndrome 2. Clinical associations and immunological phenomena. *Quart., J. Med.*, **42**, 513

111. Schaffner, F. (1975). Primary biliary cirrhosis. *Clinics Gastroenteral.*, **4**, 351

112. Reynolds, T. B., Denison, E. D., Frankl, H. D., Lieberman, F. L. and Peters, R. L. (1970). New syndrome: combination of primary biliary cirrhosis, scleroderma and hereditary haemorrhagic telangiectasia. *Gastroenterology*, **58**, 290 (Abstract).

113. Reynolds, T. B., Denison, E. K., Frankl, H. D., Lieberman, F. L. and Peters, R. L. (1971). Primary biliary cirrhosis with scleroderma, Raynaud's phenomenon and telangiectasia. *Amer. J. Med.*, **50**, 302

114. Diaz, P. A. and Schuman, B. M. (1973). Primary biliary cirrhosis with systemic sclerosis associated with Raynaud's phenomenon and telangiectasiae. *Gastroenterology*, **64**, 180 (Abstract).

115. Murray-Lyon, I. M., Thompson, R. P. H., Ansell, I. D. and Williams, R. (1970). Scleroderma and primary biliary cirrhosis. *Brit. Med. J.*, **3**, 258

116. Bartholomew, L. G., Cain, J. C., Winkelmann, R. K. and Baggenstoss,

A. H. (1964). Chronic disease of the liver associated with systemic scleroderma. *Am. J. Dig. Dis.*, **9**, 43

117. Levrat, M., Descos, L., Trepo, C., Vandanput, F., Lesbros, F., Moulin, G. and Berthelemy, C. (1973). Association of scleroderma, Sjøgren's syndrome and primary biliary cirrhosis. *Arch. Franc. Mal. App. Dig.*, **62**, 495
118. Turner-Warwick, M. (1968). Fibrosing alveolitis and chronic liver disease. *Quart. J. Med.*, **37**, 133
119. Ross, A., Heathcote, J. and Sherlock, S. (1974). A trial of azathioprine in primary biliary cirrhosis. *Gastroenterology*, **67**, 824 (Abstract)
120. Kehayoglou, A. K., Holdsworth, C. D., Agnew, J. E., Whelton, M. J. and Sherlock, S. (1968). Bone disease and calcium absorption in primary biliary cirrhosis. *Lancet*, **i**, 715
121. Ajdukiewicz, A. B., Agnew, J. E., Byers, P. D., Wills, M. R. and Sherlock, S. (1974). The relief of bone pain in primary biliary cirrhosis with calcium infusions. *Gut*, **15**, 788
122. Bulkley, B. H., Heizer, W. E., Goldfinger, S. E., Isselbacher, K. J. and Shulman, N. R. (1970). Distinctions in chronic active hepatitis based on circulating hepatitis-associated antigen. *Lancet*, **ii**. 1323
123. Mathews, J. D. and Mackay, I. R. (1970). Australia Antigen in chronic hepatitis in Australia. *Br. Med., J.*, **1**, 259
124. Vischer, T. L. (1970). Australia antigen and autoantibodies in chronic hepatitis. *Br. Med., J.*, **2**, 695
125. Berg, P. A. (1972). Hepatitis assoziiertes Antigen (HAA). Klinische und immunologische Bedeutung. *Klin. Wschr.*, **50**, 125
126. Dudley, F. J., O'Shea, M. J. and Ajdukiewicz, A. (1973). Serum autoantibodies and immunoglobulins in hepatitis associated antigen (HAA)-positive and -negative liver disease. *Gut*, **14**, 360
127. Galbraith, R. M., Eddleston, A. L. W. F., Smith, M. G. M., Williams, R., MacSween, R. N. M., Watkinson, G., Dick, H., Kennedy, L. A. and Batchelor, J. R. (1974). Histocompatibility antigens in active chronic hepatitis and primary biliary cirrhosis. *Brit. Med. J.*, **3**, 604
128. MacSween, R. N. M., Laiwah, A. A. C. Y., Busuttil, A. A., Thomas, M. A., Ross, S. K., Watkinson, G., Millman, I. and Blumberg, B. S. (1973). Australia antigen and primary biliary cirrhosis. *J. Clin. Pathol.* **26**, 335
129. Reed, W. D., Eddleston, A. L. W. F., Stern, R. B. and Williams, R. (1973). Detection of Hepatitis-B antigen by radioimmunoassay in chronic liver disease and hepatocellular carcinoma in Great Britain. *Lancet*, **ii**, 690.
130. Hadziyannis, S. J., Merikas, G., Moussouros, A. and Afroudakis, A. (1971). Hepatitis-associated antigen and tissue antibodies in active chronic hepatitis. *Digestion*, **4**, 149
131. Soloway, R. D., Summerskill, W. H. J., Baggenstoss, A. H. and Schoenfield, L. J. (1972). Lupoid Hepatitis, a nonentity in the spectrum of chronic active liver disease. *Gastroenterology*, **63**, 458

132. Eddleston, A. L. W. F. and Williams, R. (1974). Inadequate antibody response to HB Ag or suppressor T-cell defect in development of active chronic hepatitis. *Lancet*, **ii**, 1543
133. Summerskill, W. H. J. (1974). Chronic active liver disease reexamined: prognosis hopeful. *Gastroenterology*, **66**, 450
134. Van Waes, L., Segers, J., Van Egmond, J., Van Nimmen, L., Barbier, F., Wieme, R. Demeulenaere, L. (1974). Chronic liver disease and hepatitis-B antigen: a prospective study. *Brit. Med. J.*, **3**, 444
135. Lee, W. M., Reed, W. D., Mitchell, C. G., Galbraith, R. M., Eddleston, A. L. W., Zuckerman, A. J. and Williams, R. (1975). Cellular and humoral immunity to hepatitis-B surface antigen in active chronic hepatitis. *Brit. Med., J.*, **1**, 705
136. Hopf, U., Meyer zum Büschenfelde, K. H. and Freudenberg, J. (1974). Liver specific antigens of different species. 11. Localisation of a membrane antigen at cell surface of isolated hepatocytes. *Clin. Exp. Immunol.*, **16**, 117
137. Hopf, U., Meyer zum Büschenfelde, K. H. and Arnold, W. (1975). Cytophilic autoantibody in chronic active hepatitis. *Lancet*, **i**, 690
138. Dudley, F. J., Fox, R. A. and Sherlock, S. (1972). Cellular immunity and hepatitis-associated Australia antigen liver disease. *Lancet*, **i**, 723
139. Sharp, G. C., Irvin, W. S., LaRoque, R. L., Velez, C., Daly, V., Kaiser, A. D. and Holman, H. R. (1971). Association of autoantibodies to different nuclear antigens with clinical patterns of rheumatic disease and responsiveness to therapy. *J. Clin. Invest.*, **50**, 350
140. Fagraeus, A., Lidman, K. and Biberfeld, G. (1974). Reaction of human smooth muscle antibodies with human blood lymphocytes and lymphoid cell lines. *Nature*, **252**, 246

CHAPTER 11

The role of immunity and hypersensitivity in gut and liver disease: a comparison

RALPH WRIGHT

The immunology of the gastrointestinal tract and liver is especially interesting for a number of reasons. Anatomically the gastrointestinal tract provides an extensive surface area of the body which is in direct contact with the external environment. Because of its function as an absorptive surface for nutrients, it would not be surprising if the gut were to be permeable to antigenic protein molecules and regulatory mechanisms are necessary to contain such potentially dangerous absorption of antigenic materials. An understanding of the normal immunological mechanisms could clearly be relevant to an understanding of the pathogenesis of the immune response to pathogenic viral, bacterial and parasitic infections and to allergic reactions resulting from dietary antigen absorption. In addition the gastrointestinal tract is affected by a number of diseases of uncertain aetiology in whose pathogenesis immunological mechanisms appear to be important. These include atrophic gastritis, celiac disease, ulcerative colitis and Crohn's disease. Furthermore, abnormalities of the gut are prominent in rare disorders in which there are major immunological deficiencies such as hypogammaglobulinaemia. This suggests that more subtle immunological defects could be a factor in the pathogenesis of some of the diseases of unknown aetiology mentioned above.

The relevance of the normal immunological function of the liver to immune mediated liver disease is less apparent. The concept of the liver as an organ strategically placed between the gut and the antibody-forming organs elsewhere to help to control antigen absorption has only been emphasized relatively recently. Of special interest in liver disease is the possible interplay between viral infection and autoimmune phenomena and research in this area may have relevance not only to liver disease itself but to an understanding of immunopathological mechanisms elsewhere in the body.

Many of the topics mentioned above have been covered comprehensively in earlier chapters. The purpose of the present chapter will be to attempt to summarize and highlight the areas which appear to me to be of special interest.

There have been considerable advances in our understanding of the origin and functions of the lymphoid tissue of the gut and of secretory immunoglobulins. These have been fully covered in Chapters 1 and 2. Studies of the gut as a lymphoid organ were partly stimulated by attempts to demonstrate a mammalian equivalent of the avian bursa of Fabricius. As is apparent from Parrot's paper, no single collection of lymphoid tissue in the mammalian gut has a similar function. She emphasizes the dynamic state of much of the lymphoid tissue in the gut. A constant traffic of lymphoid cells occurs between aggregated lymphoid tissue such as Peyer's patches and appendix and the lamina propria and intra-epithelial lymphocytes. It is now clear that the latter are not effete cells being dumped in the intestinal lumen but part of a thymus-dependent immune system reacting to intralumenal antigens. Large numbers of intra-epithelial lymphocytes are present in the dome area of the Peyer's patches and appendix in close proximity to the gut lumen and it is suggested that they form the affector arm of the immune response to ingested antigens. Both T and B cell areas have been demonstrated in the appendix and Peyer's patches but they do not contain antibody forming cells. There is good evidence however, that they are a source of IgA precursors.

Intralumenal antigen is the stimulus to the formation of IgA and there is general agreement that IgA is the predominant immunoglobulin in external secretions and that IgA secreting cells outnumber those producing other immunoglobulins by about 5 to 1. After the addition of a secretory component to dimeric IgA, the 11S secretory IgA passes into the lumen. What remains uncertain is the precise route whereby these IgA secreting cells reach the lamina propria and the mechanism whereby secretory IgA passes into the intestinal lumen. It seems likely, however, that most IgA precursors arise locally in the gut, for example in Peyer's patches and the appendix, migrate to mesenteric lymph nodes or more widely in the body and then return to the lamina propria. Some may pass directly to the villi. Although T-cell dependent these IgA immunoblasts differentiate into B-cells and once having reached the lamina propria they probably remain there. There is increasing evidence that T-immunoblasts migrate to T-areas in Peyer's patches and the lamina propria and that intra-epithelial lymphocytes are T-blasts. Although intralumenal antigen is a major stimulus to the increase in immunoblasts it does not seem to be the sole explanation for the intriguing observation that immunoblasts home selectively to the intestine since this can be observed in germ-free animals. Characterization of the lymphocytes in the gut has provided evidence that, in addition to a local antibody response to ingested antigens, a cell-mediated immune response occurs. The relative importance in health of the local immune system in the prevention of antigen absorption compared to non-specific factors such as intestinal mucus, enzymes, and epithelial cell permeability remains uncertain.

The importance of the local immune system notably secretory IgA in the control of pathogenic organisms including viruses, bacteria and parasites are reviewed in Chapter 4. Specific local antibody production provides immunity in poliomyelitis and certain other viral infections but its role in bacterial and parasitic infection is less clear. In bacterial infections, alternative mechanisms may be operative such as the coating of bacteria by IgA with prevention of their adsorption to the intestinal mucosa.

Despite these advances in our knowledge of the normal immunological apparatus in the gut, there is little objective evidence for the possibility that defects in the specific local immune response might commonly predispose to the development of gastrointestinal disease. Most information is provided by studies of patients with selective IgA deficiency or other more severe forms of immunodeficiency. These are reviewed in Chapter 3. Patients with selective IgA deficiency have an increase in antibody titres to dietary antigens suggesting that there is at least a partial failure to prevent antigen absorption. There is good evidence, however, that IgM can compensate for secretory IgA deficiency and despite an increased incidence of pernicious anaemia, celiac disease and possibly inflammatory bowel disease in patients with immunoglobulin deficiency, there is little evidence that a quantitative or qualitative defect in the secretory immune system plays a significant role in the pathogenesis of these diseases in their more usual form or in the pathogenesis of gastrointestinal infection.

The situation becomes very different once the mucosal barrier to intraluminal antigen becomes defective as in inflammatory bowel disease and celiac disease. Whatever the primary defect damaging the mucosal surface, which need not be immunological, the subsequent massive absorption of antigen could clearly overcome the normal barriers and rapidly have a profound effect on immune responses. In most of these diseases there is a striking increase in immunocytes and, depending on the particular disease, the infiltrate may include the deposition of immune complexes, granuloma formation or an eosinophil response. The only disease in which a specific potential antigen has been defined is celiac disease and even here the smallest polypeptide which has been shown to be toxic to the mucosa is itself too small to be antigenic although it might act as a haptene. Nevertheless, because a potential antigen is available for study challenge experiments in patients with celiac disease who have responded to a gluten-free diet provide a useful model both *in vivo* and *in vitro*. Early studies of dietary antibodies in serum and jejunal juice were disappointing as they showed that the reactions were not specific for gluten and that antibodies were formed to a wide variety of dietary proteins. Furthermore, the antibodies disappeared following healing of the mucosa on a gluten-free diet and it is now generally accepted that they are a secondary phenomenon. Although it is still possible that the reticulin antibody plays a role in pathogenesis, it is likely that it may be similarly explained.

Claims of specific cell-mediated immunity to gluten antigen must equally be treated with caution since, for technical reasons, they are most difficult to control and interpret. Although there is good evidence that an Arthus-type reaction occurs in the mucosa within 12 hours of challenge, so rapid are the immunological responses in the gut that the mucosal reaction could be a secondary phenomenon to non-immunological toxic damage to the epithelium. Despite the heavy infiltrate of immunocytes into the mucosa it has only been possible to demonstrate specific gluten antibody production in occasional cells although the technical problems are serious. Interesting recent claims of specific IgA gluten antibody production by celiac biopsies *in vitro*, referred to in Chapter 5, will require critical assessment.

In atrophic gastritis and inflammatory bowel disease discussed by Jewell in Chapter 6, the situation is even more confused. Despite their usefulness as a marker of pernicious anaemia, intrinsic factor antibodies seem unlikely to be important in the pathogenesis of the gastric lesion and although it is possible that the parietal cell antibody is cytotoxic, available evidence is flimsy. Claims of *in vitro* cell-mediated reactions to gastric antigens pose the usual problems of interpretation and are compounded by lack of purified antigen; nevertheless, if one accepts the concept of organ-specific autoimmune disease the gastritis associated with pernicious anaemia fulfils most of the criteria and may depend on other advances in this general area.

In inflammatory bowel disease the immunological phenomena described are even more difficult to interpret particularly the studies of lymphocyte cytotoxicity. Clues to a possible transmissible agent in Crohn's disease must clearly be vigorously followed. However, in both ulcerative colitis and Crohn's disease the possibility that they represent an abnormal immune response to exogenous dietary antigens or haptenes or to endogenous organisms which are usually non-pathogenic remains an attractive hypothesis but one which would be very difficult to substantiate. As discussed in earlier chapters, the interplay between normal immunological responses and endogenous bacterial flora is poorly understood but may be highly relevant to inflammatory bowel disease. The role of non-specific factors such as mucus secretion and disturbances of motility or vascular permeability may be crucial and may explain the link between relapses in these disorders and psychological factors so impressive to the clinician.

In celiac disease and inflammatory bowel disease study of the extra-intestinal manifestations may be most rewarding from an immunological point of view. The splenic atrophy commonly associated with celiac disease and possibly also with inflammatory bowel disease may have an immunological basis but currently defies explanation. An understanding of the pathogenesis of the arthropathy, uveitis, cutaneous manifestations and liver disease associated with inflammatory bowel disease may be possible even though that of the bowel lesion itself remains unresolved. The question posed several years ago as to whether they represent true complications of the intestinal disease or indicate that they are multi-system disorders remains unresolved, but the deposition of absorbed immune complexes in sites remote from the bowel remains a strong possibility.

The vexed topic of gastrointestinal food allergy is dealt with by Ferguson in Chapter 5. Leaving aside the problem of celiac disease the best studied example is milk allergy in infancy. This should provide a useful model for assessing the role of reaginic, Arthus-type and cell-mediated immune reactions to milk protein in producing the intestinal damage, but is limited by difficulty in conducting challenge experiments in children. It will also provide an opportunity for assessing the value of skin tests and tests for specific IgE antibody in serum and intestinal secretions.

Disaccharidase deficiency, disturbances of intestinal motility and psychological disorders may all mimic gastrointestinal allergy. This makes the assessment of elimination diets and challenge experiments extremely difficult to interpret in the absence of specific immunological tests. This is particularly true of ulcerative colitis where despite clinical and histological evidence favouring allergy, e.g. to milk in some patients, laboratory proof is lacking.

It is only relatively recently that the role of the liver in normal immunological responses has been fully recognized. Although the liver is a source of developing lymphoid cells in the fetus, there is no evidence that it has any function as a lymphoid organ in health in adults. Bjørneboe and Prytz present a comprehensive review of the immunological function of the reticulo-endothelial system of the liver in Chapter 7. They examine the mechanism of phagocytosis by the mononuclear phagocyte system and, in particular, the function of Kupffer cells in the liver in the sequestration and elimination of antigens. There is good experimental evidence that Kupffer cells behave differently from other macrophages when taking up antigens, in that they may not induce antibody formation. It has been suggested that these cells destroy sequestered antigen or that they do not process them for antibody formation by lymphoid cells. It has also been suggested that the Kupffer cells may induce a state of tolerance to antigens by this process of sequestration. The interesting Chase–Sulzberger phenomenon, the development of tolerance to orally administered haptens, is discussed in Chapters 2 and 7. There is indirect experimental evidence to suggest that the liver, probably Kupffer cells, may play an active role in this phenomenon. However, it is possible that the absorption of antigen from the gut or its release into the portal system may be different in animals made tolerant by the oral route and may be a partial explanation.

The mechanisms of the hyperglobulinaemia observed in liver disease has received much attention recently. It is still undecided whether patients with liver disease have an enhanced capacity to produce circulating antibodies but it is unlikely that this is a crucial factor in the development of the hyperglobulinaemia. At present defective function of Kupffer cells seems the more likely explanation. This is based on the demonstration of raised antibody titres to enterobacteria in patients with chronic liver disease and the increase in serum globulin levels and *E. coli* antibody titres which occur following portacaval shunt in man and experimentally in the rat. What is not clear is whether simple bypass of Kupffer cells by antigen is the mechanism or whether impaired function of Kupffer cells due to alterations in blood flow, saturation by excessive antigen load or damage by endotoxin is responsible. Increased circulating endotoxin in liver disease may also be a factor by acting as a stimulant of B cells. Another factor may be excessive bacterial overgrowth in the intestine in liver disease. However, as Bjørneboe and Prytz point out there is little direct evidence of increased bacterial antigen absorption in patients with liver disease. It is interesting, however, to contrast the marked hyperglobulinaemia which appears in patients with liver disease with the relatively minor changes which occur in inflammatory bowel disease and celiac disease where increased antigen absorption from the small intestine or the damaged colon occurs. This may be due to the remarkable capacity of Kupffer cells, which are presumably normal in these diseases, to sequester antigen or antigen–antibody complexes. It seems likely that immune responses to many antigens other than the gut-associated bacteria contribute to the hyperglobulinaemia, including an autoimmune response to damaged liver cells.

The striking elevation of antibody titres to viruses including measles and rubella, seen particularly in chronic active hepatitis, is more difficult to explain. Increased susceptibility to re-infection with viraemia, failure of Kupffer cells to degrade these antigens with their subsequent release, or continuing infection in the Kupffer cell are among a number of possible explanations but they are difficult to test.

At present there is no explanation for the differences in immunoglobulin levels in different forms of chronic liver disease, IgA predominating in the alcoholics, IgM in primary biliary cirrhosis and IgG in chronic active hepatitis. There is also no evidence that the hyperglobulinaemia is harmful or that immune complexes of non-specific antigens are a factor in the pathogenesis of the chronic liver disease, although it is possible that they may be deposited elsewhere and produce certain extra-hepatic manifestations.

Bjørneboe and Prytz speculate on the possibility that a defect of hepatic phagocytic function may be a factor in the development and progression of cirrhosis. They postulate that, as a result, there is a low grade chronic infection of the liver and advocate re-examination of the use of antibiotics in the treatment of cirrhosis. Although I agree that defective phagocytic function may be a factor in the development of the septicaemia which occasionally complicates cirrhosis, I find it difficult to accept that chronic bacterial infection of the liver plays a significant part in the progression of the cirrhosis.

A more interesting possibility which has received little attention is that failure of Kupffer cells to contain a viral infection may govern the severity of hepatitis A and B infections and determine chronicity. The replication of viruses in Kupffer cells with spill-over to involve parenchymal cells is a well-known phenomenon in animal virus infections, but there is no direct evidence for this possibility in man. *In vivo* or *in vitro* techniques for assessing macrophage function in man are urgently required but at present are primitive.

The relationship of viral hepatitis and autoimmunity to chronic liver disease are discussed by MacSween and Berg, Paronetto and Eddleston. It is clearly established that heptatitis B infection can progress to chronic liver disease but the mechanisms of the tissue damage remains speculative. Despite the direct demonstration of immune complexes of HBsAg and antibody in serum by electron microscopy they have not been unequivocally demonstrated in hepatocytes. Paronetto contrasts the failure to demonstrate immune complexes in the liver, in part attributable to the avid ability of Kupffer cells to ingest such complexes, with their ready demonstration in extrahepatic sites such as the kidneys.

Depression of T-lymphocyte function with a decrease in the absolute number of T-lymphocytes is observed in acute viral hepatitis as in other viral infections. They usually return to normal on recovery but remain decreased if there is progression to chronic liver disease. As with gastrointestinal inflammatory disorders, however, it is not known if this has implications with regard to pathogenesis or whether it merely implies traffic of lymphocytes into the affected organs. It is well established that patients who have impaired cell-mediated immunity are liable to become carriers of the antigen and although results have been conflicting, there is some evidence that a cell-mediated immune response to the HBsAg is necessary to clear the antigen; there is no direct evidence that a defective or enhanced type IV response to the surface antigen is responsible for the liver damage.

Thus, despite the fact that the core particles of hepatitis B can be identified in the nucleus of the hepatocyte and the HBsAg in the cytoplasm, and despite reproducible techniques for detecting HBs antibody and HBc antibody in serum, the pathogenesis of the hepatic injury remains uncertain. It is possible that studies of the *e* antigen, discussed by Eddleston in Chapter 9, which appears to correlate with infectivity and chronic activity of hepatitis B infection may provide a clue. Currently it would seem that the *e* antigen, Dane particles and DNA polymerase activity often occur together in serum but it is not clear whether the *e* antigen is viral or host determined. The availability of the chimpanzee as an animal model may also facilitate an understanding of the immunopathological mechanisms involved.

The wide spectrum of autoantibodies described in liver disease has stimulated interest in the possibility that autoimmune mechanisms may be implicated in the pathogenesis of chronic active hepatitis and primary biliary cirrhosis. It seems unlikely that smooth muscle, mitochondrial or antinuclear antibodies have any direct bearing on pathogenesis and it might therefore be questioned whether it is relevant to rigidly sub-divide chronic active liver disease on that basis. Nevertheless, the classification adopted by MacSween and Berg is the best that can be used at present. More relevant than the autoantibodies is the contrast between the rarity of other putative autoimmune diseases in the HBsAg positive chronic active hepatitis, and their frequency in the typical lupoid type of hepatitis.

Eddleston has postulated, on the basis of leukocyte migration inhibition studies using HBsAg and liver specific lipoprotein, that the HB antigen negative chronic active hepatitis is initiated by hepatitis B which then disappears from the serum, the liver injury being perpetuated by an autoimmune response. This hypothesis, however, remains speculative. If correct, other markers of previous infection with hepatitis B such as antibody to the core of the Dane particle should be present in such patients. Clearly, the possibility that persistence of hepatitis A or a 'non-A, non-B' virus may be responsible for some cases of HBsAg negative chronic active hepatitis will be examined once an appropriate serological technique for testing such viruses becomes available.

Other interesting models for the possible induction of autoimmunity are the rare cases of chronic active liver disease reported after an adverse reaction to drugs such as oxyphenisatin and methyl-dopa. Also of considerable interest is the pseudo-lupus erythematosus syndrome described by MacSween and Berg.

The possibility that chronicity in liver disease may be due to an antibody dependent lymphocyte cytotoxicity is discussed by Paronetto and by Eddleston. Both groups using different systems have demonstrated such cytotoxicity for liver cells using lymphocytes from patients with chronic active hepatitis. Eddleston and associates had previously shown leukocyte migration inhibition to a liver specific lipoprotein and they suggest that lymphocyte mediated cytotoxicity is directed against this liver specific lipoprotein. The use of leukocyte migration inhibition as an index of cell-mediated immunity to liver specific liproproteins or biliary antigens should be regarded with the same reservations as were expressed about its use in gastrointestinal disease.

As Eddleston points out, the diseases in which these autoimmune phenomena have been described have a high frequency of the histocompatability antigen HLA-8 and he postulates that this may be related to defective suppressor T cell function with antibody mediated autoimmune liver damage occurring either directly or by the activation of K cells. This hypothesis fits in well with current immunological theories of autoimmune induced tissue damage but firm experimental evidence is not yet forthcoming and, like so many immunological theories, it might prove ephemeral.

Although the accidental discovery of the Australia antigen as a marker for hepatitis B infection provided a powerful stimulus for research in this area, and the development of a vaccine seems likely, much remains to be learnt about the pathogenic mechanisms involved. It provides scope for both encouragement and caution with regard to the possibility that unidentified infective agents may be responsible for disorders of the gastrointestinal tract such as Crohn's disease and ulcerative colitis.

Index